Evidence-Based Implant Dentistry

Evidence-Based Implant Dentistry

Editor: Preston Bailey

AMERICAN
MEDICAL PUBLISHERS
www.americanmedicalpublishers.com

AMERICAN
MEDICAL PUBLISHERS
www.americanmedicalpublishers.com

Cataloging-in-publication Data

Evidence-based implant dentistry / edited by Preston Bailey.
p. cm.
Includes bibliographical references and index.
ISBN 979-8-88740-115-7
1. Dental implants. 2. Mouth--Surgery. 3. Implants, Artificial. 4. Dentures.
5. Dentistry. I. Bailey, Preston.
RK667.I45 E95 2023
617.693--dc23

American Medical Publishers,
41 Flatbush Avenue,
1st Floor, New York,
NY 11217, USA

ISBN 979-8-88740-115-7 (Hardback)

Contents

Preface

In my initial years as a student, I used to run to the library at every possible instance to grab a book and learn something new. Books were my primary source of knowledge and I would not have come such a long way without all that I learnt from them. Thus, when I was approached to edit this book; I became understandably nostalgic. It was an absolute honor to be considered worthy of guiding the current generation as well as those to come. I put all my knowledge and hard work into making this book most beneficial for its readers.

The branch of medicine that comprises the study, diagnosis, prevention, and treatment of diseases, disorders, and conditions of the oral cavity is defined as dentistry. Implant dentistry is a subspecialty within dentistry which is involved in procedures connected to dental implants. These implants are used for supporting the recovery of a missing tooth by installing an artificial tooth root. Osseointegration, a biological process, is the basis of dental implants. The implant fixture is first placed to ensure that it will osseointegrate, and then a dental prosthetic is attached. The position and angle of adjacent teeth helps in determining the position of implants, through lab simulations, or computed tomography with CAD/CAM simulations and surgical guides known as stents. The final prosthetic can be either fixed, where the denture or teeth cannot be removed from the mouth, or removable, where the prosthetic can be removed. An abutment is attached to the implant fixture in both the cases. This book is a valuable compilation of topics, ranging from the basic to the most complex advancements in the field of implant dentistry. It is a resource guide for experts as well as students.

I wish to thank my publisher for supporting me at every step. I would also like to thank all the authors who have contributed their researches in this book. I hope this book will be a valuable contribution to the progress of the field.

Editor

1

Bacterial Leakage Along the Implant-Abutment Interface

Cássio do Nascimento and
Rubens Ferreira de Albuquerque Jr.
Faculty of Dentistry of Ribeirão Preto,
Department of Dental Materials and Prosthodontics
Brazil

1. Introduction

Titanium implants have been successfully and increasingly used for the substitution of dental elements in the treatment of total or partial edentulism, exhibiting success rates frequently above 90%, since the earliest reports on this technique in the 1960 decade (Lang et al., 2004; Pjetursson et al., 2007; Jung et al., 2008). When treatment failures are calculated based on patients who lost implants and not on implant lost by the population in general, success rates may be considerably lower (Lambrecht et al., 2003; Stavropoulos et al., 2007; Esposito et al., 2010).

Excessive premature loading, occlusal trauma and poor bone support are considered the main factors associated with early implant loss (Esposito et al., 2000; Piattelli et al., 2003). Recent reports demonstrated that microorganisms in the oral cavity, especially the ones involved in periodontal diseases, together with unfavorable occlusal factors are considered as the main causes of unsuccessful treatment with implants (Mombelli & Lang, 1998; Covani et al., 2006).

A direct correlation between presence of microorganisms and disease of the peri-implant tissues has been demonstrated. Gram-negative, anaerobic species like *Fusobacterium spp, Prevotella spp* and spirochetes are frequently found in large quantities in affected sites. In contrast, healthy sites are predominantly colonized by Gram-positives (Mombelli & Lang, 1998; Quirynen et al., 2006). Periodontitis in proximity to implants and presence of periodontal pathogenic bacteria in the peri-implant sulci are considered risk factors to the success of dental implants (Mombelli et al., 1995; Mombelli & Décaillet, 2011). Surface characteristics, physical properties, as well as biological factors involved in this type of treatment may facilitate bacterial colonization and growth of potentially pathogenic microorganisms at the implant sites (Mombelli et al., 1995; Jansen et al., 1997; Covani et al., 2005).

Another risk factor to the peri-implant tissues is the presence of marginal discrepancies between prosthetic crowns and implants abutments, although it is a controversial issue. The assessment of these discrepancies varies largely depending on the material employed for crown fabrication, type of cement, measuring methods, etc. Studies using human extracted teeth have reported marginal discrepancies ranging from 5 to 430 μm (Abbate et al., 1989; Felton et al., 1991; Valderrama et al., 1995; Kosyfaki et al., 2010). The highest values, varying from 110 to 160 μm, are frequently associated to feather–edge cast gold crowns (Marxkors,

1980; Diedrich & Erpenstein 1985). In contrast, clinical evaluation of ceramic crowns have shown smaller discrepancies, ranging from 32-145 μm (May et al., 1998; Boening et al., 2000; Kokubo et al., 2005). Acceptable discrepancies between abutments and fixed prosthesis should not be higher than 120 μm (Jemt & Book, 1996; Kosyfaki et al., 2007), although some authors report success in patients having misfits of around 30 to 200 μm (Boeckler et al., 2005).

The great majority of current implant systems contain two parts connected by screws, the intraosseous cylinder and the abutment, showing, as a result, an interface and empty spaces between the components. Localization levels of the implant-abutment interface in relation to the alveolar bone crest during implant placement, as well as the type of connection may vary between the different implant systems. Depending on the system, the implant-abutment interface is positioned either at the bone or gingival level. In bone level systems, a second screw, or cementing agent, connects the prosthetic structure to the abutment, thus introducing a second union interface. Gingival level implant systems have the implant-abutment interface many times covered by the prosthetic structure, which results externally in a single implant-prosthesis interface that are positioned about the gingival level. Frequently, the implant and abutment connection surfaces are machine made while prosthetic structures may be machined or cast. In general, more regular surfaces and precise marginal adaptations can be achieved with machined components in comparison with in comparison with cast ones. On the other hand, independent parts connected by screws are prone to micro-movements, which may alter the adaptation between components and inevitably originate hollow spaces (Steinebrunner et al., 2005). In some systems the abutment is connected to the implant using a cementing agent, which fills the existing interfacial gaps (Piattelli et al., 2001; Scarano et al., 2005). Jansen et al. (1997) have demonstrated that the presence and sizes of gaps between implants and abutments may vary according to the type of connections and the structural characteristics of the abutments. Vertical marginal discrepancies between implant and abutment of approximately 0 to 10 μm (Jansen et al., 1997; Bondan et al., 2009) and horizontal average discrepancies of 60 μm (Byrne et al., 1998; Kano et al., 2007) have been observed. Even wider variations were found when methodological differences are considered, particularly in comparisons involving unitary and multiple prosthetic elements. Although considerably smaller than the spaces between implants and cast or synterized ceramic crowns, discrepancies between machined components are still larger than the corpuscular dimensions of various bacterial species.

The hollow spaces between implant and abutments may act as reservoir for commensal and/or pathogenic bacteria, especially anaerobic or microaerophilic species, representing a potential source of tissue inflammation. Hence, microbial colonization of the interfacial gaps may ultimately result in bone resorption (Quirynen et al., 1990; Quirynen et al., 1994; Mombelli et al., 1995).

Several *in vivo* and *in vitro* studies have shown bacterial leakage through the implant-abutment interface, either from the external sites to the inner parts of the implants or vise-versa (Quirynen et al.,1994; Jansen et al., 1997; Rimondini et al., 2001; Steinebrunner et al.,2005; Callan et al., 2005; do Nascimento et al., 2009a; Cosyn et al. 2009; Aloise et al., 2010). Other studies, have demonstrated the leakage of dyes and/or bacterial endotoxins through the implant-abutment interface (Gross et al., 1999; Piattelli et al 2001).

Bacterial contamination of two-part dental implants has been well described in non-loading conditions but several questions remain on the biomechanical principles that control the whole system during masticatory function (Brunsky et al. 2000). Lack of component

adaptation and passive connection are potential causes of mechanical damages, like screw loosening and fracture, as well as the development of mucositis and peri-implantitis due to biofilm retention (Quirynen et al., 1994; Mombelli et al., 1995).
Mechanical loading of the prosthetic abutments is another factor that may affect adaptation of implant and components and in consequence, leakage of microorganisms through the implant-abutment junction. Reports by Steinebrunner et al. (2005) indicate that bacterial penetration between implants and abutments connected by screws varies according to the number of loading cycles applied to the abutment. The leakage of microorganisms and fluids to the inner parts of the implants is considerably increased by load application, which generates micro-movements and interfacial gaps (Khraisat et al., 2006).
Bacterial species harboring the internal surfaces of the implants and components is not surprising, since the size of oral bacterial species ranges in average from 1.1 to 1.5 μm in length and 2 to 6 μm in diameter. Smaller species like spirochetes (diameter of 0.1 to 0.5 μm) may also be found in the oral microbiota (Jansen et al., 1997).
The presence of bacterial contamination of implants and components has traditionally been detected by conventional microbiological cultures, which have inherent deficiencies, particularly in the identification of fastidious species and strict anaerobes (Rolph et al., 2001; Moraes et al., 2002).
The last two decades witnessed the development and extensive use of new molecular techniques to detect, identify and quantify microbial species dwelling in the oral cavity. These rapid, sensitive and specific techniques revealed an enormous, hitherto unknown, microbiota. (Sakamoto et al., 2005; Haffajee et al. 2009). Improvements in new implants systems are being rapidly developed, for instance in their connection mechanism, surface treatment and physicochemical properties.
Considering the increased use of dental implants in restorative dentistry and recognizing the impact of bacterial leakage along the implant-abutment interface on the health of peri-implant tissues, this chapter intends to review and discuss the literature on the subject.

2. Biofilms and bacterial colonization of dental implants

2.1 Biofilm formation

Bacterial colonization of the the oral cavity in humans starts at birth and remains constant through life (Carlsson et al., 1970; Rosan & Lamont, 2000). A saliva film is initially formed composed basically of a cell-free matrix and proteins. Subsequently, bacterial colonization of this film is followed by selective adhesion on the different substrates (Gibbons, 1984). Large quantities of lactobacillus spp, responsible for biofilm adhesion, and streptococcus spp (mainly *S. sanguinis, S.oralis, S.mitis* and *S. sobrinus*),which promote biofilm growth, are initially found. Actinomyces spp and Gram-negative species are found in low proportion at this phase (Rosan & Lamont, 2000), and cell viability and adhesion capacity are fundamental requirements for the success and keeping of bacterial colonization (Gibbons & Van Houte, 1975).
A variety of bacterial species are transitory in the oral cavity. However, the characteristics of existing surfaces may facilitate adherence and prolong their permanence. Indeed, there are reports suggesting that some of the colonizing strains may remain stable for years while others may fluctuate (Alaluusua et al., 1994; Emanuelsson & Thorqvist, 2000). The profile of the oral microbiota is shaped, in addition to environmental factors, by significant interactions between bacterial species, inhibiting or stimulating each other (Grenier & Mainard, 1986). Bacterial antagonism with predominance of pathogenic species may be the

determinant of health or disease status of the supporting tissues (Hillman et al., 1985; Socransky et al., 1988).

According to Quirynen et al. (2002), gaps in the implant-abutment interface may act as a trap for bacteria, favoring the development of biofilm with varying composition and impact on periodontal tissues. *Agregatibacter actinomycetemcomitans, Tannerella forsythia and Porphyromonas gingivalis,* many times present in these biofilms, are pathogens intimately related to the development and maintenance of periodontitis and peri-implantitis. Other pathogens with relevant participation in these diseases are *Prevotella intermedia, Campylobacter rectus, Peptostreptococcus micros, Fusobacterium nucleatum, Eubacterium nodatum, Streptococcus intermedius* and spirochetes (Quirynen et al., 2002; Socransky & Haffajee, 2002).

Periodontal disease affects tissues that support teeth and is characterized by loss of periodontal ligament insertion, and resorption of adjacent alveolar bone. This disease has multifactorial etiology, which includes biofilms as having an essential role in its pathogenesis (Lamont & Jenkinson, 1998). The term peri-implantitis, established in the Periodontia European Workshop, 1993, characterizes diseased implant supporting tissues (Albrektsson & Isidor, 1994). The initial bacterial colonization of peri-implant sulci is characterized by an increasing number of facultative anaerobic *streptococcus,* although Gram-negatives anaerobes may be occasionally found but in smaller numbers (Monbelli et al., 1988). With time, strict gram–negative anaerobes as *Fusobacterium spp and Prevotella spp* become increasingly predominant (Mombelli & Mericske-Stern, 1990).

Several reports on the microbiota detected around dental implants were published in the last decade (Haffjee et al .,1998; Botero et al., 2005; Cosyn et al., 2009; Van Brakel, et al. 2010). Presence of potential periodontal pathogens colonizing the peri-implant grooves in unsuccessful implants has also been described (Laine et al., 2005; Shibli et al., 2007; Persson et al., 2010). Other studies suggested that periodontal pathogens and/or their metabolic products might be involved in peri-implant bone losses (Lindhe et al., 1992, Persson et al., 1996). However, information on the diversity of bacteria colonizing the internal surfaces of two-part dental implants, abutments and implant prostheses and on their correlation with periodontal and peri-implantar sulci species is still lacking. . Cosyn et al. (2009), in a short clinical evaluation, have found similarities in the microbiota of samples collected from the internal parts of implants and from their related peri-implant sulci.

Another investigations indicated that the existing oral microbiota prior to implant placement is determinant to the establishment and maintenance of the implant related microbiota.. Partially edentulous patients with a history of periodontal disease show high incidence of putative periodontal pathogens in implant sites (Mombelli et al., 1995; Quirynen et al., 2002, Quirynen et a., 1996a). Laine et al. (2005), reported that the bacterial biofilm composition in the peri-implant sulcus changes during the healing period following implantation and shows constant alterations subsequently. Pathogenic and non-pathogenic species have been found surrounding peri-implant sites (Callan et al., 2005; Quirynen et al., 2006). De Boever & De Boever (2006) suggested that periodonto-pathogenic species isolated from the implant sites during the first 6 months after placement there might be no clinical consequence. However, the presence of these pathogens in the immediate healing phase may have future consequences. Bacterial species found in the wound healing of implants that failed immediately after surgery are similar to the ones seen in acute infections (Laine et al., 2005). Lately, when the implants have been exposed to oral microorganisms for a long period, the microbial biofilm changes into a pattern similar to the one found in chronic periodontal disease (Mombelli & Lang, 1998).

2.2 Design features and marginal fit of implant components

One of the most common causes of dental implants failure is poor adaptation of implant and prosthetic components, irrespectively of the implant system and connection design. Notwithstanding the constant efforts to overcome this drawback, the hollow spaces produced by poor adaptation act as traps for bacteria of the oral cavity resulting in inflammatory reactions of the peri-implant tissues (Mombelli et al., 1995; Quirynen et al., 2002). Both the microorganism and their metabolic products may be responsible for inflammation and bone loss (Lindhe et al., 1992; Quirynen & Van Steenberghe, 1993). Ultimately, uncontrolled local inflammation may lead to generalized peri-implantitis and compromise the long-term success with dental implants (Ericsson et al. 1995).

Two-part dental implant systems with screw-retained abutments are still largely used, principally due to their well reported protocol, high success rates, and broad spectrum of indications. However, gaps and cavities in the assemblies after abutment attachment are frequently related to peri-implant tissue problems. Figure 1 illustrates the gaps resulted from attached components of an implant system. These gaps favor bacterial biofilm accumulation between components, generally in the interfaces implant-abutment, abutment-prosthesis, and on the exposed surfaces of abutments, prosthesis and implants to the oral environment. Under loading, where the abutment components are subjected to eccentric forces, the number and size of gaps can be augmented. Moreover, micro-movements of implant components during function may allow the initiation of a pumping effect that facilitates bacterial leakage through the implant-abutment interface (Steinebrunner et al., 2005). Also, the abutment screw loosening may contribute to joint instability, screw fracture, and clinical failure. Increased percentages of abutment screw loosening and the consequent increase in micro-movements between components are more common in implants with external hexagonal connections (Binon et al., 2000).

Sahin & Cehreli (2001), in a revision study, evaluated the clinical significance of the passive fit on the final marginal fit of implant-supported restorations. The authors recommend that the implant-abutment assembly should result in a passive connection, not inductive of tension in implant components and adjacent bone. However, according to the authors, this is not possible since clinical and laboratory procedures utilized in the fabrication of the super structures are not adequate. The lack of dimensional precision and may introduce strains to the fixation screws, potentially causing screw or abutment fracture.

Studies on the adaptation between implant and components have been related their failed adaptive conditions to the presence of bacterial infiltration (Jansen et al., 1997; Steinebrunner et al., 2005). Quirynen & Van Steenberghe (1993) investigated the presence of microorganisms in the internal screw threads of Branemark implants. In nine patients, the apical part of two intermediate screws installed three months before was examined through contrast phase microscopy, showing a significant quantity of microorganisms, mainly coccus (86.2%) and nonmotile rods (12.3%). Motile species (1.3%) and spirochetes (0.1%) were scarce. Another similar study observed a microbiota mainly composed of anaerobes and facultative streptococcus, Gram-positive anaerobic rods such as *Propionibacterium, Eubacterium and Actinomyces* besides Gram-negative anaerobes, including *Fusobacterium, Prevotella and Porphyromonas* (Persson et al., 1996).

Several implant systems with different designs are currently available in the market. The Figure 2 and 3 illustrate three different implants and platform connections of an implant system. They have different shapes, surfaces, sizes and distances between screw threads, as well as different types of connections between implants and abutments. The external hexagonal platform proposed by Branemark et al. (1969), was until recently the most widely used and well documented. The system has a connecting hexagonal platform acting as an anti-rotational mechanism that is, together with the connecting screw, responsible for the mechanical stability of the implant-abutment set. Despite the wide acceptance and use, the system shows an external connection concentrating considerable more strength in the threads of the abutment screw, which may lead to fractures and implant failures (Norton et al., 1997; Finger et al., 2003; Bernardes et al., 2009). This type of connection shows the highest vertical and horizontal implant-abutment discrepancies described in the literature (Binon et al., 1996).

Studies on the precision of the connection between components of different systems showed that some can be interchanged with an accuracy similar to the one observed in connections with components of the same system (Hagiwara et al., 1997; Dellow et al., 1997).

Scanning electron microscopy examinations of the implant-abutment interface, showed vertical and horizontal maladaptations between implants with external hexagonal connections and their respective abutments varying, on average, from 1 to 100 µm, (Binon et al., 1996; Jansen et al., 1997). In general, machined abutments show superior adaptation in relation to laboratory cast ones, suggesting that stricter standard controls should be held on components obtained by casting procedures (Byrne et al., 1998). The type of metal alloy in cast components has also a relevant role on the final adaptation of the assemblies. Components cast in Ni/Cr or Cr/Co are more variable in respect to the marginal dimensional stability when compared with Au or Ag/Pd alloys cast components (Binon et al., 1995; Byrne et al., 1998).

Bone crest changes around implants were studied in dogs by Hermann et al. (2001), by observing the influence of marginal gaps in the implant-abutment interface and occurrence of micro-movements. Gap sizes were in the range of 10-100 µm and micro-movements were abolished in some groups by laser welding of interfaces The results showed that resorption in crest bone was significantly influenced by movements between abutments and implants but not by gap sizes along the interface.

New connection designs were proposed to overcome the drawbacks of the hexagonal precursor system. Hexagonal platforms with larger interfacial area as well as internal connection systems with varied shapes were developed to improve adaptation and stability of the implant components. However, in contrast to the well-standardized features of the external hexagonal precursor, the internal connections are usually unique for each developer and thus difficult to standardize.

Clinical and in vitro evaluations indicate that connections between components are more stable in the internal hexagonal system, in which the larger contact area between internal implant and abutments walls favors force distribution and preserves the abutment screw (Norton et al., 1997; Mollersten et al., 1997; Binon et al., 2000; Finger et al., 2003). Microbiological studies, however, do not show significant differences between hexagonal internal or external connections, when bacterial leakage is concerned (Jansen et al., 1997; Steinebrunner et al., 2005; Duarte et al., 2006).

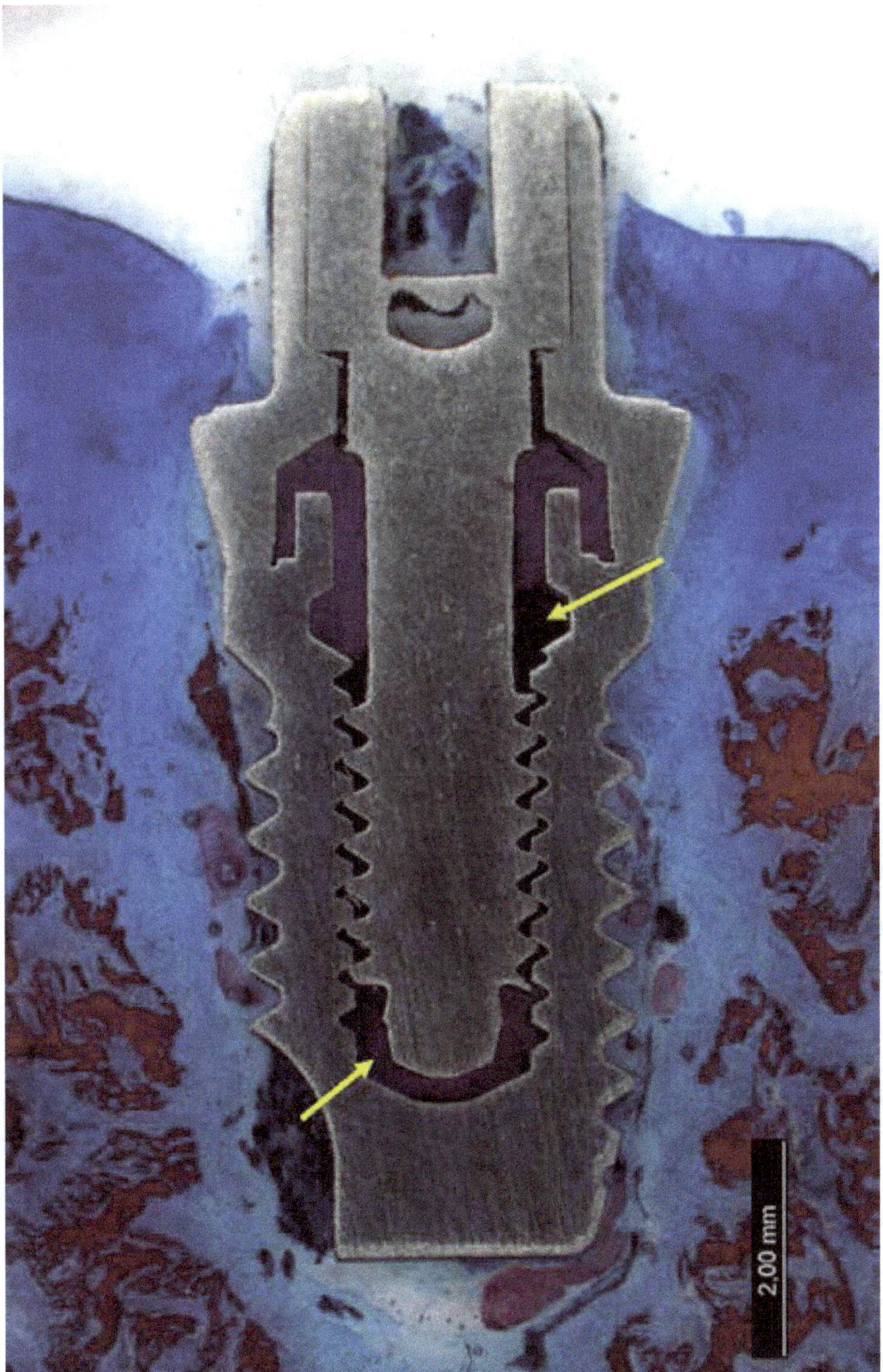

Fig. 1. Histological Photomicrograph showing the gaps and hollow spaces (arrows) resulted from the poor adaptation of the implant and prosthetic components in the two-part implant systems (MKIII TiUnit and it respective abutment, Nobel Biocare- regular external hexagonal platform with 3.75 mm in diameter and 7 mm in length).

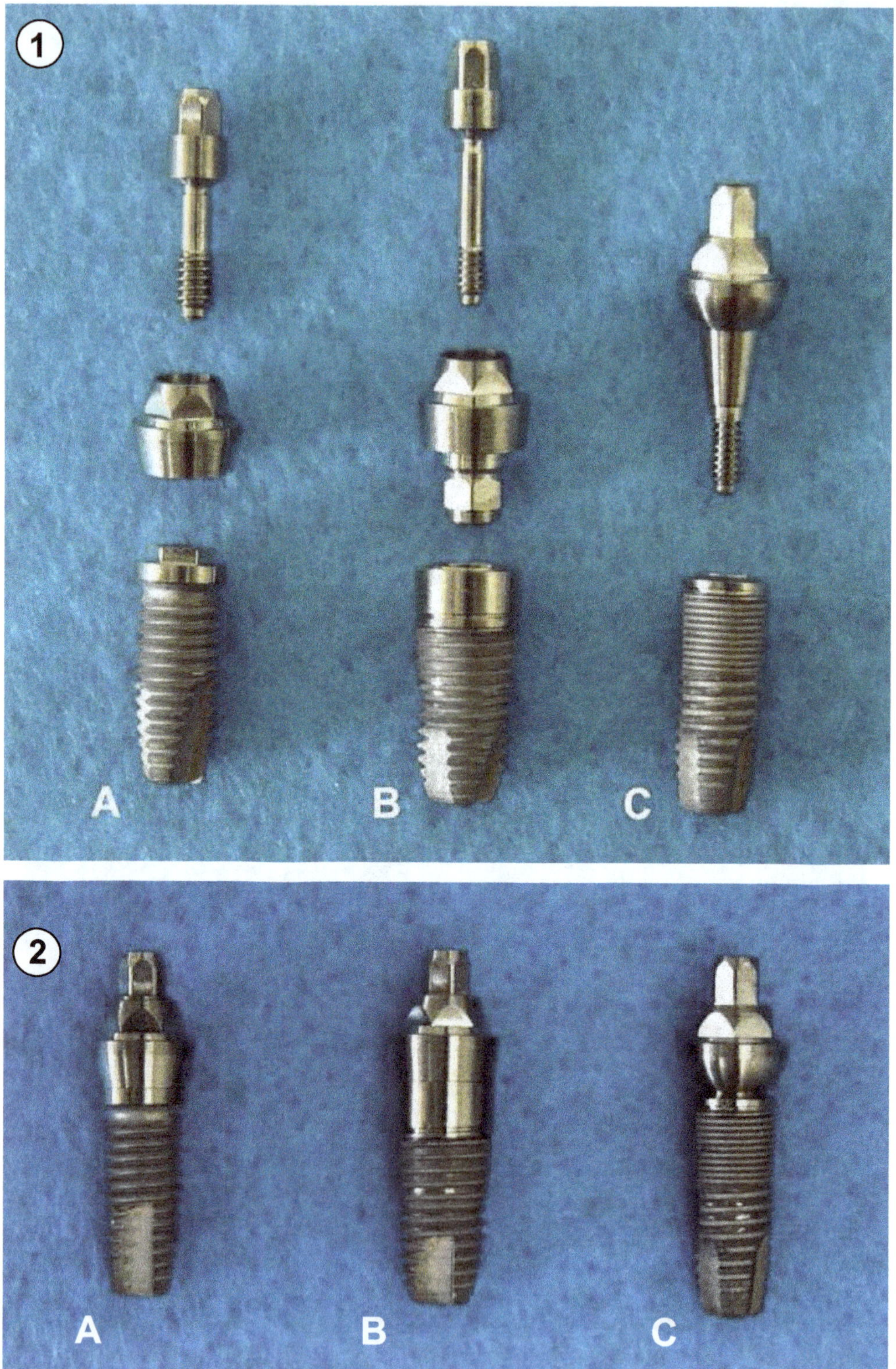

Fig. 2. Illustration showing 3 different implants and abutments before (1) and after (2) connection: (A) External Hexagonal, (B) Internal Hegonal and (C) Morse Cone.

The Morse cone connection system has recently been introduced and is becoming increasingly popular in implant dentistry. Due to its tapered design, the system is considered mechanically more stable and efficient in preventing bacterial leakage. The Morse cone connection, compared with other types, is more efficient in the dissipation of forces exerted on the prosthesis and consequently on the supporting bone tissue (Merz et al., 2000). It does not completely inhibit the passage of bacteria and fluids through the interface, but microbiological evaluations show that there is a more efficient bacterial sealing between the Morse cone implant and its abutment, revealed by lower bacterial counts in comparison to other connection systems (Pautke et al., 2009; Aloise et al., 2010). The intimate adaptation between contacting surfaces obtained with this type of connection seems to produce a frictional locking, which restrains micro-movements. Concurrently, minimized spaces at the interface seem to be related to decreased levels of bacterial contamination, probably by preventing leakage and reducing the available volume for bacterial growth. Further investigations are necessary, however, in order to determine the biomechanical behavior of these components in long-term studies, since most of these findings were obtained in short term studies.

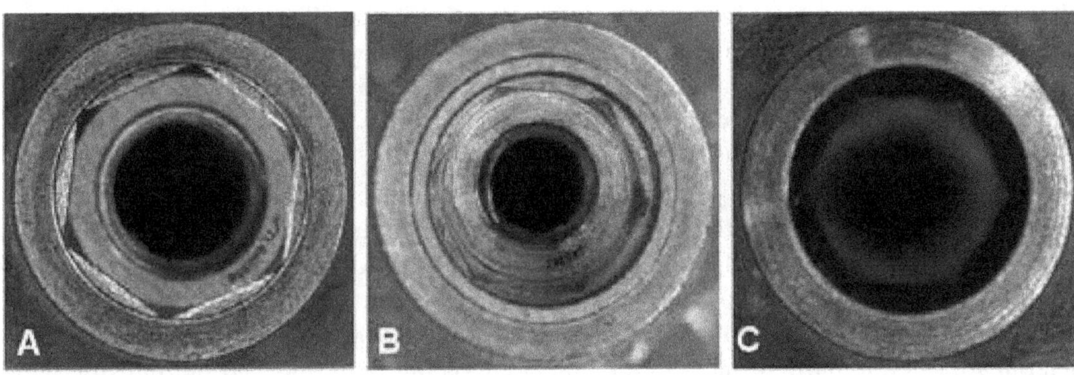

Fig. 3. Microscopy picture showing the External Hexagonal (A), Internal Hexagonal (B) and Morse Cone (C) platform.

2.3 Abutment materials

Peri-implant soft tissues act as a protection barrier between the oral cavity environment and the peri-implant bone (Welander et al., 2008). The type of material used in the abutment fabrication seems to be crucial in determining the final quality of the mucosa in contact with theabutment surface (Abrahamsson et al., 1998). It has been observed that when titanium abutments are used, the surrounding mucosais mainly composed of epithelial and connective healthy tissues. Healthy soft tissues should promote an effective barrier against the passage of microorganisms and/or their products, preserving the adjacent bone from being damaged (Welander et al., 2008).

Precious and basic metals, as well as ceramic materials, are also used in the manufacture of abutments. Ceramic materials, such as zirconium dioxide, or simply zirconia, are popular materials, increasingly used in prosthetic abutments. They are similar in color to dental structures and have potential advantages over metallic materials (Brodbeck, 2003; Watkin & Kerstein, 2008) besides other properties such as higher translucency, (Denry & Kelly, 2008), good tissue adhesion (Pessková et al., 2007), less tissue discoloring effect (Bressan et al., 2010), lower bacterial adhesion and growth (Scarano et al., 2004) and lower toxicity (Uo et al., 2003).

Zirconia has excellent mechanical properties besides being material of choice for esthetic and biological reasons. It has high resistance against fractures (Anusavice et al., 2007; Manicone et al., 2007; Denry & Kelly, 2008) which was demonstrated in short term (3-4years) *in vivo* studies with satisfactory clinical results (Glauser et al., 2004; Canullo et al., 2007; Ekfeldt et al., 2011).
Although abutments with esthetic properties are continually sought, conclusive clinical evidence of their ability to maintain healthier periimplant tissues is still lacking in the current literature (Linkevivius & Apce, 2008). Few studies have compared bacterial adhesion in metallic and non-metallic components. While some authors claim that bacterial adhesion is lower in zirconia components (Scarano et al., 2004), others show that there is no difference between zirconia and titanium components (Salihoglu et al., 2010). Results from a study in animals (Abrahamssom et al., 1998) and a recent one in humans (Van Brakel et al., 2010), indicate that zirconia and titanium abutments may exert a similar healthier effect on peri-implant tissues.
On the other hand, the use of zirconia abutments in esthetic components can be limited in cases of cemented prosthesis, due to the low adhesion of the cement to the ceramic material, although the use of recently developed primers may minimize the problem. Another recent proposal to improve the treatment outcome with implants by taking advantage of the best properties of different materials is the use of hybrid connection systems, composed of titanium abutments surrounded by a zirconia-overlaid collar. Future studies are expected to evaluate the biomechanical behavior of these systems.

2.4 Effects of surface characteristics (chemistry, free energy and roughness)

The surface physico-chemical properties of implants and abutments, like roughness, chemical treatments and free energy have an important role in the formation and maintenance of bacterial biofilms (Grossner -Screiber et al., 2001).
Bacterial adhesion to hard surfaces in the oral cavity is highly influenced by rugosity, which in turn is related to the number of colonies formed (Quirynen et al., 1996b). Scanning electron microscopy analysis of bacterial behavior on different materials used in implant and prosthetic components, indicated that rough surfaces have higher indexes of bacterial adhesion (Grossner-Schreiber et al., 2001; Amoroso et al., 2006). Implants and components showing an average roughness lower than 0.1 μm partially inhibited bacterial biofilm formation and growth after 24 hours (Rimondini et al., 1997). High surface rugosity and consequent high hydrophobic properties (low wettability) tend to favor biofilm formation and bacterial adhesion (Drake et al., 1999). Steam-autoclave sterilization of titanium increases the oxide layer thickness, accumulation of impurities on the metal surface, and hydrophobicity, as shown by Drake et al. (1999). The authors demonstrated that surfaces that were steam-autoclaved 10 times showed significantly greater CFU/mm2, specially of *S. sanguis*, than other methods of sterilization, regardless of surface roughness. .
Surface treatment of components has a relevant impact on bacterial adhesion and colonization. Titanium implants treated with titanium nitrate (TiN) or zirconia nitrate (ZrN) followed by thermal oxidation or laser irradiation produced significant reduction of biofilm formation and bacterial adhesion when compared to surfaces of polished titanium (Grosner-Schreiber et al., 2001). Other surface treatments proposed to inhibit microorganism adhesion such as, antibacterial coverings (Ge et al., 2010), electro-chemical treatments (Visai et al., 2008), and new metallic alloys (Pautke et al., 2009) still need further evaluations to warrant applicability.

Biofilm formation is directly, but less intensely, related to component surface free energy (SFE) (Burgers et al., 2010). SFE results from the interaction of cohesion and adhesion forces, responsible for the wettability property of surfaces. SFE facilitates accumulation of bacterial biofilm, by promoting firm adhesion to contact surfaces besides selecting specific bacterial species, a property intimately related to the acid-basic characteristics of bacterial cell walls. In a literature review, Quirynen & Bollen (1995) conclude that smooth surfaces with low SFE can potentially reduce the occurrence of caries and periodontitis. In contrast, rough surfaces promote plaque formation and maturation, and high-energy surfaces are known to collect more plaque and to select specific bacteria.

3. Culture and culture-independent methods focusing on oral microbiota of dental implants

Identification of microorganisms inhabiting peri-implant crevices and the internal parts of implants has been of relevant importance in respect to the outcome of the treatment with dental implants, since several studies showed a correlation between bacterial species of the oral cavity, especially those involved in periodontal diseases, and the occurrence of failure in the treatment with implants (Ong et al. 1992; Shibli et al., 2007). Periodontal pathogenic bacteria in peri-implant crevices and teeth with periodontitis close to dental implants are considered risk factors for the success of dental implants (Gouvoussis et al., 1997; Saito et al., 1997). To date, a large number of microbial species related to periodontal and peri-implant diseases have been identified and can be quantified by different methods.

3.1 Conventional cultures

Bacterial culture is a well-known method historically used to characterize the oral cavity microbiota, and considered a classical reference method in microbiology. Traditionally, culture-dependent methodologies are used to isolate, enumerate and detect probiotic organisms, especially from mixed cultures (Charteris et al., 1997). Several variables in culture technology, especially an appropriate sample collection technique and media selection, have been recognised as having a significant impact on the sensitivity and specificity of the test, mainly on the organism recovery rates and time for reporting results (Riedel & Carroll, 2010). This method constitutes an important epidemiological tool, with results that serve as a base for building an empirical therapeutic strategy. Also, this methodology is essential in the initial phase of several culture-independent techniques, where bacterial growth and isolation is necessary to DNA probes confection.

These methods are essentially designed around the recovery and (or) enumeration of viable bacteria in the contaminant media. Detection of viable bacteria is traditionally performed by implementing a means of culturing growth of individual species. The use of non-selective media such as trypticase soy agar or standard methods agar, known as the aerobic or standard plate count, is routinely applied in this methodology. In addition, in specific conditions, the increased sensitivity of these standard media has been achieved using a selective agar overlay approach designed to recover a larger proportion of bacteria from contaminant media (Specket et al. 1975; Harrigan, 1998).

Most studies describing the microbial leakage through the implant-abutment interface are based on results with conventional culture method (Jansen et al., 1997; Piatelli et al., 1999; Steinebrunner et al., 2005; Pautke et al., 2009; Aloise et al., 2010). However, an inherent limitation of microbiological cultures is that the difficulties to identify strict anaerobes, frequently associated with periodontal and peri-implant diseases, as well as fastidious species (Barbosa et al., 2009; Roças et al., 2010). It is estimated that 50% of the oral microbiota is not cultured by conventional methods and several of these species are directly related to infectious processes in the oral cavity (Arank et al., 1969; Paster et al., 2001; Parahitiyawa et al., 2010). Furthermore, non-viable cells, still able to produce aggressive compounds against peri-implant tissues are not detected by culture methods.

Despite of the efforts to optimise broth composition, enhance the growth of microorganisms and prevent contamination during procedures, the methodology is time-consuming and the microbial viability is essential to confirm the presence pathogens. Cell killing and degradation by bacteriocin as well as degradation of DNA by proteolytic enzymes and endonucleases has been demonstrated in several studies (Loyola-Rodriguez et al. 1992, Cowman & Baron 1993, Cascales et al. 2007). These substances may cause deleterious effects on the peri-implant support tissues. Therefore, despite the advantages of these familiar culture methods in detecting viable bacteria, such as ease of use and low cost, assay sensitivity is still relatively low compared with alternative methods (such as molecular-based approaches).

Quantitative bacterial measurements are widely used in microbiology. Many years of research studies using quantitative microbiology on solid media have demonstrated that such measurements provide clinically valuable information. For example, bacterial load is predictive for the occurrence of complications (Yagupsky & Nolte, 1990). However, the bacteria quantitation in conventional culture method is difficult to achieve and is rarely practised in clinical laboratories because it requires subsequent plating on solid media rather than incubation in liquid media. The time required for liquid culture bottles to become positive provides some suggestion of bacterial load, but is a weak quantitative measure and varies with the microorganisms present. Also, each bacterial must be individually evaluated with a specific media.

3.2 Culture- independent methods

In the last two decades great advances in molecular diagnostic methods were achieved, which have been extensively used in the detection and identification of microbial species inhabiting the oral cavity (Sakamoto et al., 2005; Haffajee et al., 2009; Costa et al., 2010). These techniques are more rapid, sensitive and specific when compared to the conventional culture methods. Species showing diverse phenotypic behavior may be identified by their genomic characteristics, which are not dependent on cell viability, a great advantage in studies evaluating anaerobic infections, when cell death may occur during sample collection or transportation (Whelen & Persing, 1996; Pitt & Saundres, 2000). These techniques have also promoted advances in the knowledge of the microbiota in other parts of the human body (Eckburg et al., 2005; Dethlefsen et al., 2007; Grice et al.,2008; Oakley et al., 2008) revealing a great quantity of bacterial species not cultured, whether associated or not to infectious processes (Turnbaugh et al., 2007; Mallard, 2008)

3.2.1 Checkerboard DNA- DNA hybridization

Methods based on cellular DNA characterization, used for microbial detection and quantitation have been documented in the current literature. The Checkerboard DNA hybridization technique utilizes genomic DNA probes to identify and quantify several bacterial species simultaneously in a great number of samples from the oral cavity, and has been largely employed in studies on the oral microbiota (Socransky et al., 1994). Several areas in dentistry have recently been using the technique to evaluate the composition of bacterial biofilms in health or disease conditions (Aberg et al., 2009; Teles et al., 2010; Kim et al., 2010, Vettore et al., 2010), and in studies on the association of local and systemic factors that can affect biofilm formation (Borges et al., 2009; Demmer st al., 2010). The technique is also employed to evaluate bacteria associated with endodontic lesions (Roças & Siqueira, 2010) and to verify changes in biofilm composition as a result of periodontal treatments (Haffajee et al., 2009).

More recently the DNA hybridization technique has been used to identify and quantify multiple bacterial species associated to dental implants. *In vitro* studies show that several bacterial species colonizing the internal surfaces of implants may be consistently identified and quantified (do Nascimento et al., 2009; Barbosa et al., 2009). The DNA Checkerboard method is significantly more sensitive in the bacterial detection than conventional cultures according to Loesche et al. (1992). Barbosa et al., (2009) compared the two methods in an *in vitro* study involving the investigation of *F. nucleatum*in the interior of implants with an external hexagonal connection. The microorganism counts were significantly higher with the DNA -Checkerboard method leading to the conclusion that it is more sensitive than conventional cultures and allows identification of bacteria that are viable or not. Considering that bacterial cell structure and its degradation products may act as nutrients to other opportunistic species, the identification of non viable species may be relevant to risk determination associated to peri-implant tissues.

3.2.2 PCR-based techniques

Other molecular diagnostic methods utilize amplified genetic material by the Polymerase Chain reaction (PCR). These methods are more specific and sensitive and may be useful to complete results obtained by DNA hybridization. PCR-based techniques are very sensitive and specific allowing the identification of species in the interior of implants even when they are present in very small quantities (Haffajee et al., 2009). Susceptibility of contamination due the amplification procedure is the main limitation of this method.

PCR methods involve the enzymatic synthesis of a specific DNA segment of the target species by DNA polymerase. The reaction develops the annealing and enzymatic extension of an oligonucleotide pair utilized as initiators, the so-called primers, which delimit the DNA sequence of the double strand targeted by the amplification. Three variants of the technique can be employed in dentistry to identify bacterial species in the oral cavity: PCR (conventional or qualitative), RT_PCR (Real time PCR or Quantitative PCR) and 16SrDNA-based PCR.

The high specificity of amplification by the qualitative PCR technique discriminates numerous species of microorganisms in the oral cavity, including pathogens not easily detected by other methods. However, detection is limited to the plateau reaction and it is unable to determine the precise number of bacteria present in a determined site (Higushi et al., 1992; Jervoe-Storm et al., 2005). Real-Time PCR precisely quantifies the species in the study. The number of product molecules synthesized in this technique depends directly on the number of molecules used as standards. Quantification data are collected in the exponential phase of PCR, producing a precise quantification of the number of target DNA copies when internal and external standard are used. Real Time PCR has been used as a complement to conventional cultures or DNA Checkerboard to quantify main periodontal pathogens, as for instance, *P. gingivalis, A. actinomycetemcomitans, T. denticola* and *T. forsythia.*

The sequencing of the DNA ribosome gene (rDNA) 16S, found in the bacteria genome, has recently been used to evaluate the microbial diversity of the oral cavity (Gu et al., 2009), esophagus (Macfarlane et al., 2007), stomach (Li et al., 2009), intestine (Hill et al., 2010, colon (Mäkivuokko et al., 2010) and vagina (Oakley et al., 2008). In contrast with molecular methods, which employ DNA probes, like the DNA Checkerboard, this methodology identifies large populations of non-cultured species, many times associated to the disease conditions. Through these methods it was possible to characterize the subgengival microbiota of the periodontal pouch as being composed of more than 700 diverse species isolated from different individuals. The great majority does not have a DNA totally identified and sequenced and, thus, cannot be investigated by methods using DNA probes (Roças et al., 2010).

4. Conclusions

Implant materials, connection systems, and surface properties have all relevant impact on the initial formation of biofilm and on the characteristics of the peri- and intra- implant microbiota. These factors can influence bacterial adhesion to implants and prosthetic abutments, with varied impact on the peri-implant tissues, and may interfere on the success with this type of treatment.

More stable connections, showing smaller and less frequent free spaces after component adjustments, have shown to be more efficient in containing bacterial leakage through the interfaces. Modifications of the titanium surfaces, or the surfaces of other materials used in the manufacture of implants systems, may reduce biofilm formation and consequent outcomes. Diagnostic techniques currently used to evaluate bacterial contamination of implant related structures have specific characteristics and applications, and thus, should be considered as complementary.

5. References

Abbate, M.F.; Tjan, A.H.L. & Fox, W.M. (1989). Comparison of the marginal fit of various ceramic crown systems. *Journal of Prosthetic Dentistry*, Vol.61, No.5, pp. 527-531

Aberg, C.H.; Sjödin, B.; Lakio, L.; Pussinen, P.J.; Johansson, A. & Claesson, R. (2009). Presence of Aggregatibacter actinomycetemcomitans in young individuals: a 16-year clinical and microbiological follow-up study. *Journal of Clinical Periodontology*, Vol.36, No.10, pp. 815-822

Abrahamsson, I.; Berglundh, T.; Glantz, P.O. & Lindhe, J. (1998).The mucosal attachment at different abutments. An experimental study in dogs. *Journal of Clinical Periodontology*, Vol.25, No.9, pp. 721-727

Al-Ahmad, A.; Wiedmann-Al-Ahmad, M.; Faust, J.; Bächle, M.; Follo, M.; Wolkewitz, M.; Hannig, C.; Hellwig, E.; Carvalho, C. & Kohal, R. (2010). Biofilm formation and composition on different implant materials in vivo. *Journal of Biomedical Materials Ressearch Part B: Applied Biomaterials,* Vol.95, No.1, pp.101-109

Alaluusua, S. & Malmivirta, R. (1994). Early plaque accumulation--a sign for caries risk in young children. *Community Dentistry and Oral Epidemiology*, Vol.22, No.(5 Pt 1), pp. 273-276

Albrektsson, T. & Isidor, F. (1994). Consensus report of session IV. In: Lang N.P, Karring, T (eds.), *Proceedings of the 1st European Workshop on Periodontology,* 365-369, Quintessence Publishing, London

Aloise, J.P.; Curcio, R.; Laporta, M.Z.; Rossi, L.; da Silva, A.M. & Rapoport, A. (2010). Microbial leakage through the implant-abutment interface of Morse taper implants in vitro. *Clinical Oral Implants Research*, Vol.21, No.3, pp. 328-35

Amoroso, P.F.; Adams, R.J.; Waters, M.G. & Williams, D.W. (2006). Titanium surface modification and its effect on the adherence of Porphyromonas gingivalis: an in vitro study. *Clinical Oral Implants Research*, Vol.17, No.6, pp. 633-637

Anusavice, K.J.; Kakar, K. & Ferree, N. (2007). Which mechanical and physical testing methods are relevant for predicting the clinical performance of ceramic-based dental prostheses? *Clinical Oral Implants Research*, Vol.18, No.3, pp. 218–231

Arank, A.; Syed, S.A.; Kenney, E.B. & Freter, R. (1969). Isolation of anaerobic bacteria from human gingiva and mouse cecum by means of a simplified glove box procedure. *Applied Microbiology*, Vol.17, No.4, pp. 568-576

Barbosa, R.E.; do Nascimento, C., Issa, J.P.; Watanabe, E.; Ito, I.Y. & de Albuquerque Juniot, R.F. (2009). Bacterial culture and DNA Checkerboard for the detection of internal contamination in dental implants. *Journal of Prosthodontics*, Vol.18, No.5, pp. 376-381

Bernardes, S.R.; de Araujo, C.A.; Neto, A.J.; Simamoto Junior, P. & das Neves, F.D. (2009). Photoelastic analysis of stress patterns from different implant-abutment interfaces. *International Journal of Oral and Maxillofacial Implants*, Vol.24, No.5, pp. 781-789

Binon, P.P. (1995). Evaluation of machining accuracy and consistency of selected implants, standard abutments, and laboratory analogs. *International Journal of Prosthodontics*, Vol.8, No.2, pp. 162-178

Binon, P.P. (1996). The effect of implant/abutment hexagonal misfit on screw joint stability. *International Journal of Prosthodontics*, Vol.9, No.2, pp. 149-160

Binon, P.P. (2000). Implants and components: entering the new millennium. *International Journal of Oral and Maxillofacial Implants*, Vol.15, No.1, pp. 76-94

Boeckler, A.F.; Stadler, A. & Setz, J.M. (2005). The significance of marginal gap and overextension measurement in the evaluation of the fit of complete crowns. *Journal of Contemporary Dental Practice*, Vol.15, No.4, pp. 26-37

Boening, K.W.; Wolf, B.H.; Schmidt, A.E.; Kästner, K. & Walter, M.H. (2000). Clinical fit of Procera AllCeram crowns. *Journal of Prosthetic Dentistry*, Vol.84, No.4, pp. 419-424

Bondan, J.L.,;Oshima, H.M.; Segundo, R.M.; Shinkai, R.S.; Mota, E.G. & Meyer, K.R. (2009). Marginal fit analysis of premachined and castable UCLA abutments. Acta Odontolica Latinoamericana, Vol.22, No.2, pp. 139-42

Borges, M.A.; De Figueiredo, L.C.; De Brito Junior, R.B.; Faveri, M. & Feres, M. (2009). Microbiological composition associated with vitamin D receptor gene polymorphism in chronic periodontitis. *Brazilian Oral Research*, Vol.2, No.23, pp. 203-208

Botero, J.E.; González, A.M.; Mercado, R.A.; Olave, G. & Contreras, A. (2005). Subgingival microbiota in peri-implant mucosa lesions and adjacent teeth in partially edentulous patients. *Journal of Periodontology*, Vol.76, No.9, pp. 1490-1495

Brånemark, P.I.; Adell, R.; Breine, U.; Hansson, B.O.; Lindström, J. & Ohlsson, A. (1969). Intra-osseous anchorage of dental prostheses. I. Experimental studies. *Scandinavian Journal of Plastic and Reconstrutive Surgery*, Vol.3, No.2, pp. 81-100

Bressan, E.; Paniz, G.; Lops, D.; Corazza, B.; Romeo, E. & Favero, G. (2010). Influence of abutment material on the gingival color of implant-supported all-ceramic restorations: a prospective multicenter study. *Clinical Oral Implants Research*, InPress

Brodbeck, U. (2003). The ZiReal Post: A new ceramic implant abutment. *Journal of Esthetic and Restorative Dentistry*, Vol.15, No.1, pp. 10-23

Brunski, J.B.; Puleo, D.A. & Nanci, A. (2000). Biomaterials and biomechanics of oral and maxillofacial implants: current status and future developments. *International Journal of Oral and Maxillofacial Implants*, Vol.15, No.1, pp. 15-46

Bürgers, R.; Gerlach, T.; Hahnel, S.; Schwarz, F.; Handel, G. & Gosau, M. (2010). In vivo and in vitro biofilm formation on two different titanium implant surfaces. *Clinical Oral Implants Research*, Vol.21, No.2, pp. 156-164

Byrne, D.; Houston, F.; Cleary, R. & Claffey, N. (1998). The fit of cast and premachined implant abutments. *Journal of Prosthetic Dentistry*, Vol.80, No.2, pp. 184-192

Callan, D.P.; Cobb, C.M. & Williams, K.B. (2005). DNA probe identification of bacteria colonizing internal surfaces of the implant-abutment interface: a preliminary study. *Journal of Periodontology*, Vol. 76, No.1, pp. 115-120

Carlsson, J.; Grahnen, H.; Jonsson, G. & Wikner, S. (1970). Establishment of Streptococcus sanguis in the mouths of infants. Archives of Oral Biology, Vol.15, No.12, pp. 1143–1148

Canullo, L. (2007). Clinical outcome study of customized zirconia abutments for single-implant restorations. *The International Journal of Prosthodontics*, Vol.20, No.5, pp. 489–493

Cascales, E.; Buchanan, S.K.; Duché, D.; Kleanthous, C.; Lloubès, R.; Postle, K.; Riley, M.; Slatin, S. & Cavard, D. (2007). Colicin biology. *Microbiology and Molecular Biology Reviews*, Vol.71, No.1, pp. 158-229

Charteris, W.P.; Kelly, P.M.; Morelli, L. & Collins, J.K. (1997). Selective detection, enumeration and identification of potentially probiotic *Lactobacillus* and *Bifidobacterium* species in mixed bacterial populations. International Journal of Food Microbiology, Vol.35, No.1, pp. 1–27

Cosyn, J.; Van Aelst, L.; Collaert, B.; Persson, G.R. & De Bruyn, H. (2009). The Peri-Implant Sulcus Compared with Internal Implant and Suprastructure Components: A Microbiological Analysis. *Clinical Implant Dentistry and Related Research*, InPress

Covani, U.; Marconcini, S.; Crespi, R. & Barone, A. (2006). Bacterial plaque colonization around dental implant surfaces. *Implant Dentistry*, Vol.15, No.3, pp. 298-304

Cowman, R.A. & Baron, S.S. (1993). Comparison of aminopeptidase activities in four strains of mutans group oral streptococci. *Infection and Immunity*, Vol.61, No.1, pp. 182-186

De Boever, A.L. & De Boever, J.A. (2006). Early colonization of non-submerged dental implants in patients with a history of advanced aggressive periodontitis. *Clinical Oral Implants Research*, Vol. 17, No.1, pp. 8–17

Dellow, A.G.; Driessen, C.H. & Nel, H.J. (1997). Scanning electron microscopy evaluation of the interfacial fit of interchanged components of four dental implant systems. *The International Journal of Prosthodontics*, Vol.10, No.3, pp. 216-221

Demmer, R.T.; Papapanou, P.N.; Jacobs Jr, D.R. & Desvarieux, M. (2010). Evaluating clinical periodontal measures as surrogates for bacterial exposure: The Oral Infections and Vascular Disease Epidemiology Study. *BMC Medical Research Methodology*, Vol.7, pp. 10-12

Denry, I. & Kelly, J.R. (2008). State of the art of zirconia for dental applications. *Dental Materials*, Vol.24, No.3, pp. 299–307.

Dethlefsen, L.; McFall-Ngai, M. & Relman, D.A. (2007). An ecological and evolutionary perspective on human-microbe mutualism and disease. *Nature*, Vol.449, No.7164, pp. 811-818

Diedrich, P. & Erpenstein, H. (1985). Scanning electron optical analysis of the marginal space of in vivo incorporated shoulder crowns and inlays. *Schweiz Monatsschr Zahnmed*, Vol.95, No.7, pp. 575-86

do Nascimento, C.; Barbosa, R.E.; Issa, J.P.; Watanabe, E.; Ito, I.Y. & Albuquerque Junior, R.F. (2009a). Bacterial leakage along the implant-abutment interface of premachined or cast components. *International Journal of Oral and Maxillofacial Surgery*, Vol.37, No.2, pp. 177-180

do Nascimento, C.; Barbosa, R.E.; Issa, J.P.; Watanabe, E.; Ito, I.Y. & Albuquerque Junior R.F. (2009). Use of checkerboard DNA-DNA hybridization to evaluate the internal contamination of dental implants and comparison of bacterial leakage with cast or pre-machined abutments. *Clinical Oral Implants Research*, Vol.20, No.6, pp. 571-577

Drake, D.R.; Paul, J. & Keller, J.C. (1999). Primary bacterial colonization of implant surfaces. *International Journal of Oral and Maxillofacial Implants*, Vol.14, No.2, pp. 226-232

Duarte, A.R.; Rossetti, P.H.; Rossetti, L.M.; Torres, S.A. & Bonachela, W.C. (2006). In vitro sealing ability of two materials at five different implant-abutment surfaces. *Journal of Periodontology*, Vol.77, No.11, pp. 1828-1832

Eckburg, P.B.; Bik, E.M.; Bernstein, C.N.; Purdom, E.; Dethlefsen, L.; Sargent, M.; Gill, S.R.; Nelson, K.E. & Relman, D.A. (2005). Diversity of the human intestinal microbial flora. *Science*, Vol.308, No.5728, pp. 1635-1638

Ekfeldt, A.; Fürst, B. & Carlsson, G.E. (2011). Zirconia abutments for single-tooth implant restorations: a retrospective and clinical follow-up study. *Clinical Oral Implants Research*, InPress

Emanuelsson, I.R. & Thornqvist, E. (2000). Genotypes of mutans streptococci tend to persist in their host for several years. *Caries Research*, Vol.34, No.2, pp. 133-139

Ericsson, I.; Persson, L.G.; Berglundh, T.; Marinello, C.P.; Lindhe, J. & Klinge, B. (1995). Different types of inflammatory reactions in peri-implant soft tissues. *Journal of Clinical Periodontology*, Vol.22, No.3, pp. 255-261

Esposito, M.; Thomsen, P.; Ericson, L.E.; Sennerby, L. & Lekholm, U. (2000). Histopathologic observations on late oral implant failures. *Clinical Implant Dentistry and Related Research*, Vol.2, No.1, pp. 18-32

Esposito, M.; Grusovin, M.G.; Chew, Y.S.; Coulthard, P. & Worthington, H.V. (2009). Interventions for replacing missing teeth: 1- versus 2-stage implant placement. *Cochrane Database Systematic Reviews*, Vol.18, No.3, pp. CD006698

Esposito, M.; Worthington, H.V.; Loli, V.; Coulthard, P. & Grusovin, M.G. (2010). Interventions for replacing missing teeth: antibiotics at dental implant placement to prevent complications. *Cochrane Database Systematic Reviews*, Vol.7, No.7, pp. CD004152

Felton, D.A.; Kanoy, B.E.; Bayne, S.C. & Wirthman, G.P. (1991). Effect of in vivo crown margin discrepancies on periodontal health. *Journal of Prosthetic Dentistry*, Vol.65, No.3, pp. 357-364

Finger, I.M.; Castellon, P.; Block, M. & Elian, N. (2003). The evolution of external and internal implant/abutment connections. *Practical Procedures & Aesthetic Dentistry*, Vol.15, No.8, pp. 625-632

Ge, X.; Leng, Y.; Bao, C.; Xu, S.L.; Wang, R. & Ren, F. (2010). Antibacterial coatings of fluoridated hydroxyapatite for percutaneous implants. *Journal of Biomedical Materials Researcs A*, Vol.95, No.2, pp. 588-599

Gibbons, R.J. & van Houte, J. (1975). Dental caries. *Annual Review of Medicine*, Vol.26, pp. 121-136

Gibbons, R.J. (1984). Adherent interactions which may affect microbial ecology in the mouth. *Journal of Dental Research*, Vol.63, No.3, pp. 378-385

Glauser, R.; Sailer, I.; Wohlwend, A.; Studer, S.; Schibli, M. & Schärer, P. (2004). Experimental zirconia abutments for implant-supported single-tooth restorations in esthetically demanding regions: 4-year results of a prospective clinical study. *The International Journal of Prosthodontics*, Vol.17, No.3, pp. 285-290.

Gouvoussis, J.; Sindhusake, D. & Yeung, S. (1997). Cross-infection from periodontitis sites to failing implant sites in the same mouth. *International Journal of Oral and Maxillofacial Implants*, Vol.12, No.5, pp. 666-673

Grenier, D. & Mayrand, D. (1986). Nutritional relationships between oral bacteria. *Infection and Immunity*, Vol.53, No.3, pp. 616-620

Grice, C.A.; Tays, K.L.; Savall, B.M.; Wei, J.; Butler, C.R.; Axe, F.U.; Bembenek, S.D.; Fourie, A.M.; Dunford, P.J.; Lundeen, K.; Coles, F.; Xue, X.; Riley, J.P.; Williams, K.N.; Karlsson, L. & Edwards, J.P. Identification of a potent, selective, and orally active leukotriene a4 hydrolase inhibitor with anti-inflammatory activity. *Journal of Medicinal Chemistry*, Vol.51, No.14, pp. 4150-4169

Grössner-Schreiber, B.; Griepentrog, M.; Haustein, I.; Müller, W.D.; Lange, K.P.; Briedigkeit, H. & Göbel, U.B. (2001). Plaque formation on surface modified dental implants. An in vitro study. *Clinical Oral Implants Research*, Vol.12, No.6, pp. 543-551

Gross, M.; Abramovich, I. & Weiss, E.I. (1999). Microleakage at the abutment-implant interface of osseointegrated implants: a comparative study. *International Journal of Oral and Maxillofacial Implants*, Vol.14, No.1, pp. 94-100

Gu, F.; Li, Y.; Zhou, C.; Wong, D.T.; Ho, C.M.; Qi, F. & Shi, W. (2009). Bacterial 16S rRNA/rDNA. Profiling in the Liquid Phase of Human Saliva. *Open Dentistry Journal*, Vol.3, pp. 80-84

Haffajee, A.D.; Cugini, M.A.; Tanner, A.; Pollack, R.P.; Smith, C.; Kent Jr, R.L. & Socransky, S.S. (1998). Subgingival microbiota in healthy, well-maintained elder and periodontitis subjects. *Journal of Clinical Periodontology*, Vol.25, No.5, pp. 346-353

Haffajee, A.D.; Yaskell, T.; Torresyap, G.; Teles, R. & Socransky, S.S. (2009). Comparison between polymerase chain reaction-based and checkerboard DNA hybridization techniques for microbial assessment of subgingival plaque samples. Journal of Clinical Periodontology, Vol.36, No.8, pp. 642-649

Hagiwara, Y.; Suzuki, Y. & Igarashi, T. (1997). Three dimensional compatibility of implant components by using scanning laser microscope. *Journal of Dental Research*, Vol.76, pp. 427

Harrigan, W. (1998). Laboratory methods in food microbiology. 3rd ed. Academic Press, San Diego, Calif. pp. 43–70

Hermann, J.S.; Schoolfield, J.D.; Schenk, R.K.; Buser, D. & Cochran, D.L. (2001). Influence of the size of the microgap on the crestal bone changes round titanium implants. A histometric evaluation of unloaded non-submerged implants in the canine mandible. *Journal of Periodontology*, Vol.72, No.10, pp. 1372-1383

Hill, D.A.; Hoffmann, C.; Abt, M.C.; Du, Y.; Kobuley, D.; Kirn, T.J.; Bushman, F.D. & Artis, D. Metagenomic analyses reveal antibiotic-induced temporal and spatial changes in intestinal microbiota with associated alterations in immune cell homeostasis. *Mucosal Immunology*, Vol.3, No.2, pp. 148-158

Hillman, J.D.; Yaphe. B.I. & Johnson, K.P. (1985). Colonization of the human oral cavity by a strain of Streptococcus mutans. *Journal of Dental Research*, Vol.64, No.11, pp. 1272-1274

Higuchi, Y.; Miyahara, Y.; Kawano, M.; Tsurudome, M.; Matsumura, H.; Kusagawa, S.; Komada, H.; Nishio, M. & Ito, Y. (1992). Sequence analysis of the large (L) protein of simian virus 5. *Journal of General Virology*, Vol.73, No.4, pp. 1005-1010

Jansen, V.K.; Conrads, G. & Richter, E.J. (1997). Microbial leakage and marginal fit of the implant-abutment interface. *International Journal of Oral and Maxillofacial Implants*, Vol.12, No.4, pp. 527-540

Jemt, T. & Book, K. (1996). Prosthesis misfit and marginal bone loss in edentulous implant patients. *International Journal of Oral and Maxillofac Implants*, Vol.11, No.5, pp. 620-625

Jervøe-Storm, P.M.; Koltzscher, M.; Falk, W.; Dörfler, A. & Jepsen, S. (2005). Comparison of culture and real-time PCR for detection and quantification of five putative periodontopathogenic bacteria in subgingival plaque samples. *Journal of Clinical Periodontology*, Vol.32, No.7, 778-783

Jung, R.E.; Pjetursson, B.E.; Glauser, R.; Zembic, A.; Zwahlen, M. & Lang, N.P. (2008). A systematic review of the survival and complication rates of implant supported single crowns (SCs) after an observation period of at least 5 years. *Clinical Oral Implants Research, Vol.*19, No.2, pp. 119-130

Kano, S.C.; Binon. P.P. & Curtis, D.A. (2007). A classification system to measure the implant-abutment microgap. *International Journal of Oral and Maxillofacial Implants*, Vol.22, No.6, pp. 879-885

Karl, M.; Graef, F.; Heckmann, S. & Taylor, T. (2009). A methodology to study the effects of prosthesis misfit over time: an in vivo model. *International Journal of Oral and Maxillofacial Implants*, Vol.24, No.4, pp. 689-694

Kim, K.; Heimisdottir, K.; Gebauer, U. & Persson, G.R. (2010). Clinical and microbiological findings at sites treated with orthodontic fixed appliances in adolescents. *American Journal of Orthodontics and Dentofacial Orthopedics*, Vol.137, No.2, pp. 223-228

Kokubo, Y.; Ohkubo, C.; Tsumita, M.; Miyashita, A.; Vult von Steyern, P. & Fukushima, S. (2005). Clinical marginal and internal gaps of Procera AllCeram crowns. *Journal of Oral Rehabilitation*, Vol.32, No.7, pp. 526-530

Kosyfaki, P.; del Pilar Pinilla Martín, M. & Strub, J.R. (2010). Relationship between crowns and the periodontium: a literature update. *Quintessence International*, Vol.41, No.2, pp. 109-126

Khraisat, A.; Baqain, Z.H.; Smadi, L.; Nomura, S.; Miyakawa, O. & Elnasser, Z. (2006). Abutment rotational displacement of external hexagon implant system under lateral cyclic loading. *Clinical Implant Dentistry and Related Research*, Vol.8, No.2, pp. 96-99

Laine, P.; Salo, A.; Kontio, R.; Ylijoki, S.; Lindqvist, C. & Suuronen, R. (2005). Failed dental implants - clinical, radiological and bacteriological findings in 17 patients. *Journal of Craniomaxillofacial Surgery*, Vol.33, No.3, pp. 212-217

Lambrecht, J.T.; Filippi, A.; Künzel, A.R. & Schiel, H.J. (2003). Long-term evaluation of submerged and nonsubmerged ITI solid-screw titanium implants: a 10-year life table analysis of 468 implants. *International Journal of Oral and Maxillofacial Implants*, Vol.18, No.6, pp. 826-834

Lamont, R.J. & Jenkinson, H.F. (1998). Life below the gum line: pathogenic mechanisms of Porphyromonas gingivalis. *Microbiology and Molecular Biology Reviews*, Vol.62, No.4, pp. 1244-1263

Lang, N.P.; Berglundh, T.; Heitz-Mayfield, L.J.; Pjetursson, B.E.; Salvi, G.E. & Sanz, M. (2004). Consensus statements and recommended clinical procedures regarding implant survival and complications. *International Journal of Oral and Maxillofacial Implants*, Vol.19, pp. 150-154

Leonhardt, A.; Berglundh, T.; Ericsson, I. & Dahlén, G. (1992). Putative periodontal pathogens on titanium implants and teeth in experimental gingivitis and periodontitis in beagle dogs. *Clinical Oral Implants Research*, Vol.3, No.3, pp.112-119

Li, X.X.; Wong, G.L.; To, K.F.; Wong, V.W.; Lai, L.H.; Chow, D.K.; Lau, J.Y.; Sung, J.J. & Ding, C. (2009). Bacterial microbiota profiling in gastritis without Helicobacter pylori infection or nonsteroidal anti-inflammatory drug use. *PLoS One*, Vol.4, pp. e7985

Lindhe, J.; Berglundh, T.; Ericsson, I.; Liljenberg, B. & Marinello, C. (1992). Experimental breakdown of peri-implant and periodontal tissues. A study in the beagle dog. *Clinical Oral Implants Research*, Vol.3, No.1, pp. 9-16

Linkevicius, T. & Apse, P. (2008). Influence of abutment material on stability of peri-implant tissues: a systematic review. *International Journal of Oral and Maxillofacial Implants*, Vol.23, No.3, pp. 449-456

Loesche, W.J. (1968). Importance of nutrition in gingival crevice microbial ecology. *Periodontics*, Vol.6, No.6, pp. 245-249

Loyola-Rodriguez, J.P.; Morisaki, I.; Kitamura, K. & Hamada, S. (1992). Purification and properties of extracellular mutacin, a bacteriocin from Streptococcus sobrinus. *Journal of General Microbiology*, Vol.138, No.2, pp. 269-274

MacFarlane, S.; Furrie, E.; Macfarlane, G.T. & Dillon, J.F. (2007). Microbial colonization of the upper gastrointestinal tract in patients with Barrett's esophagus. *Clinical Infectious Diseases*, Vol.45, No.1, pp. 29-38

Mäkivuokko, H.; Tiihonen, K.; Tynkkynen, S.; Paulin, L. & Rautonen, N. (2010). The effect of age and non-steroidal anti-inflammatory drugs on human intestinal microbiota composition. British Journal of Nutrition, Vol.103, No.2, pp. 227-234

Manicone, P.F.; Rossi, I.P. & Raffaelli, L. (2007). An overview of zirconia ceramics: basic properties and clinical applications. *Journal of Dentistry*, Vol.35, No.11, pp. 819–826

Marxkors, R. (1980). Marginal seal of cast crowns. *Deutsche Zahnarztl Zeitschrift*, Vol.35, No.9, pp. 913-95

May, K.B.; Russell, M.M.; Razzoog, M.E. & Lang, B.R. (1998). Precision of fit: the Procera All Ceram crown. Journal of Prosthetic Dentistry, Vol.80, pp. 394–404

Merz, B.R.; Hunenbart, S. & Belser, U.C. (2000). Mechanics of the implant-abutment connection: an 8-degree taper compared to a butt joint connection. *International Journal of Oral and Maxillofacial Implants*, Vol.15, No.4, pp. 519-526

Möllersten, L.; Lockowandt, P. & Lindén, L.A. (1997). Comparison of strength and failure mode of seven implant systems: an in vitro test. *Journal of Prosthetic Dentistry*, Vol.78, No.6, pp. 582-591

Mombelli, A.; Buser, D. & Lang, N.P. (1988). Colonization of osseointegrated titanium implants in edentulous patients. Early results. *Oral Microbiology and Immunology*, Vol.3, No.3, pp. 113-120

Mombelli, A. & Mericske-Stern, R. (1990). Microbiological features of stable osseointegrated implants used as abutments for overdentures. *Clinical Oral Implants Research*, Vol.1, No.1, pp. 1-7

Mombelli, A.; Marxer, M.; Gaberthüel, T.; Grunder, U. & Lang, N.P. (1995). The microbiota of osseointegrated implants in patients with a history of periodontal disease. *Journal of Clinical Periodontology*, Vol.22, No.2, pp. 124-130

Mombelli, A. & Lang, N.P. (1998). The diagnosis and treatment of peri-implantitis. *Periodontology 2000*, Vol.17, pp. 63-76

Mombelli, A. & Décaillet, F. (2011) The characteristics of biofilms in peri-implant disease. *Journal of Clinical Periodontology*, Vol.38, No.11, pp. 203-213

Moraes, S.R.; Siqueira Jr, J.F.; Colombo, A.P.; Rocas, I.N.; Ferreira, M.C. & Domingues, R.M. (2002). Comparison of the effectiveness of bacterial culture, 16S rDNA directed polymerase chain reaction, and checkerboard DNA-DNA hybridization for detection of Fusobacterium nucleatum in endodontic infections. *Journal of Endodontics*, Vol.28, No.2, pp. 86-89

Mullard, A. (2008). Microbiology: the inside story. *Nature*, Vol.453, No.7195, pp. 578-580

Norton, M.R. (1997). An in vitro evaluation of the strength of an internal conical interface compared to a butt joint interface in implant design. *Clinical Oral Implants Research*, Vol.8, No.4, pp. 290-298

Oakley, B.B.; Fiedler, T.L.; Marrazzo, J.M. & Fredricks, D.N. (2008). Diversity of human vaginal bacterial communities and their association with clinically defined bacterial vaginosis. *Applied in Environmental Microbiology*, Vol.74, No.15, pp. 4898–4909

Ong, G.; Soh, G. & Chong, Y.H. (1992). Periodontal status of institutionalized elderly in Singapore. *Community Dentistry in Oral Epidemiology*, Vol.20, No.6, pp. 382-383

Parahitiyawa, N.B.; Scully, C.; Leung, W.K.; Yam, W.C.; Jin, L.J. & Samaranayake, L.P. (2010). Exploring the oral bacterial flora: current status and future directions. *Oral Diseases*, Vol.16, No.2, pp. 136-145

Paster, B.J.; Boches, S.K.; Galvin, J.L.; Ericson, R.E.; Lau, C.N.; Levanos, V.A.; Sahasrabudhe, A. & Dewhirst, F.E. (2001). Bacterial diversity in human subgingival plaque. *Journal of Bacteriology*, Vol.183, No.12, pp. 3770–3783

Pautke, C.; Kolk, A.; Brokate, M.; Wehrstedt, J.C.; Kneissl, F.; Miethke, T.; Steinhauser, E.; Horch, H.H. & Deppe, H. (2009). Development of novel implant abutments using the shape memory alloy nitinol: preliminary results. *International Journal of Oral and Maxillofacial Implants*, Vol.24, No.3, pp. 477-483

Persson, L.G.; Lekholm, U.; Leonhardt, A.; Dahlén, G. & Lindhe, J. (1996). Bacterial colonization on internal surfaces of Brånemark system implant components. *Clinical Oral Implants Research*, Vol.7, No.2, pp. 90-95

Persson, G.R.; Samuelsson, E.; Lindahl, C. & Renvert, S. (2010). Mechanical non-surgical treatment of peri-implantitis: a single-blinded randomized longitudinal clinical study. II. Microbiological results. Journal of Clinical Periodontology, Vol.37, No.6, pp. 563-573

Pessková, V.; Kubies, D.; Hulejová, H. & Himmlová, L. (2007). The influence of implant surface properties on cell adhesion and proliferation. *Journal of Material Science and Material Medicine*, Vol.18, No.3, pp. 65-73

Piattelli, A.; Scarano, A.; Paolantonio, M.; Assenza, B.; Leghissa, G.C.; Di Bonaventura, G.; Catamo, G. & Piccolomini, R. (2001). Fluids and microbial penetration in the internal part of cement-retained versus screw-retained implant-abutment connections. *Journal of Periodontology*, Vol.72, No.9, pp. 1146-1150

Piattelli, A.; Scarano, A.; Favero, L.; Iezzi, G.; Petrone, G. & Favero, G.A. (2003). Clinical and histologic aspects of dental implants removed due to mobility. *Journal of Periodontology*, Vol.74, pp. 385-390

Pitt, T.L. & Saunders, N.A. (2000). Molecular bacteriology: a diagnostic tool for the millennium. *Journal of Clinical Pathology*, Vol.53, No.1, pp. 71-75

Pjetursson, B.E.; Brägger, U.; Lang, N.P. & Zwahlen M. (2007). Comparison of survival and complication rates of tooth supported fixed partial dentures and implant supported fixed partial dentures and single crowns. *Clinical Oral Implants Research, Vol.*18, pp. 97-113

Quirynen, M. & Listgarten, M.A. (1990). Distribution of bacterial morphotypes around natural teeth and titanium implants ad modum Brånemark. *Clinical Oral Implants Research*, Vol.1, No.1, pp. 8-12

Quirynen, M. & van Steenberghe, D. (1993) Bacterial colonization of the internal part of two-stage implants. An in vivo study. *Clinical Oral Implants Research*, Vol.4, No.3, pp. 158-161

Quirynen, M.; Bollen, C.M.; Eyssen, H. & van Steenberghe, D. (1994). Microbial penetration along the implant components of the Brånemark system. An in vitro study. *Clinical Oral Implants Research*, Vol.5, No.4, pp. 239-244

Quirynen, M. & Bollen, C.M. (1995). The influence of surface roughness and surface-free energy on supra- and subgingival plaque formation in man. A review of the literature. *Journal of Clinical Periodontology*, Vol.22, No.1, pp. 1-14

Quirynen, M.; Papaioannou, W. & Van Steenberghe, D. *(*1996a*)* Intraoral transmission and the colonization of oral hard surfaces. *Journal of Periodontology*, Vol.67, No.10, pp. 986–993

Quirynen, M.; Bollen, C.M.; Papaioannou, W.; Van Eldere, J. & van Steenberghe, D. (1996b). The influence of titanium abutment surface roughness on plaque accumulation and gingivitis: short-term observations. *International Journal of Oral and Maxillofacial Implants*, Vol.11, No.2, pp. 169-178

Quirynen, M.; De Soete, M. & van Steenberghe D. (2002). Infectious risks for oral implants: a review of the literature. *Clinical Oral Implants Research*, Vol.13, No.1, pp. 1-19

Quirynen, M.; Avontroodt, P.; Soers, C.; Zhao, H.; Pauwels, M. & van Steenberghe, D. (2004). Impact of tongue cleansers on microbial load and taste. *Journal of Clinical Periodontology*, Vol.31, No.7, pp. 506-510

Quirynen, M.; Vogels, R.; Alsaadi, G.; Naert, I.; Jacobs, R. & van Steenberghe, D. (2005). Predisposing conditions for retrograde peri-implantitis, and treatment suggestions. *Clinical Oral Implants Research*, Vol.16, No.5, pp. 599-608

Quirynen, M.; Vogels, R.; Peeters, W.; van Steenberghe, D.; Naert, I. & Haffajee, A. (2006). Dynamics of initial subgingival colonization of 'pristine' peri-implant pockets. *Clinical Oral Implants Research*, Vol.17, No.1, pp. 25-37

Riedel, S. & Carroll, K.C. (2010). Blood cultures: key elements for best practices and future directions. Journal of Infection and Chemotherapy, Vol.16, No.5, pp. 301-316

Rimondini, L.; Farè, S.; Brambilla, E.; Felloni, A.; Consonni, C.; Brossa, F. & Carrassi, A. (1997). The effect of surface roughness on early in vivo plaque colonization on titanium. *Journal of Periodontology*, Vol.68, No.6, pp. 556-562

Rimondini, L.; Marin, C.; Brunella, F. & Fini, M. (2001). Internal contamination of a 2-component implant system after occlusal loading and provisionally luted reconstruction with or without a washer device. *Journal of Periodontology*, Vol.72, No.12, pp. 1652-1657

Rôças, I.N. & Siqueira JR, J.F. (2010). Distribution of Porphyromonas gingivalis fim. A genotypes in primary endodontic infections. *Oral Surgery Oral Medecine Oral Pathology Oral Radiology and Endodontics*, Vol.109, No.3, pp. 474-478

Rolph, H.J.; Lennon, A.; Riggio, M.P.; Saunders, W.P.; MacKenzie, D.; Coldero, L. & Bagg, J. (2001). Molecular identification of microorganisms from endodontic infections. *Journal of Clinical Microbiology*, Vol.39, No.9, pp. 3282-3289

Rosan, B. & Lamont, R.J. (2000). Dental plaque formation. *Microbes and Infection*, Vol.2, No. 13, pp. 1599-1607

Sahin, S. & Cehreli, M.C. (2001). The significance of passive framework fit in implant prosthodontics: current status. *Implant Dentistry*, Vol.10, No.2, pp. 85-92

Saito, A.; Hosaka, Y.; Sekiguchi, K.; Kigure, T.; Isobe, S.; Shibukawa, Y.; Sumii, H.; Ito, T.; Nakagawa, T. & Yamada, S. (1997). Responses of peri-implant tissues to undisturbed plaque formation in dogs: clinical, radiographic, and microbiological findings. *Bulletin of Tokyo Dental College*, Vol.38, No.1, pp. 13-20

Sakamoto, M.; Umeda, M. & Benno, Y. (2005). Molecular analysis of human oral microbiota. Journal of Periodontal Research, Vol.40, No.3, pp. 277-285

Salihoglu, U.; Boynuegri, D.; Engin, D.; Duman, A.N.; Gokalp, P. & Balos, K. (2011). Bacterial adhesion and colonization differences between zirconium oxide and titanium alloys: an in vivo human study. *International Journal of Oral and Maxillofacial Implants*, Vol.26, No.1, pp. 101-107

Scarano, A.; Piattelli, M.; Caputi, S.; Favero, G.A. & Piattelli, A. (2004). Bacterial adhesion on commercially pure titanium and zirconium oxide disks: an in vivo human study. *Journal of Periodontology*, Vol.75, No.2, pp. 292–296

Scarano, A.; Assenza, B.; Piattelli, M.; Iezzi, G.; Leghissa, G.C.; Quaranta, A.; Tortora, P. & Piattelli, A. (2005). A 16-year study of the microgap between 272 human titanium implants and their abutments. *Journal of Oral Implantology*, Vol.31, No.6, pp. 269-275

Shibli, J.A.; Vitussi, T.R.; Garcia, R.V.; Zenóbio, E.G.; Ota-Tsuzuki, C.; Cassoni, A.; Piattelli, A &, d'Avila, S. (2007). Implant surface analysis and microbiologic evaluation of failed implants retrieved from smokers. *Journal of Oral Implantology*, Vol.33, No.4, pp. 232-238

Socransky, S.S. 7 Manganiello, S.D. (1971). The oral microbiota of man from birth to senility. *Journal of Periodontology*, Vol.42, No.8, pp. 485-496

Socransky, S.S.; Haffajee, A.D. & Dzink, J.L. (1988). Relationship of subgingival microbial complexes to clinical features at the sampled sites. *Journal of Clinical Periodontology*, Vol.15, No.7, pp. 440-444

Socransky, S.S.; Smith, C.; Martin, L.; Paster, B.J.; Dewhirst, F.E. & Levin, A.E. (1994). Checkerboard DNA–DNA hybridization. *Biotechniques*, Vol.17, No.4, pp. 788-792

Socransky, S.S. & Haffajee, A.D. (2002). Dental biofilms: difficult therapeutic targets. *Periodontol 2000,* Vol.28, 12-55

Speck, M.; Ray, B. & Read Jr, R. (1975). Repair and enumeration of injured coliforms by a plating procedure. *Applied Microbiology,* Vol.29, No.4, pp. 549–550

Stavropoulos, A.; Karring, T. & Kostopoulos, L. (2007). Fully vs. partially rough implants in maxillary sinus floor augmentation: a randomized-controlled clinical trial. *Clinical Oral Implants Research,* Vol.18, No.1, pp. 95-102

Steinebrunner, L.; Wolfart, S.; Bössmann, K. & Kern, M. (2005). In vitro evaluation of bacterial leakage along the implant-abutment interface of different implant systems. *International Journal of Oral and Maxillofacial Implants,* Vol.20, No.6, pp. 875-81

Teles, R.; Sakellari, D.; Teles, F.; Konstantinidis, A.; Kent, R.; Socransky, S.S. & Haffajee, A. (2010). Relationships among gingival crevicular fluid biomarkers, clinical parameters of periodontal disease, and the subgingival microbiota. *Journal of Periodontology,* Vol.81, No.1, pp. 89-98

Turnbaugh, P.J.; Ley, R.E.; Hamady, M.; Fraser-Liggett, C.M.; Knight, R.; Gordon, J.I. (2007). The human microbiome project. *Nature,* Vol.449, No.7164, pp. 804-810

Uo, M.; Sjögren, G.; Sundh, A.; Watari, F.; Bergman, M. & Lerner, U. (2003). Cytotoxicity and bonding property of dental ceramics. *Dental Materials,* Vol.19, No.6, pp. 487-492

Valderrama, S.; Van Roekel, N.; Andersson, M.; Goodacre, C.J.; & Munoz, C.A. (1995). A comparison of the marginal and internal adaptation of titanium and goldplatinum-palladium metal ceramic crowns. The International Journal of Prosthodontics, Vol.8, No.1, pp. 29-37

Van Brakel, R.; Cune, M.S.; Van Winkelhoff, A.J.; De Putter, C.; Verhoeven, J.W. & Van Der Reijden, W. (2010). Early bacterial colonization and soft tissue health around zirconia and titanium abutments: an in vivo study in man. *Clinical Oral Implants Research,* InPress

Vettore, M.V.; Leão, A.T.; Leal, M.D.O.C.; Feres, M.; De Figueiredo, L.C. & Sheiham, A. (2010). Periodontal bacterial load: a proposed new epidemiological method for periodontal disease assessment. *Journal of Contemporary Dental Practice,* Vol.11, No.1, pp. In Press

Visai, L.; Rimondini, L.; Giordano, C.; Del Curto, B.; Sbarra, M.S.; Franchini, R.; Della Valle, C. & Chiesa, R. (2008). Electrochemical surface modification of titanium for implant abutments can affect oral bacteria contamination. *Journal of Applied Biomaterials & Biomechanics,* Vol.6, No.3, pp. 170-177

Watkin, A. & Kerstein, R.B. (2008). Improving darkened anterior peri-implant tissue color with zirconia custom implant abutments. *Compendium of Continuing Education in Dentistry,* Vol.29, No.4, pp. 238-240

Welander, M.; Abrahamsson, I. & Berglundh, T. (2008). The mucosal barrier at implant abutments of different materials. *Clinical Oral Implants Research,* Vol.19, No.7, pp. 635-641

Whelen, A.C. & Persing, D.H. (1996). The role of nucleic acid amplification and detection in the clinical microbiology laboratory. *Annual Review of Microbiology,* Vol.50, pp. 349-373

2

Dental Reconstruction Using Secondary Bone Graft Followed by Implant Placement in Alveolar Cleft of Patients with Cleft Lip and/or Palate

Tetsu Takahashi
Division of Oral and Maxillofacial Reconstructive Surgery,
Kyushu Dental College
Japan

1. Introduction

Alveolar cleft is the major problem during the formation of the ideal dental arch and dental reconstruction in cleft lip and/or palate (CLP) patients. In 1972, Boyne and Sands introduced secondary autogenous particulate cancellous bone and marrow (PCBM) grafting for the treatment of alveolar and residual palatal clefts (Boyne and Sands, 1972) Nowadays, a golden standard protocol for the dental reconstruction of patients with CLP is to perform bone grafting (BG) before canine eruption and subsequent orthodontic closure of the dental arch without using prosthesis, as described in previous reports. (Abyholm, et al., 1981; Enemark, et al., 1985; Bergland, et al., 1986). However, because of the excessively long treatment period or a wide interdental space resulting from several congenitally missing teeth, prosthodontic treatment such as bridgework or denture is sometimes necessary.
Verdi et al. firstly reported the use of osseointegrated implant for dental rehabilitation in patients after the repair of the alveolar cleft (Verdi et al., 1991). Since then, numerous reports indicated that the use of dental implants placed in grafted alveoli after repair of an alveolar cleft using a secondary BG with particulate PCBM is a viable option for the dental reconstruction of patients with cleft lip or palate (CLP) (Ronchi et al., 1995; Takahashi T et al., 1997; Jasma et al., 1999; Härtel et al., 1999; Dempf et al., 2002). Since 1993, we have used this treatment procedure in patients with graft alveolar clefts. (Takahashi et al., 1997, 2008). In this chapter, dental reconstruction using secondary BG followed by dental implant placement in alveolar cleft of patients with CLP is described. The main purpose of this chapter to demonstrate the surgical procedure, long-term clinical outcome, and the impact on the preservation of the grafted alveoli after implant placement of this treatment procedure.

2. Use of dental implants for dental reconstruction in clp patients with grafted alveolar cleft

2.1 Secondary alveolar bone grafting for osseous reconstruction of the alveolar and palatal cleft

The management of the dentoalveolar cleft is a significant challenge for the surgeon. Timing is generally described as "primary," "secondary," and "delayed." Primary bone grafting is generally defined as that taking place before eruption of the primary dentition or before 1 year of age. Secondary bone grafting is that performed after developing of the permanent dentition, and delayed bone grafting takes place after eruption of the permanent canine. Historically, primary bone grafting was used from 1950 to 1968, and was found to inhibit normal growth and to impede later treatment using orthopedic forces of arch expansion. Nowadays, early secondary (5 to 6 years of age) or secondary (7 to 11 years of age) before canine eruption is recommended for osseous reconstruction followed by orthodontic dental arch closure. The erupting tooth stimulates alveolar and graft bone growth and produces a more normal-appearing canine eminence. Late bone grafting is not recommended because root resorption and graft failure sometimes observed when bone grafts are placed after eruption of the canine and when the bone graft is placed in contact with exposed tooth root surfaces. As bone graft source, the standard bone graft is autogenous particulate cancellous bone and marrow (PCBM) from the ilium. This bone is highly cellular, making it both resident to infection and able to heal rapidly. The graft materials are clinically and radiographically indistinguishable from alveolar bone by 3 months after operation and function as alveolar bone. Orthodontic treatment, thus, could be started 3 months after bone grafting. The purposes of bone grafting to the alveolar cleft are (1) closure of the oronasal fistula; (2) stabilization of the expanded arch, and in the case of bilateral clefts, of the premaxilla; (3) bone to support the canine eruption; (4) improved bone and periodontal status for the central incisor and lateral, if present; (5) support for the ala of the nose; and (6) a more normal appearance of the alveolar process, teeth, and gingival of the anterior maxilla. Now, another important purpose of bone grafting should be added to the list. Seventh purpose of bone grafting to the alveolar cleft would be to give osseous support for dental implant placement.

2.2 Problems related to the dental reconstruction of the grafted alveolar cleft

Although golden standard procedure of dental reconstruction in CLP patients is to perform bone grafting between the ages of 7 and 11 years, followed by orthodontic closure of the cleft dental gap without the use of a prosthesis, CLP is often associated with congenital absence of the lateral incisor adjacent to the cleft. Many patients therefore require prostheses such as a denture or bridge, particularly when the cleft-dental gap might not result in a good occlusion relationship between the upper and lower jaws. For such patients, we propose the option of dental reconstruction with dental implants after repair of the alveolar cleft by autogenous PCBM grafting.

2.3 Subjects and methods

2.3.1 Subjects

Twenty-one (7 male, 14 female) patients with CLP underwent implant placement between February 1993 and May 1995. Thirteen of the patients had unilateral cleft lip and palate (UCLP), and three had unilateral cleft lip and alveolus (UCLA). The mean age at first implant surgery was 19.1 ± 4.7 years (range: 13.9 to 33.6 years).

2.3.2 Bone grafting

Surgical procedure was shown in Fig 1 (Fig. 1a and 1b).

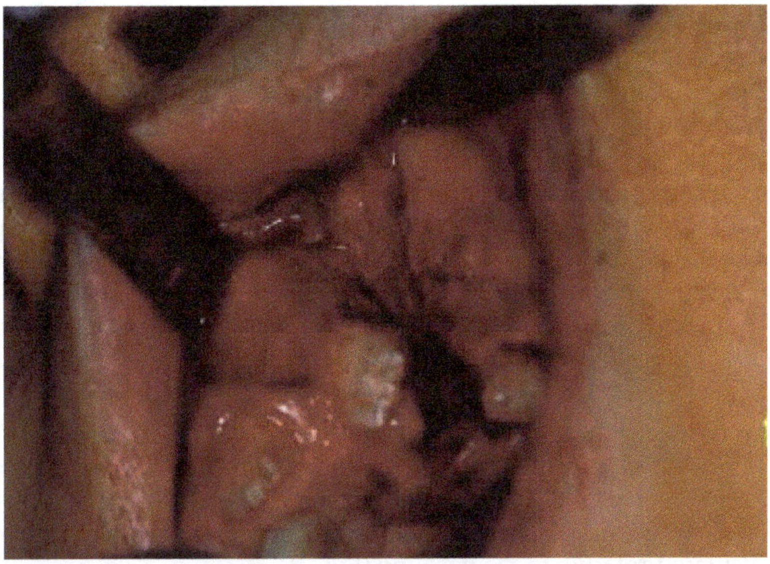

a: closure of the nasal mucosa at the cleft site

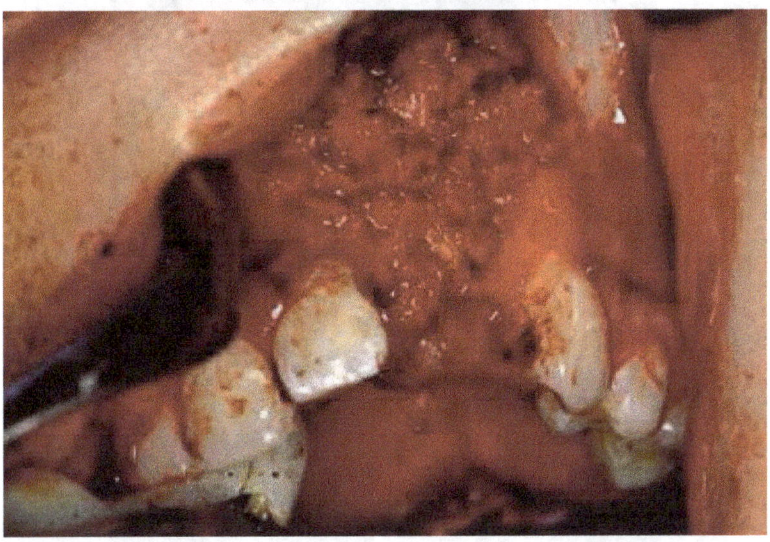

b: PCBM filled in the cleft gap

Fig. 1. Secondary bone grafting of alveolar cleft

All patients received autogenous particulate cancellous bone and marrow (PCBM) grafts from the ilium beaten 8.3 and 31.7 years of age under general anesthesia. Epinephrine 1:00, 000 is administered in the labial tissues to reduce bleeding. Incisions are made, and the labial flaps are reflected on either side of the cleft and these two incisions connected by sharp and blunt dissection deep to the orbicularis oris muscle on the nasal mucosa. This dissection is extended superiorly to the level of the floor of the nose. The nasal mucosa is reflected from the bone of the cleft and extended to the palatal tissues. Subperiosteal reflections of the palatal tissues on either side of the cleft are performed from the gingival margin to the depth of the palate. The reflection of mucosa through the alveolar cleft is completed. The nasal mucosa that passes through the cleft and is attached to the palatal tissues is separated from the palatal mucosa to the depth of the palate. If a palatal fistula extends further posteriorly, the separation and reflection are carried to the posterior end of the fistula. Then, nasal mucosa is closed with 4-0 Vicryl. The edges of he palatal fistula are freshened and closed with 4-0 Vicryl. Specifically, the very end of the fistula is closed using through-and-through suture using 4-0 Vicryl. PCBM is packed firmly from the level of the floor of the nose to the crest of the ridge. Releasing incisions are made through the periosteium of the posterior buccal flap, allowing anterior and inferior advancement. The labial and palatal flaps are closed with sutures. For the subsequent implant placement, the most important point of BG bed preparation is the level of the floor of the nose. The level of the floor of the nose at the BG bed should be the same level of the contra-lateral side. If inferior nasal turbinate is obstructive for the preparation of the floor of the nose, it should be removed. Usually, inferior nasal turbinate is easily removed without any bleeding.

2.3.3 Evaluation of the grafted alveoli around the implants

The marginal bone level around the implants was evaluated radiologically as previously described. (Takahashi et al., 2008). Using the reference points of the dimension of the implants, especially the fixture length and screw pitch (0.6 mm), the marginal crest level of the bone was calculated relative to the baseline (Fig. 2).

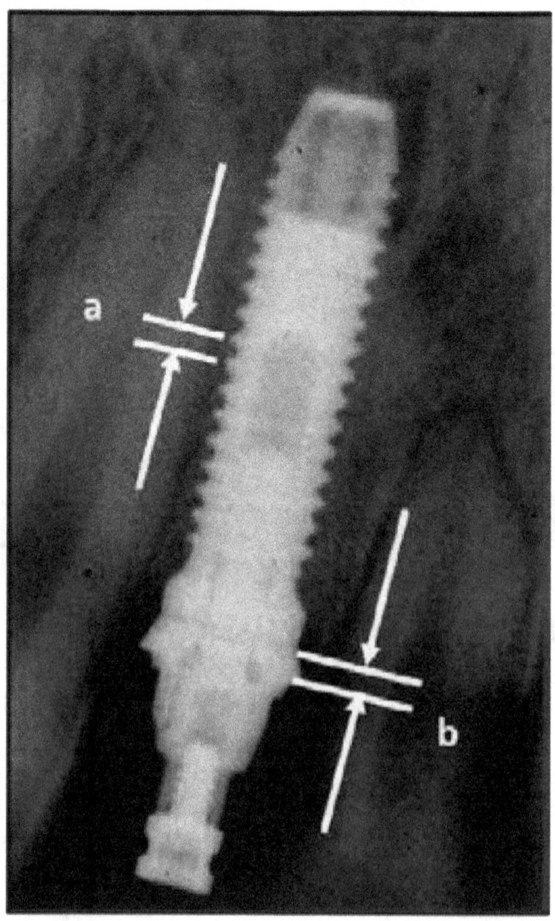

Fig. 2. **Measuring the marginal bone level.** a, A screw pitch (0.6 mm); b, baseline to bone level (marginal bone level) (Takahashi T, et al. Oral Surg Oral Med Oral Pathol Oral Radiol Endod2008: 105: 297-302)

An average of the mesial and distal values was used. All assessments were performed at three stages after abutment connection, at 1 (stage I), 3 (stage II), and 6 (stage III) years after abutment connection.

2.3.4 Evaluation of the marginal interdental alveolar bone height (IABH)

The interdental alveolar bone height (IABH) was estimated and was indicated by 4 score values (Fig. 3). (Enemark, et al., 1987).

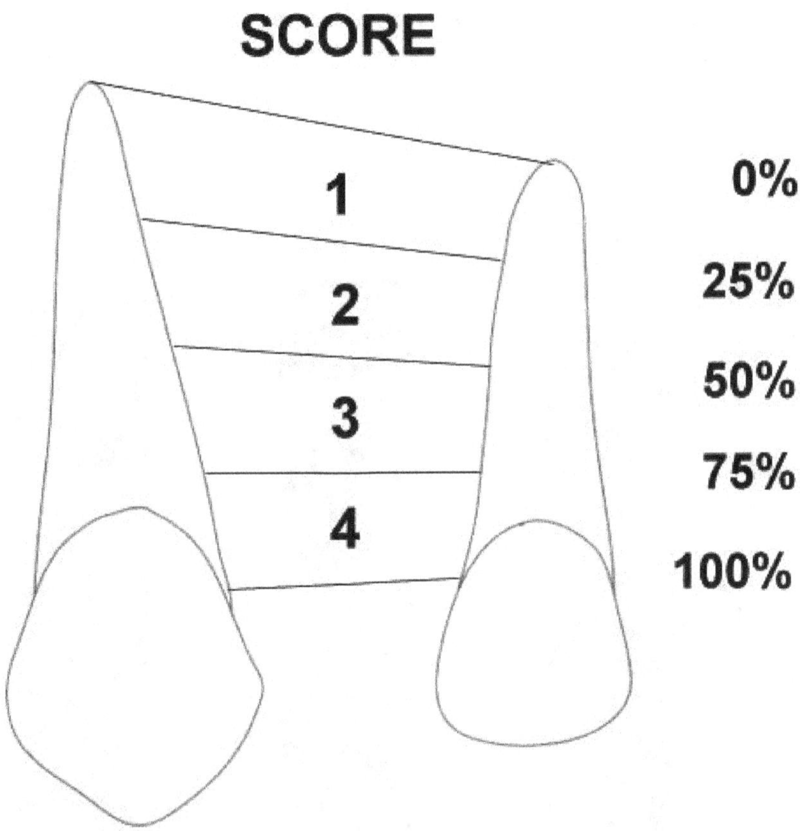

Fig. 3. Score of interdental alveolar bone height (IABH)

Briefly, The extent of the vertical bone height was determined in relation to the interdental bone height and assessed on a 4-point scale: score 4= 0 % to 25 % bone loss, score 3= 25 % 50% bone loss, score 2= 50 % to 75 % bone loss, score 1= 75% to 100 % bone loss. All assessments were performed 1, 6, 12, 24, 36, and 72 months after implant placement.

2.4 Clinical outcomes in a long-term follow-up

A total of 23 implants were placed in bone-grafted alveoli in 21 patients between February 1993 and May 1995. One patient was lost to follow-up, two implants were lost in one patient, and three implants in three patients were still temporary restoration because of the prolonged orthodontic treatment. The implant length ranged from 10 to 18 mm; the most frequently used length was 15 mm. The duration from bone grafting to first implant surgery ranged from 1.4 to 10.2 years (mean: 5.0 ± 2.7 years). In five patients with insufficient IABH, which was evaluated as Score 1 or 2, a chin bone-onlay graft (CBOG) was used during implant placement as described later. Two of these patients had wound dehiscence, and the exposed chin bone was partially lost. Ultimately, however, all five implants were osseointegrated, and the alveolar bone height was increased in these patients. The follow-up period ranged from 7.2 to 9.4 years (mean period: 8.6 ± 0.6 years). Twenty implants placed in 19 patients survived, and the overall rate of implant survival was 90.9%. IABH was reduced in 2 of 16 (12.5%) of the implant-placed grafted alveoli, in which score 4 was reduced to score 3, and score 3 was reduced to score 2, 6 years after implant placement, respectively. In other 14 cases, there was no change in score of IABH up to 6 years after implant placement (Fig. 4). These results clearly suggested that placement implants in the grafted alveoli would maintain alveolar bone height in the region.

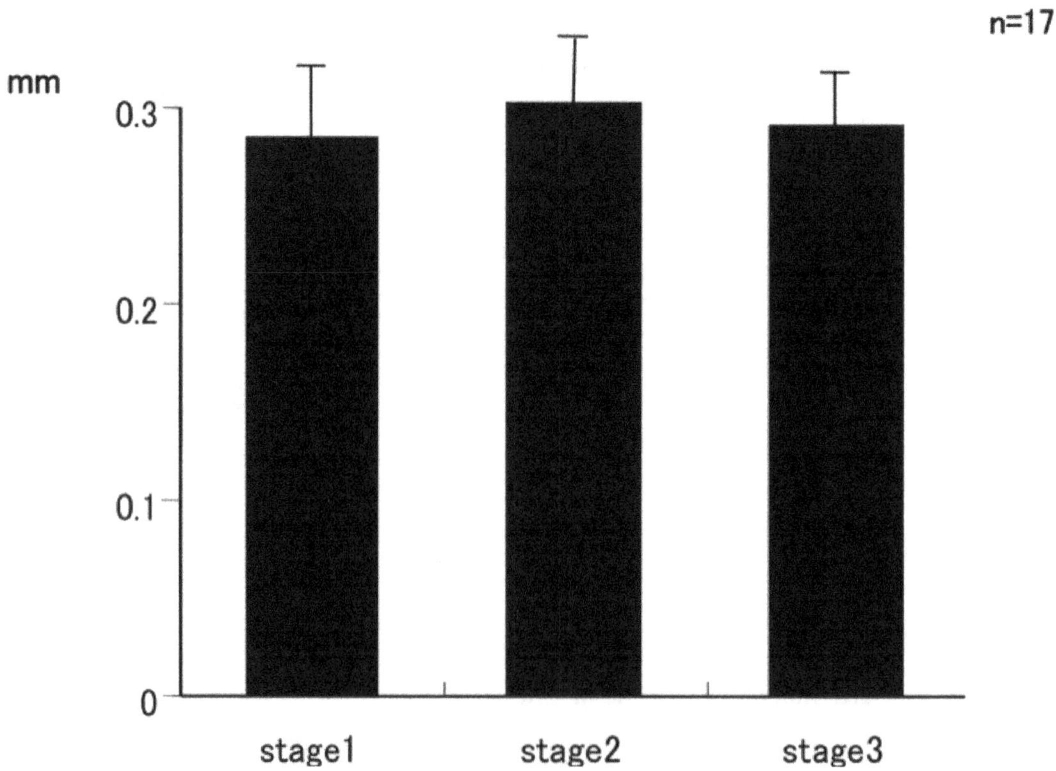

Fig. 4. Marginal bone loss around the implant

The mean marginal bone levels were 0.29 ± 0.18, 0.29 ± 0.19, and 0.28 ± 0.15 mm at stages I to III, respectively. In addition, there was no mobility of the implants and was no pain, swelling, or inflammation around the peri-implant tissue. Clinically, all the implants were functioning in excellent condition 7.2 to 9.4 years after implant placement. A long-term follow-up of a typical case was shown in Figure 5a-c and Figure 6a-c. These data satisfied the implant success criteria according to Albrektsson et al., (Albrektsson, et al., 1986), who stipulated that the vertical bone loss should be less than 0.2 mm annually after the first year of implant service. In addition, our long-term follow-up study showed that the use of dental implants placed in the grafted alveoli is an excellent treatment modality for the dental rehabilitation of patients with alveolar clefts and congenitally missing teeth.

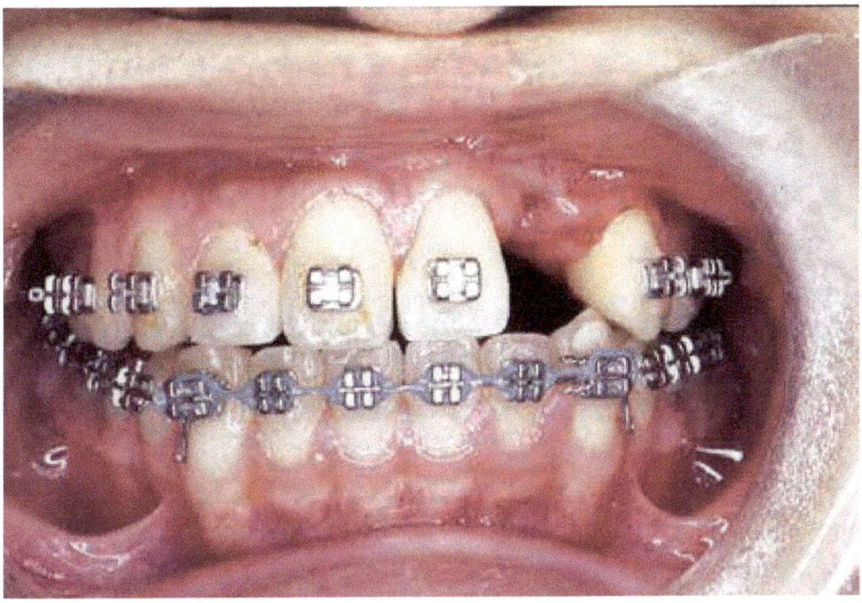

a: After orthodontic alignment and space making for an implant placement of the grafted alveolar cleft.

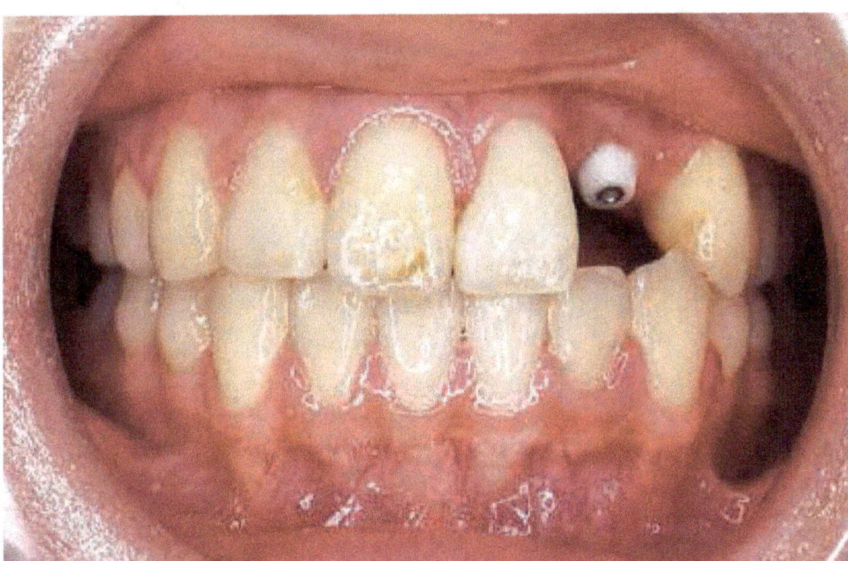

b: Postoperative view after implant placement

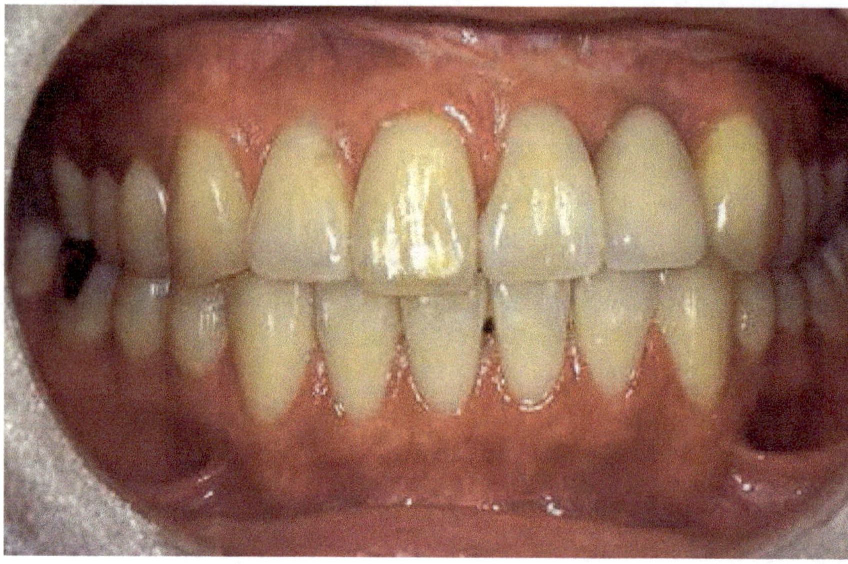

c: 13 years after implant placement

Fig. 5. A Long-term follow-up in a unilateral cleft lip and palate (UCLP) patient.

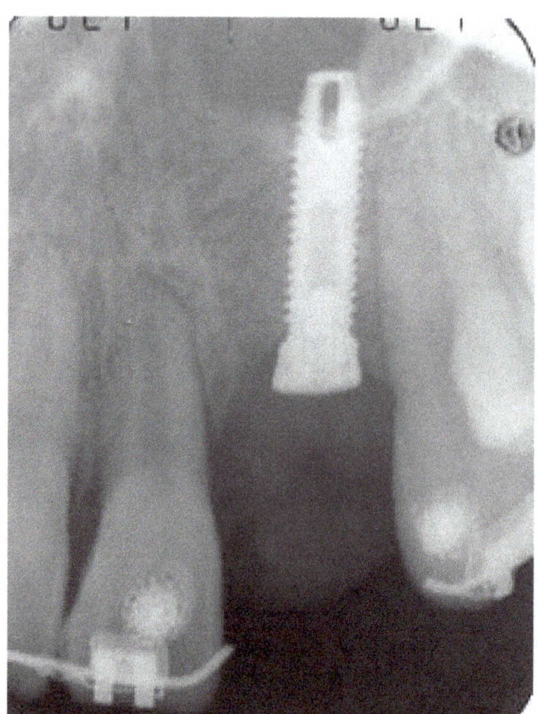

a: Periapical radiograph immediately after implant placement

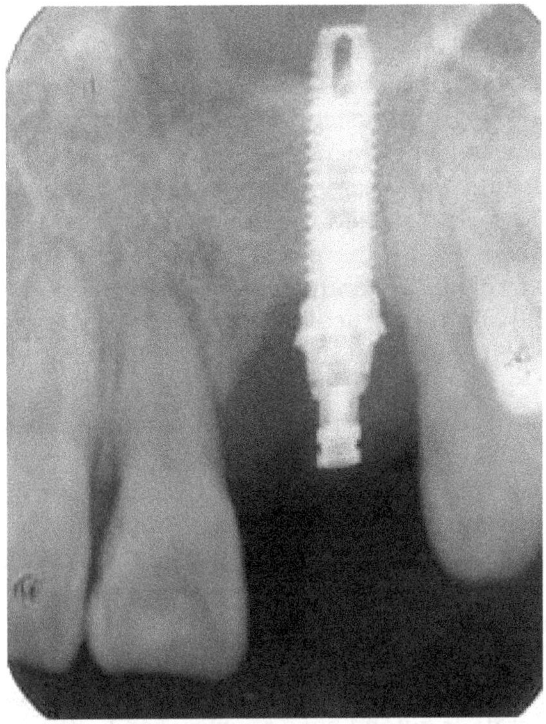

b: Periapical radiograph years after implant placement (marginal bone level: -1.0 mm).

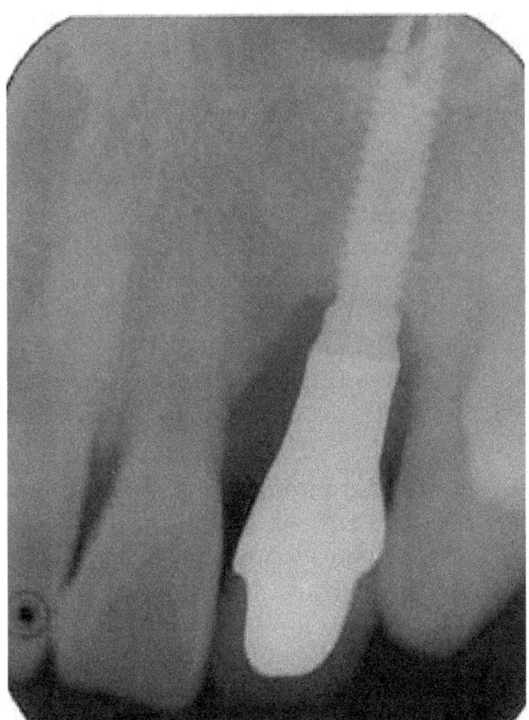

c: 13 years after implant placement (marginal bone level: -1.0 mm)

Fig. 6. Radiological evaluation of the long-term follow up in a UCLP patient.

2.5 Timing for BG and for implant placement

Generally, secondary BG is recommended to perform before canine eruption. (Enemark, et al., 1985; Bergland, et al., 1986). The reasons for this are the better clinical results seen in younger individuals, and the greater osteogeneic activity in younger than older patients. It was shown that there was a tendency to an inverse correlation between IABH and age at the time of BG (Takahashi, et al., 1999). Therefore, from the clinical point of view, secondary BG for alveolar clefts should be performed when the patient is young. On the other side, generally implant placement before the growth spurt is assumed to be contraindication. (Lekholm, 1993) because implants are immobile similar to ankylotic teeth (Adell, et al., 1981; Shapiro and Kokich, 1988) and do not accompany other parts of the jaw bone during rapid growth in the adolescence. Adhering to this rule, the time lag between BG and implant placement is required. Actually, the mean duration from BG to implant placement was 4.6 ±2.5 years. It is well known that the grafted alveoli undergoes resorption 3-dimensionally (Van der Meji, et al., 1994), and the interdental alveolar bone height (IABH) also decreases (Takahashi et al., 1999). The mean net bone height 1 month after BG was approximately 17 mm, and the mean width 1 month after BG was 12. 9 mm, both of which were enough for the implant placement. However, almost half of the grafted alveoli required another bone graft within 24 months after the original bone graft to increase IABH level for implant placement (Takahashi et al., 1999).

None the less, the grafted alveoli with PCBM are suitable for implant placement. If the grafted alveoli do not have sufficient bone volume and IABH, another bone augmentation procedure such as onlay graft or guided bone regeneration (GBR) should be considered. The flow chart of the dental reconstruction of alveolar cleft using PCBM BG and implant placement was shown in Fig. 7. According to this flow chart, BG with PCBM should be performed followed by orthodontic teeth movement and space making for an implant bed in adult CLP patient with un-repaired alveolar cleft. Subsequently, implant placement should be performed within 2 years after BG to avoid another bone augmentation procedure (Fig. 7a). If the patient is young and is on the line of multi-disciplinary team approach, secondary BG to the alveolar cleft should be performed between 7 to 11 years of age before canine eruption. Orthodontic dental arch closure without prosthodontic treatment should be the primary choice as golden standard procedure for dental reconstruction of the grafted alveolar cleft. However, in cases of excessively long treatment period or a wide interdental space resulting from several congenitally missing teeth, use of dental implant placement in the grafted alveoli should be considered after the growth spurt (Fig. 7b) as an alternative treatment protocol. Please keep in mind that another bone augmentation procedure may be required for implant placement in the grafted alveoli as will be discussed later.

2.6 Bone augmentation procedure for implant placement in grafted alveoli

For the dental reconstruction of the grafted alveoli, insufficient bone volume and IABH seems to be a limiting factor for implant placement. Therefore, another bone augmentation procedure is sometimes necessary. Generally speaking, the treatment modality depends on the shape and the volume of the residual grafted alveoli. Small defect could be repaired by GBR (Buser et al., 1990) as a simultaneous augmentation procedure with implant placement. Sometimes however, greater bone volume is necessary for esthetic and functional dental reconstruction in the maxillary anterior region of the grafted alveoli. A various augmentation procedures including onlay bone graft (Fukuda et al., 1998, 2000), titanium mesh and particulate bone graft (Von Arx, et al., 1996; Miyamoto et al., 2011) and alveolar distraction osteogenesis (ADO) (Buis, et al., 2001) could be available for bone augmentation.

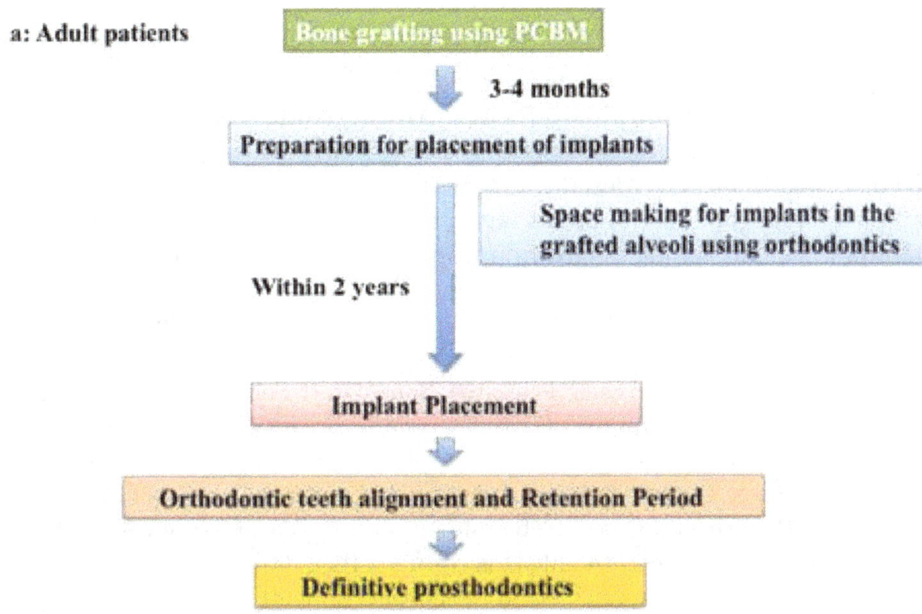

Flow Chart of Dental reconstruction of the alveolar cleft using BG and dental implant

a: Adult patients

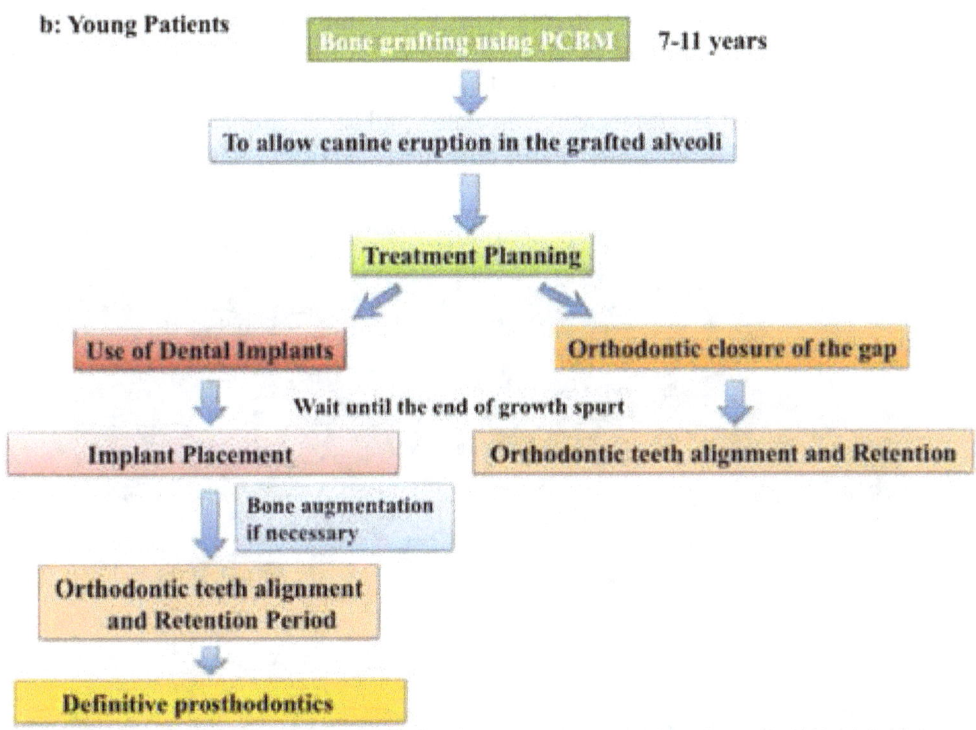

Flow Chart of Dental reconstruction of the alveolar cleft using BG and dental implant

b: Young patients

Fig. 7. Flow Chart of Dental reconstruction of the alveolar cleft using BG and dental implant

2.6.1 Chin bone onlay graft

Onlay grafting provides for appropriate alveolar bone height and width in patients with alveolar local bone defects. We have been using chin bone onlay grafting with simultaneous implant placement in patients with insufficient IABH (Fukuda et al., 1998 and 2000). Surgical procedures are as follows. At the grafted alveolus with insufficient IABH, the gingival on top of the alveolar ridge is incised. Mesially and distally to the alveolus, releaf incisions are made buccally. A buccal mucoperiosteal flap is raised to expose the nasal floor. The thickness of the chin bone graft needed, i.e. the height from top to bottom of the inter-dental alveolar bone margin is calculated using calipers. Drilling for implant installation is performed following a surgical protocol, without perforating the nasal mucosa. In the mandibular symphysis region, a vestibular sulcus incision is made through the mucosa. The periosteium is elevated to allow a hand-driven instrument (Leibinger® Fritsch™ Bone Graft Set; Leibinger GmbH, Freiburg, Germany) to be introduced. The tip of a self-tapping implant is inserted into the chin bone without penetration of the lingual cortical bone. The instrument is rotated around the placed implant perpendicularly to the chin bone surface until the labial cortical bone plate has been passed through to the cancellous bone. The implant and monocorticocancellous bone complex are removed by rotating the instrument. This complex (Fig. 8a) is then placed at the prepared recipient site, and the implant is inserted in the cortical bone of the nasal floor (Fig. 8b). Small gap between the complex and the alveolus are filled with cancellous bone chips obtained from the donor site. The periosteium of the mucoperiosteal flap is incised to allow this flap to cover the complex without any tension, and the wound is closed. Six months later, the abutment connection was performed, and prosthetic rehabilitation was completed with a single-unit implant-supported prosthesis. In 7 patients with CLP, simultaneous chin bone onlay graft (CBOG) was performed for implant placement. Although four of the seven patients had an uneventful course, three had some wound dehiscence and exposed chin bone underwent partial (2 cases) or total necrosis (one case). Ultimately, all seven implants were integrated, and the alveolar bone height had increased in all patients except one. A typical case is shown in Fig. 8 (Fig. 8a-d) .

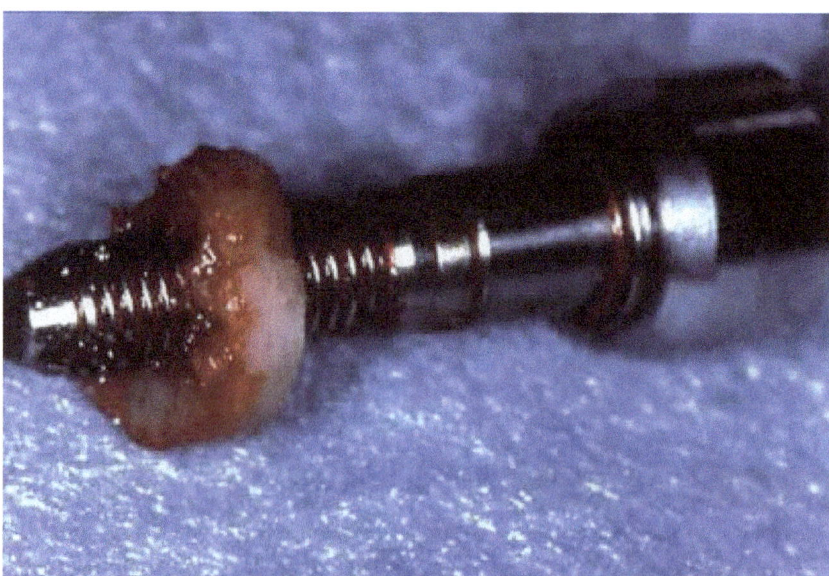

a: Fixture and corticocancellous chin bone complex

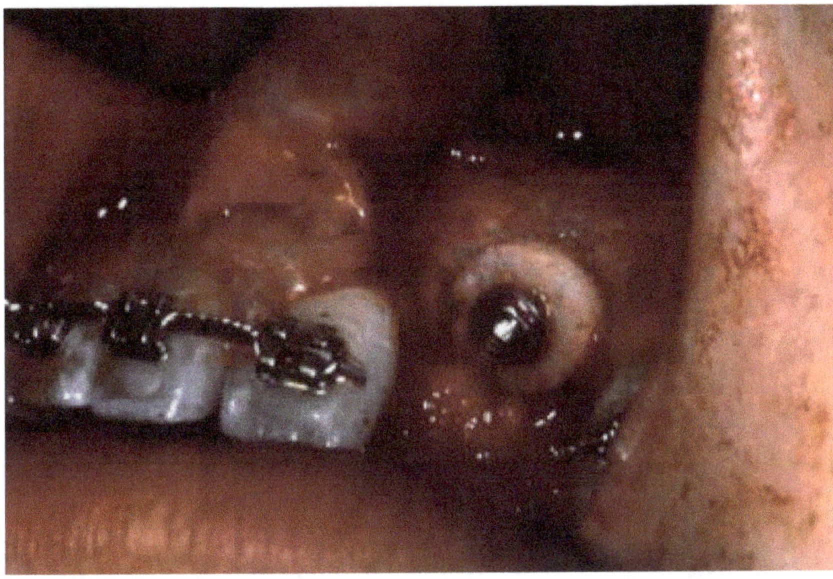

b: Clinical appearance after placement of complex

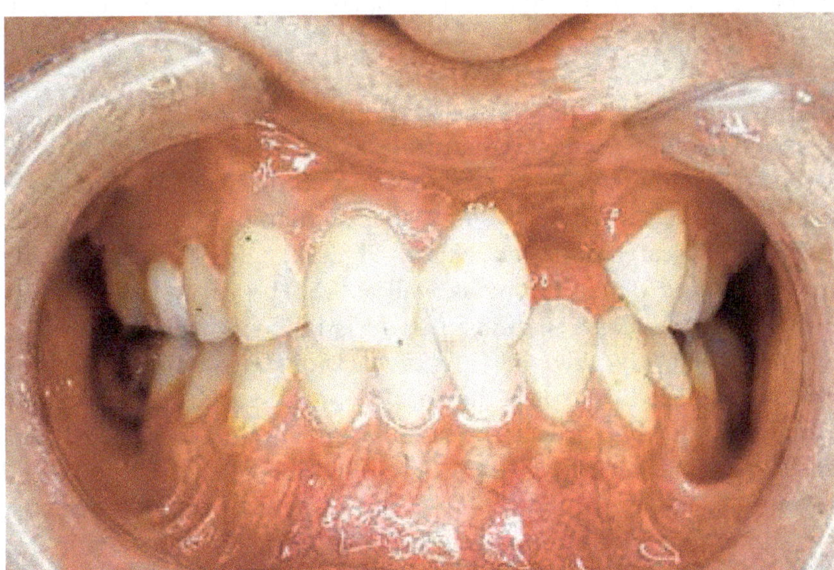

c: Intra-oral view after secondary BG with PCBM followed by completion of orthodontic alignment of maxillary arch.

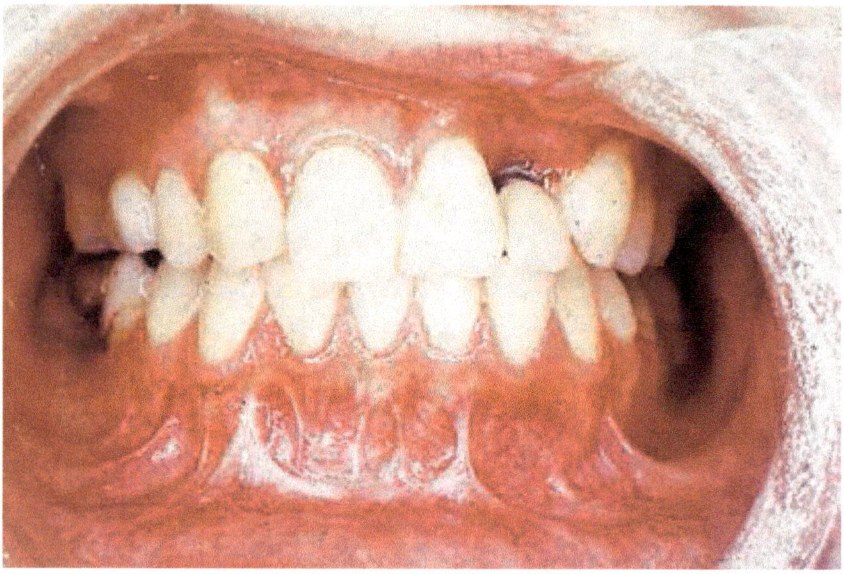

d: Occlusal view showing final prosthesis rehabilitation. Interdental alveolar bone height (IABH) was increased by CBOG. (Takahashi T, et al. J Oral Maxillofac Surg 1997: 55: 576-583)

Fig. 8. Augmentation procedure using chin bone onlay graft (CBOG) for dental implant placement

2.6.2 Titanium mesh and particulate bone graft

The titanium mesh technique is one alternative, based on bone grafting with a stiff occlusive titanium membrane. Titanium meshes were used according to the shape of the defects. Harvested bone was set on the defects and a shaped titanium mesh was fixed with small titanium screws. A typical case is shown in Fig.9a-e. In this case, grafted alveolus underwent resorption and bone volume as well as IABH was decreased. For the surgical procedure, at the grafted alveolus with insufficient IABH, crestal incision was always used. Mesially and distally to the alveolus, relief incisions are made buccally. A buccal mucoperiosteal flap is raised to expose the nasal floor. Decortication of the drill holes was performed by using round burr to ensure vascular nutrition of the grafted bone. Titanium mesh (0.1- or 0.2-mm thickness; M-TAM, Stryker Leibinger GmbH & Co., USA) were trimmed to ensure to cover the bone grafts. Autogenous particulate bone grafts were obtained from intraoral, mainly from mandibular retromolar region with a scraper (mx-grafter; Maxilon Laboratories, Inc., Hollis, NH, USA). Bone grafts are filled in the recipient site. Then, the titanium mesh was stabilized with several small titanium screws buccally and palatally. With sufficient saline irrigation for a clean surgical field, tension free 5-0 nylon sutures were placed across the incision on the periosteal membrane over the mucoperiosteal flap. A staged approach was used for implant installation.

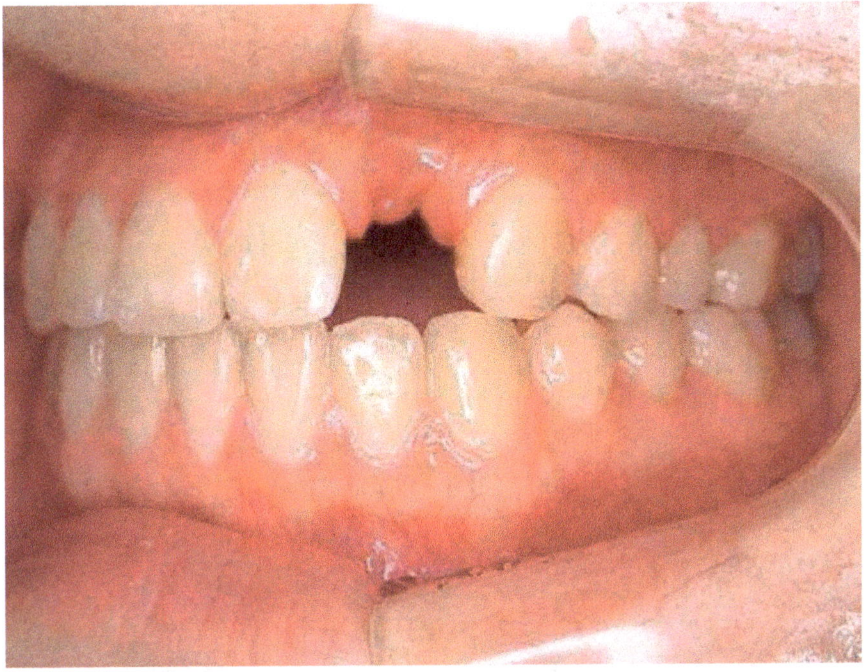

a: Preoperative view after secondary GB with PCBM followed by completion of orthodontic alignment of maxillary arch.

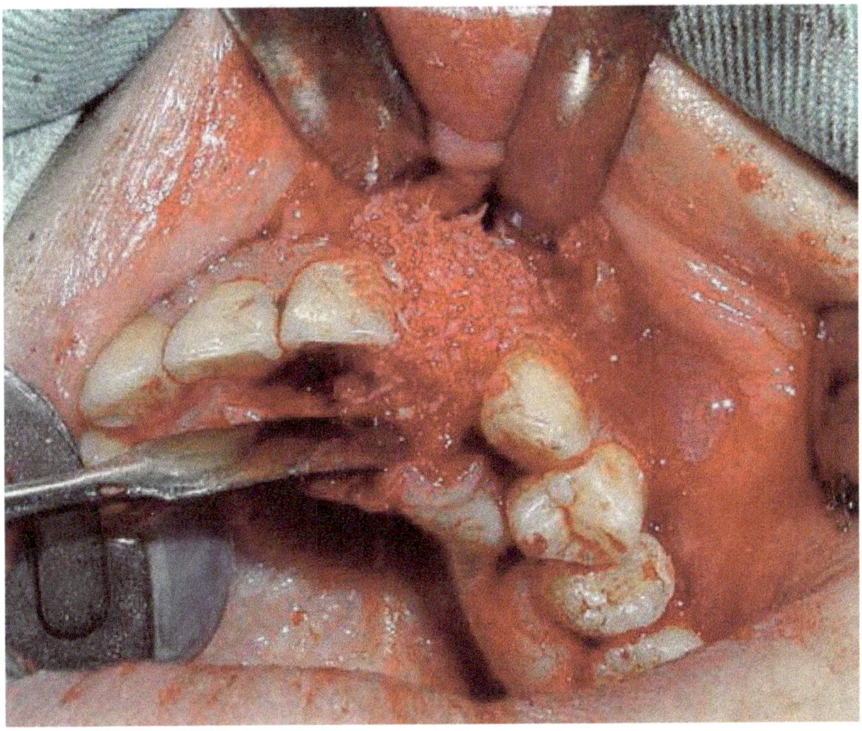

b: Bone graft (BG) using particulate bone harvested from mandibular ramus.

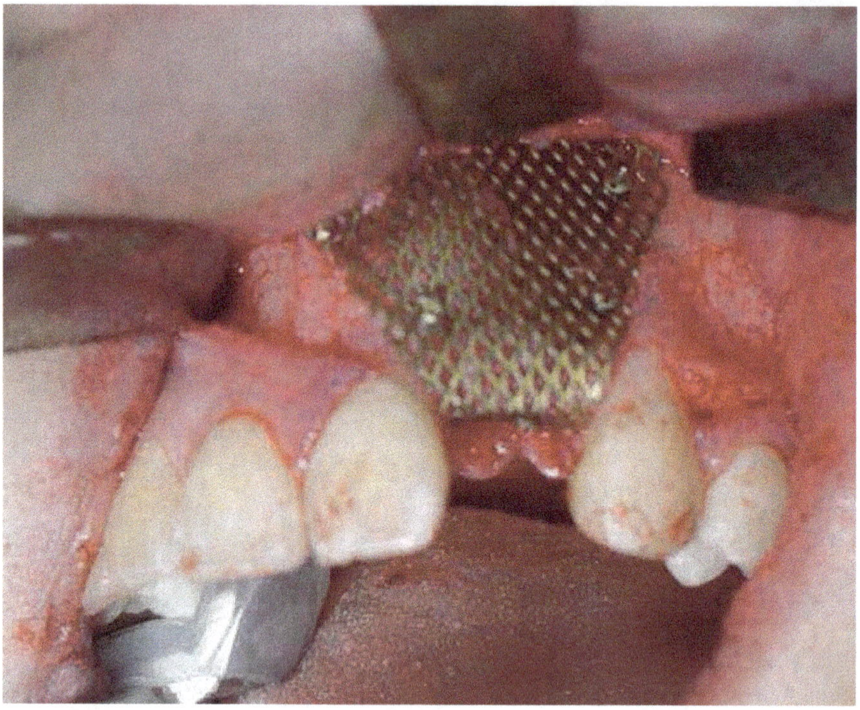

c: Intra-oral view after secondary BG with PCBM followed by completion of orthodontic alignment of maxillary arch.

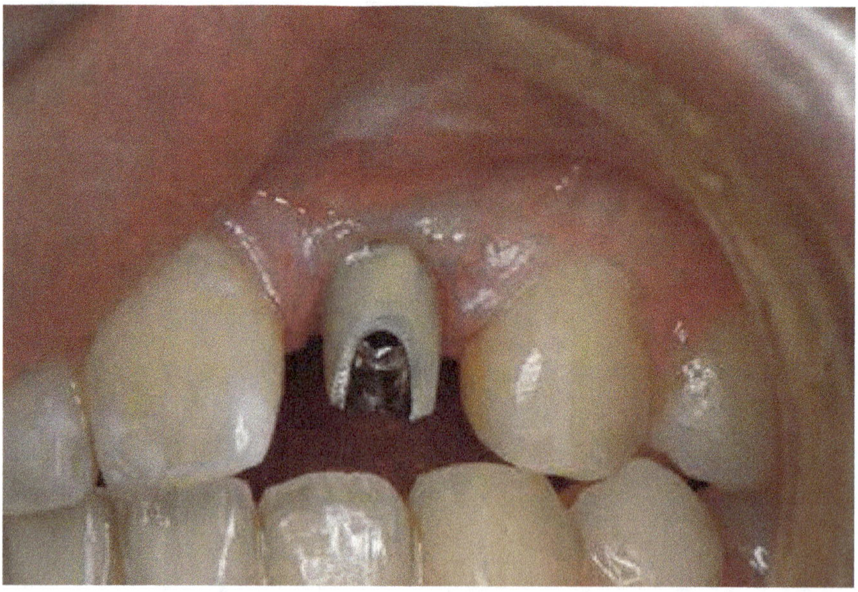

d: After implant placement and abutment connection

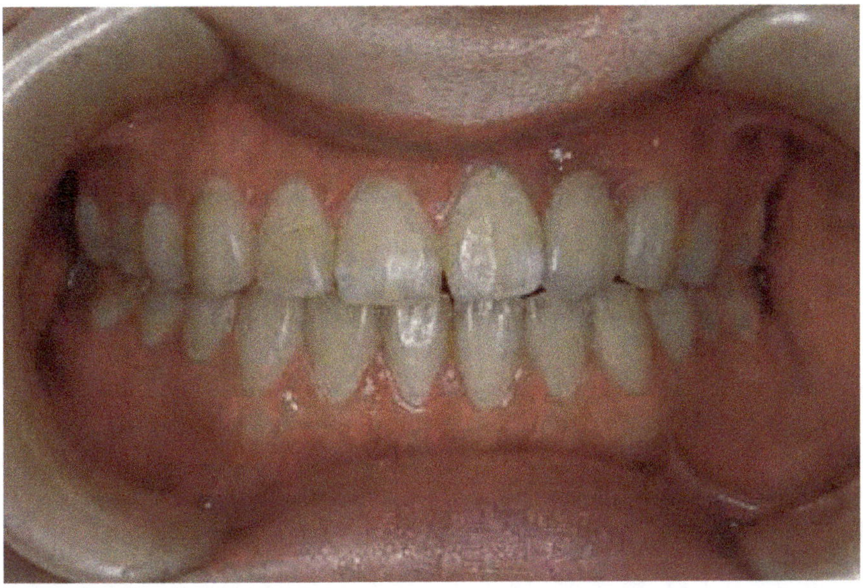

e: Occlusal view showing final prosthesis rehabilitation. IABH was increased by titanium mesh and BG.

Fig. 9. Augmentation procedure using titanium mesh for dental implant placement

A major complication of the titanium mesh technique is mesh exposure during healing period. Mesh exposure would result in infection, which can jeopardize the results. Therefore, two-stage approach is strongly recommended. Usually, implant placement is suitable 6 months after the titanium mesh and particulate autogenous and bone graft.

2.6.3 Alveolar distraction Osteogenesis

Alveolar distraction Osteogenesis (ADO) is another alternatives of augmentation in the insufficient grafted alveoli. The advantages of ADO include avoiding autogenous bone harvest, and simultaneous soft tissue expansion. However, ADO is very technically sensitive, and many complications are reported. Disadvantages of DO are difficulty in vector control, the exposure of distraction device, necessary for long treatment time. Nonetheless, since the mucosa around the grafted alveoli is abundant in scar tissue, and is difficult in soft tissue cover, the soft tissue expansion by ADO seems to be a big advantage. Clinical data concerning the use of ADO in the grafted area are lacking, and further study will be necessary for ADO.

2.7 Preservation of the grafted bone after implant placement

Our study demonstrated that the IABH did not change for up to 6 years after implant placement. Actually, in this study, IABH was reduced only in 2 of 16 (12.5%) of the implant-placed grafted alveoli. Furthermore, the marginal bone level at 6 years averaged 0.28 mm, showing extremely low resorption around the implant. Although no linear measurement of the IABH bone loss of the grafted alveoli was made in this study, these results clearly demonstrate that implant placement in grafted alveoli maintain the grafted bone after secondary PCBM.

The reason of the maintenance of the implant-placed grafted alveoli in a long-term follow-up may be achieved through functional loading of the grafted bone. Dempt et al. suggested that the endosseous implants into the grafted alveoli not only closed the gap, but exert functional stimulation of the transplanted bone by mastication (Dempf, et al., 2002). Our data support this hypothesis.

3. Conclusion

This study further confirmed that the use of dental implants placed in the alveoli after PCBM grafting is an excellent treatment modality for the dental rehabilitation of patients with alveolar clefts and congenitally missing teeth and that it is a great tool for preventing grafted bone resorption after cleft repair with secondary BG. However, the grafted alveoli undergo bone resorption in time-dependent manner. Therefore, the loss of width and height of the bone bridge must also be considered for implant installation. If the grafted alveoli do not have sufficient bone volume and IABH, another bone augmentation procedure such as onlay graft, GBR, or titanium mesh and cancellous bone graft technique should be considered.

4. References

Abyholm FE, Bergland O, Semb G. (1981). Secondary bone grafting of alveolar clefts: surgical/orthodontic treatment enabling a non-prosthetic rehabilitation in cleft lip and palate patients. *Scand J Plastic Reconstru Surg,* Vol. 15, No. 2, pp. 127-140. ISSN 0284-4311

Adell R, Lekholm U, Brånemark P-I. (1981). A 15-years sudy of osseointegrated implants in the treatment of the edentulous jaw. *Int J Oral Maxillofac Surg,* Vol. 10, No. 6, (Dec 1981), pp. 387-416, ISSN 0901-5027

Albrektsson T, Zarb G, Worthington P, Eriksson AR. (1986). The long-term efficacy of currently used dental implants: a review and proposed criteria of success. *Int J Oral Maxillofac Implants,* Vol. 1, No.1 (Summer 1986), pp. 11-25, ISSN 0882-2786

Bergland O, Semb G, Abyholm FE. (1986). Elimination of the residual alveolar cleft by secondary bone grafting an dsubsequent orthodontic treatment. *Cleft Palate Craniofac J,* Vol. 23, No. 2, pp. 175-205, ISSN 1545-1569

Boyne P.; Sands ND. (1972). Secondary bone grafting of residual alveolar and palatal clefs. *J Oral Maxillofac Surg,* Vol. 30, No.2, (Feb 1972) pp. 87-96, ISSN 02782391

Buis J, Rousseau P, Soupre V, Martinez H, Diner PA, Vazquez MP. (2001). "Distraction" of grafted alveolar bone in cleft case using endosseous implant. *Cleft Palate Craniofac J* Vol, 38, No. 4, (Jul 2001), pp. 405-409, ISSN 1545-1569

Buser D, Brägger U, Lang NP, Nyman S. (1990). Regeneration and enlargement of jaw bone using guided tissue regeneration. *Clin Oral Implant Res,* Vo.7, No. 2, pp. 22-32, ISSN 0905-7161

Dempf R, Teltrow T, Kramer FJ, Hausamen JE. (2002). Alveolar bone grafting in patients with complete clefts: a comparative study between secondary and tertiary bone grafting. *Cleft Palate Craniofac J,* Vol. 39, NO. 1 (Jan 2002), pp. 18-25, ISSN 1545-1569

Enemark H, Krants-Simonsen E, Shramm JE. (1985). Secondary bone grafting in unilateral cleft lip palate patients: indications and treatment procedure. *Int J Oral Surg*, Vol. 14, No. 1(Feb 1985), pp. 2-10, ISSN 1998-0134

Enemark H, Sindet-Pedersen S, Bundgaard M. (1987). Long-term results after secondary bone grafting of alveolar clefts. *J Oral Maxillofac Surg*, Vol. 45, No. 11, (Nov 1987), pp. 913-919, ISSN 02782391

Fukuda M, Takahashi T, Yamaguchi T, Kochi S. (1998). Placement of endosteal implants combined with chin bone onlay graft for dental reconstruction in patients with grafted alveolar clefts. *Int J Oral Maxillofac Surg*, Vol. 27, No. 6, (Dec 1998), pp. 440-444, ISSN 0901-5027

Fukuda M, Takahashi T, Yamaguchi T. (2000). Bone grafting technique to increase interdental alveolar bone height for placement of an implant. *Br J Oral Maxillofac Surg*, Vol. 38, No. 1 (Feb 2000), pp. 16-18, ISSN 0266-4356

Härtel J, Pögl C, Henkel KO, Gundlach KK. (1999). Dental implants in alveolar cleft patients: a retrospective study. *J Craniomaxillofac Surg*, Vol. 27, No. 6, pp. 354-357, ISSN 1010-5182

Jansma J, Raghoebar GM, Batenburg RH, Stellingsma C, van Oort RP. (1999). Bone grafting of cleft lip and palate patients for placement of endosseous implants. *Cleft Palate Craniofac J*, Vol. 36, No. 1, pp. 67-72, ISSN 1545-1569

Lekholm U (1993). The use of osseointegrated implants in growing jaws. Int Oral Maxillofac Implants, Vol. 8, No. 3, pp. 243-244, ISSN 0882-2786

Miyamoto I, Kodama K, Funaki K, Yamauchi K, Yamashita Y, Takahashi T (2011). Reconstruction of the alveolar ridge by titanium mesh and particulate autongenous bone: three dimensional evaluation by computed tomography at the point of bone defect. *Clin Implant Dent Relat Res*, in press (Epub ahead of print). ISSN 1708-8208

Ronchi P, Chiapasco M, Frattini D. (1995). Endosseous implants for prosthetic rehabilitation in bone grafted alveolar clefts. *J Craniomaxillofac Surg*, Vol. 23, No. 6 (Dec 1995), pp. 382-386, ISSN 1010-5182

Shapiro PA, Kokich VG. Uses of implants in orthodontics. (1988). *Dent Clin North Am*, Vol. 32, Vol. 3, (Jul 1988), pp. 539-550, ISSN 0011-8532

Takahashi T, Fukuda M, Yamaguchi T, Kochi S. (1997). Use of endosseous implants for dental reconstruction of patients with grafted alveolar clefts. *J Oral Maxillofac Surg*, Vol. 55, No. 6, pp. 576-583, ISSN 5506-0008

Takahashi T, Fukuda M, Yamaguchi T, Kochi S. (1999). Placement of endosseous implants into bone-grafted alveolar clefts: assessment of bone bridge after autogenous particulate cancellous bone and marrow graft. *Int J Oral Maxillofac Implants*, Vol. 14, No.1 (Jan-Feb 1999), pp. 86-93, ISSN 0882-2786

Takahashi T, Inai T, Kochi S, Fukuda M, Yamaguchi T, Matsui K, Echigo S, Watanabe M. (2008). Long-term follow-up of dental implants placed in a grafted alveolar cleft: evaluation of alveolar bone height. *Oral Surg Oral Med Oral Pathol Oral Radiol Endod*, Vol.105, No. 3, (March 2008), pp. 297-302, ISSN 1079-2104

Van der Meji AJ, Baart JA, Prahl-Andersen B, Valk J, Kostense PJ, Tuinzing DB. (1994). Computed tomography in evaluation of early secondary bone grafting. *Int J Oral Maxillofac Surg*, Vol. 23, No. 3, pp. 132-136, ISSN 0901-5027

Verdi FJ, Slanzi GL, Cohen SR, Powell R. (1991). Use of the Branemark implant in the cleft palate patient. *Cleft Palate Craniofac J*, Vol. 28, No. 3, pp. 301-303, ISSN 1545-1569

von Arx, Hardt N, Wallkamm B. (1996). TIME technique: a new method for localized alveolar ridge augmentation prior to placement of dental implants. Int J Oral Maxillofac Implants. Vol. 11, No. 3, (May-Jun 1996), pp. 387-394, ISSN 0882-2786

3

Computer Aided Techniques Developed for Diagnosis and Treatment Planning in Implantology

Elnaz Moslehifard
Department of Prosthodontics,
Tabriz University of Medical Sciences, Tabriz,
Iran

1. Introduction

The wide spread application of dental implants with high success rates has made them a common treatment modality in the past two decades. Despite of the predictability of the osseointegration of dental implants, the surgeon has to overcome anatomic limitations as well as restorative demands to achieve precision in planning and surgical positioning of implants. It is essential that the implants are placed properly to ensure a successful operation outcome.

Dental implants are an expected treatment modality for either the restoration of partially and completely edentulous patients or other applications such as anchorage tool in orthodontics (Moslehifard et al, 2011). Successful provision of dental implants to patients lost their teeth and in most occasions their surrounding bone relies on careful gathering of clinical and radiological information achieved with an interdisciplinary communication and detailed planning. Treatment planning is crucial for the success of dental implants.

In osseointegration of dental implants, planning and surgical positioning of implants must be carried out accurately in spite of several inherent limitations. Capabilities of the clinicians, i.e. the surgeon and prosthodontics, play a crucial rule in achieving optimum surgical and prosthetic procedures. The predictability of success is increased when the implants are placed properly. The optimum placement makes it possible to have implants and prosthetic components under establishment of favorable forces. At the early stages of evolution of the implant surgery, clinicians would place implants in regions of maximum bone volume without fully considering where the crown eventually would be placed. Biomechanics, esthetics and maintenance can be compromised if the implant location does not align properly with the crown, ultimately resulting in substandard outcomes, including failure (Worthington et al, 2010).

Several techniques have been developed in years and are currently available in the planning procedure of implant placement during the clinical settings. Palpation of the ridge, use of an osteometer, diagnostic casts and evaluation of the relationship between the jaws, and the use of simple radiographs are the most well established methods beside other advanced methods (Kopp et al, 2003; Fortin et al, 2003).

2. Importance of pre-surgical assessment

The success of any therapeutic treatment depends upon a variety of parameters including careful selection of suitable patients for each treatment, formation of a treatment plan and careful implementation of a gentle treatment procedure. If operator strictly adheres to these principles, any operator-induced damage can be significantly prevented. For instance, the selection of patient and treatment planning is the critical step in the prevention of iatrogenically induced damage during implant treatment. Therefore, a great amount of careful attention should be taken at the pre-surgical era before going through the implementation of the treatment/patient selected.

At the preliminary stages of pre-surgical examinations, the anatomical structures such as vertical height of bone, ridge width, bone quality, vital structures and any bony defects or pathologies are important to learn. It would be also necessary to estimate the number of implants to be placed and their angulations using surgical templates as a useful aid in the orientation of the implant. Bone sites are considered as another issue to address in the presurgical study and should be determined reasonably in quality and quantity. In the other hand, the anatomical limitations for the placement of implants may propagate some damages to the maxillary sinus, mental nerve and inferior alveolar nerve, if not properly introduced in the therapeutic treatment process. Once the anatomical purview of the patient/treatment is established, it is generally recommended to perform the treatment planning in a partially edentulous patient in a manner which does not cause any damage to the adjacent teeth. This may be, for example, obtained when a minimum specified edentulous space retains between the adjacent tooth and fixture. However, there should be a minimum of one millimeter clearance between the apex of the fixture and the superior wall of the inferior alveolar canal. Nevertheless, those cases that are planned with allograft and membranes are less predictable compared to straight forward cases.

During the surgery, vital structures like maxillary sinus, mental nerve and inferior alveolar nerves should not be encroached. The damage occurred in nerves can cause numbness and tingling sensation. The encroachment into maxillary sinus can cause development of oroantral communication. If implants are inserted closely to the maxillary sinus after a poor oral hygiene, it may provide a route to spread infection from the mouth. Once the maxillary dental implant is infected, sinusitis occurs readily due to the spread of inflammation. The perforation of the membranous lining of maxillary sinus occurs commonly during sinus lift operations. The floor of mouth contains branches of submental and sublingual and mylohyoid arteries that may lead to life threatening complications. Damage occurrence to arteries, especially in the floor of the mouth has been reported in the literature (Shenoy et al,. 2006). It can result in most cases in fatal hemorrhage. The branch of the sublingual or facial artery may be situated in immediate contact with the lingual periosteum. This close proximity can explain why even a small perforation could cause severe bleeding (Givol et al,. 2000). Mason et al. (Mason & Triplett, 1990) reported a case of fetal hemorrhage arising from the dental implant placement in the mandible due to damage to sublingual artery. Injury to the mandibular canal results in paralysis or numbness of the chin and corner of the mouth. Furthermore, sudden loss of tooth vitality within a whole quadrant can occur, since the neurovascular bundle within the mandibular canal also supplies the teeth. The damage to the mandibular canal during the placement of implants (or extraction of third molars), therefore, develops one of the major issues for which legal actions may be taken against dentists. The major cause of this pitfall is submandibular fossa, which is a depression on the medial surface of the body of the mandible inferior to the mylohyoid line. Submandibular gland is lodged in this fossa.

Studies by Bavitz et al. (Bavitz et al,. 1994) and Hofchneider et al (Hofchneider et al, 1999) indicated that submental and sublingual arteries may locate closely to the lingual cortical plate, from the floor of the mouth. It should be pointed out that the edentulous mandible is even shorter and, therefore, the perforations occurred are deeper in the floor of the mouth. Most of the reports of the floor of the mouth and sublingual hemorrhage have been iatrogenic in nature. Sharp instruments such as rotating dental disks and burs have slipped off mandibular teeth causing injury to the floor of the mouth and even laceration of the sublingual artery. Niamtu (Niamtu &Richmond, 2001) reported a case of near fatal airway obstruction after routine implant placement, secondary to sublingual bleeding and hematoma. The submental artery may be located against the usually concave medial body of the mandible in older edentulous patients. The horizontal wall of the submandibular fossa considered in this study has been above the mandibular nerve in all the subjects. Considering the anatomic variations, the risk of perforation is high, especially when the fossa is very deep. When delayed severe bleeding can be taking place, it is prudent to closely follow any patient with a significant penetrating trauma to the floor of the mouth. This includes injuries from iatrogenic dental treatment(s) (Niamtu &Richmond, 2001). In one study (Parnia et al,. 2010) the depth of submandibular fossa was more than 2 mm in 80% of the subjects. This situation raises the risk of perforation of lingual cortical plate, injury to the terminal branches of sublingual artery during implant placement and hemorrhagic accidents, which are critical and life-threatening. Therefore, precise evaluation of morphology and dimensions of submandibular fossa is of utmost importance before implant surgery in the posterior areas of mandible.

The mandibular inter-mental area is assumed to be a safe area for implant insertion and is considered in many other surgical procedures. It is essential to understand the anatomy of the region to avoid occurring injuries to the neurovascular bundles. Provided that the inferior alveolar or mental nerve is damaged during the preparation of an osteotomy, sensory dysfunction may appear due to nerve damage in the foraminal area. All-on-four procedure which has been recently developed, permits a quick placement of 4 dental implants in the interforaminal area of the lower jaw associated with a fixed bridge during only one appointment. The mental foramen is a strategically important landmark during osteotomy procedures. The inferior alveolar nerve may extend beyond the mental foramen as an intraosseous anterior loop. The location of foramen, as well as, the possibility that an anterior loop of the mental nerve may be present mesial to the mental foramen need to be considered before implant surgery to prevent mental nerve injury. The mandibular canal contains the inferior alveolar nerve and blood vessels and is divided into mental and incisive segments between the roots of premolars. The mental canal deviates toward the mental foramen. However, the incisive canal continues below the incisor teeth where it is generally divided into a plexus of nerve branches until its main trunk is lost (Greenstein& Tarnow, 2000). In this area lingual foramen is also present that is located in the midline, leveled with or superior to the genial tubercles. The foramen has a branch of the incisive artery that anastomosis with the lingual artery (McDonnell et al,. 1994).

In the establishment of a zone of safety (in millimeters) in implant placement, both the available bones coronal and anterior to the foramen are quite important. Any improper implant insertion anterior to the mental canal can cause oedema of the epineurium. This may spread to the main mental branch, leading to neurosensory disturbances. Some authors have reported the evidences of discomfort, pain, and disturbance of sensation after implant insertion into the inter-mental area (Abarca et al,. 2006). Rosenquist assumed that implant failure and neurosensory dysfunction were partly due to the large diameter of the mandibular incisive canal. In this report, it was found that incisive bundle causes implant failure, by migrating of soft tissue around the implant, thus preventing osteointegration (Rosenquist, 1996). In addition, sensory disturbances of the mental nerve region may arise after endosseous implants are installed in the mandibular interforaminal region because of damage to anatomical structures in this area (Wismeijer et al,. 1997).

Other landmarks are anterior loop and incisive canal. The possibility of the presence of the anterior loop does not necessarily mean that implants can be safely placed close to the mental foramen. The sensory disturbances of the lower lip have been reported due to the direct trauma to the anterior looping of the mental nerve. Incisive canal is a continuation of the mandibular canal anterior to the mental foramen. The canal contains the incisive bundle that innervates the teeth in the anterior segment. Its precise anatomy and intermedullary content is important during implant insertion. One possible result from traumatizing the neurovascular bundle is sensory disturbance. Kohavi and Bar-Ziv (Kohavi& Bar-Ziv, 1996) described a case where pain and discomfort resulted from implants placed in the intermental area. CT images revealed that the implants were placed through a large lumen of the incisive canal (Bavitz et al,. 1993). Another factor might also be related to indirect trauma to the incisive canal bundle, causing hematoma in the closed chamber that may produce pressure on the mental nerve. Thus the canal could play an important role in successful osseointegration and prevention of postoperative sensory disturbances.

The lingual foramen is situated in the midline, leveled with or superior to the genial tubercles. A pilot study by Mc Donnell (Mc Donnell et al,. 1994) revealed an incidence of 49% of the lingual foramen on periapical radiographs of the mandibular incisor region in adult population. The study suggested that the lingual foramen was a consistent finding to the lingual side of the mandible in the midline, being present in over 99% of the dried specimen examined. The foramen was definitely visible in 81% and 82% in Makris (Makris et al, 2010) based on CBCT and Jacobs (Jacobs et al,. 2002) based on CT studies, respectively. The lingual artery has sufficient size to present difficulty in control of hemorrhage intraosseously or in soft tissue. Also in view of its position it could be a factor in implant placement in the midline.

Sufficient knowledge of performing implant surgeries should be available to manage arterial hemorrhage and other medical emergencies. Accurate radiographic imaging is indispensable for the selection of appropriate implant size and placement and is an invaluable guide for surgery.

3. Imaging objectives

Over the past decade, there has been a diverse progress in using noninvasive technology to visualize human internal structures in their true form and shape. The discovery of X-ray gave birth to radiology in years. Its outcome developed in dentistry is that the pre-surgical radiographic examinations for the treatment with osseointegrated implant give detailed information on the potential area for implantation. The presence of lesions and anatomical landmarks is known as the confining conditions and structures that may influence the placement of osseous implants. The radiographic examinations should also provide evaluation of morphology, angulations of the alveolar ridge, and quantity and quality of the alveolar bone (Tyndall & Brooks, 2000). The global objective of this phase of treatment is to develop and to implement a treatment plan for the patient that enables restoration of the patient's function and esthetics by the application of accurate and strategic requirements being transformed physically into a three-dimensional diagnostic template. This enables the implant team to identify the specific sites of prospective implant surgery in the imaging examinations. The specific objectives of pre-prosthetic imaging are to (1) identify disease, (2) determine bone quantity, (3) determine bone density, (4) identify critical structures at the proposed implant regions, and (5) determine the optimum position of implant placement relative to occlusal loads (Misch, 2005).

Initially, implants were placed by use of simple periapical and panoramic radiographs (Sarment et al,. 2003). Pre-surgical imaging can provide important information in osseointegrated dental implant treatment. Placement of implants has been performed by use of simple periapical and panoramic radiographs for years (Kopp et al,. 2003). However, surgical templates have attracted much interest in obtaining more precise placement of implant on the surgical site. Because both the final restorative prosthesis, i.e. the biomechanical and aesthetic requirements, and the internal anatomy, i.e. bone volume and position of vital structure, are to be taken into account (Fortin et al,. 2003 ; Misch, 2005).

Proper radiographic assessment is an essential aspect of dental implant planning. Different imaging methods have been used to evaluate bone quantity and anatomic structures in relation to the proposed implant site, ranging from conventional 2-dimentional radiographs (panoramic and periapical radiographs) to more complex 3-dimentional modalities, such as computerized tomography (CT) or cone beam computerized tomography (CBCT).

Some clinicians may solely evaluate the edentulous site on periapical and/or panoramic radiographs. The results of these radiographic evaluations can be enhanced at the time of scanning by the application of a radiographic template with radiopaque markers or materials. Different radiopaque markers, including metal balls and tubes, gutta-percha, and barium sulfate, have been used to delineate the position and/ or the contour of the proposed restoration, but little or no information exist about the restoration contour of the proposed restoration, or it can decrease the quality of the image by increasing the scatter artifact (Zahran & Fenton, 2010). The main drawback of both techniques for implant treatment is that the images are two-dimensional. Studies have shown that only 17% of panoramic radiographs reveal true osseous height on dried specimens (Richtert, 1989). In the posterior mandibular region the buccolingual location of the mandibular canal and submandibular fossa are of utmost importance because there is a potential risk of causing damage to the inferior alveolar nerve and submental and sublingual arteries during surgery. The mental foramen is an important landmark where implant placing must be performed in the foraminal region of the mandibular arch. To prevent the mental nerve injury during implant surgery, it is necessary to define the location and also whether an anterior loop of the mental nerve may become mesial to the mental foramen. Sensory dysfunction due to nerve damage in the foraminal area could occur provided that the inferior alveolar or mental nerve is damaged during osteotomy. Since improper placement of implant in the intermental area causes pain and discomfort, reported in several cases, a zone of safety (in millimeter) for implant placement must be determined. However, neither the panoramic nor the periapical films can provide correct information (Parnia et al,. 2010).

4. Pre- prosthetic imaging

4.1 Intraoral radiography

4.1.1 Periapical radiography

Periapical radiographs are the images of a limited region of mandibular or maxillary alveolus. Periapical radiographs may suffer from distortion and magnification. The long cone paralleling technique eliminates distortion as long as it limits the magnification to less than 10%. The opposing landmark of available bone in implant dentistry is beyond lingual muscle attachments in the mandible or beyond the palatal vault in the maxilla. As such, the image most often must be foreshortened to visualize the opposing cortical plate. As a result, the actual available bone height may be difficult to determine. In terms of the objectives of preprostetic imaging, periapical radiography is (1) a useful high-yield modality for ruling out local bone or dental disease; (2) of limited value in determining quantity because the image is magnified, may be distorted, and does not depict the third dimension of bone width; (3) of limited value in determining bone density or mineralization (the lateral cortical plates prevent accurate interpretation and cannot differentiate subtle trabecular bone changes); and (4) of value in identifying critical structures but of little use in depicting the spatial relationship between the structures and the proposed implant sit (Misch,2005; Goaze &White, 1992).

4.1.2 Occlusal radiography

Occlusal radiographs have minimal application in implant dentistry. Cross-sectional occlusal radiographs of the mandible give some information about the buccolingual dimension of the mandible, but this information is only accurate in comparison to the inferior aspect of the body, not the width of the alveolar ridge where the implant is to be placed. The use of cross-sectional occlusal radiographs can be helpful when evaluating the position of the implant within the jaw following placement; this applies to both the mandible and maxilla (Mansour &Dudhia, 2008).

4.2 Extraoral radiography

4.2.1 Cephalometeric radiography

Lateral cephalometric radiographs provide accurate information about the available bone in the mid-sagittal region of the maxilla and mandible. Because of the long film-focal distances used in cephalometric radiography the resultant image has minimal magnification. The cross-sectional dimensions and morphology of the ridge are shown accurately in the midsagittal plane of the anterior maxilla and mandible.

4.2.2 Panoramic radiography

Panoramic radiography is a curved plane tomographic radiographic technique used to depict the body of the mandible, maxilla, and the lower one half of the maxillary sinuses in a single time. This modality is the most useful diagnostic modality properly utilized in implant dentistry. However, for quantitative pre-prosthetic implant imaging, panoramic radiography is not the most diagnosing way (Grondahl K, 1996; Dove& McDavid, 1993). When using panoramic imaging for diagnosis, one of the most frequent problems in the panoramic radiography is the loss of definition that happens when either the patient is improperly positioned in the machine or the curve of the mandible does not match the focal trough predetermined by the manufacturer (Truhlar et al,. 1993). One early study has shown that only 17% of panoramic radiographs represent true osseous height on dried specimens (Klinge et al,. 1989). Accordingly, due to inexorable changes in the magnification on horizontal dimensions, panoramic image does not match the real dimension. The vertical magnification is approximately 10% and horizontal magnification is approximately 20% and varies depending on the anatomical location, the position of the patient and the focus object distance, and the relative location of the rotation center of the X-ray system. Traditional panoramic radiography is a high-yield technique for demonstrating dental and bone disease. However, panoramic radiography (1) does not demonstrate bone quality/mineralization, (2) is quantitatively misleading due to lack of high magnification and third dimension cross-sectional view, and (3) is of some use in demonstrating critical structures but of little use in depicting the spatial relationship between the structures and dimensional quantitation of the implant site. For the evaluation of the recipient sites and the determination of optimum implant dimension, diagnostic templates having 5-mm ball bearing and being worn by the patient during the panoramic x-ray examination enable the dentist to determine the amount of magnification in the radiograph (Misch, 2005). The development of computer technology applied to radiology has allowed the manipulation of image such as converting the conventional radiographs into scanned images to display readily on a monitor. The scanned images can enhance interpretation, for resources such as brightness and contrast control, colorization, and inversion effects which may be applied to radiographic images (Sakakura et al,. 2004).

4.2.3 Computed tomography

Three-dimensional radiographic imaging was first conceived in the early 20th century and was proved by calculating an infinite number of projections of image of a three-dimensional object. The original purpose of the use of CT scanner was to examine the human cranium (Hounsfield, 1973). Early devices provided 1 cm thick axial cross-sectional images. Until 1980s technical developments resulted in obtaining 1.5 to 2 mm thick images. For several years, the technique was used to diagnose the lesions of the head and neck and for the evaluation of the anatomic structures of patients who were to undergo craniofacial surgery (Iplikcioglu et al,. 2002). CT scans have become one of the most frequently used imaging techniques for pre-operative evaluation of the jaws before implant treatment. The first commercially developed program was DentaScan (General Electric,Milwaukee, Wis), which produced "dentistry-friendly" images (Schwarz et al,. 1987).

CT produces axial images of a patient's anatomy. Axial images are produced perpendicular to the long axis of the body. CT images are inherently three-dimensional. The original imaging computer can create secondary images from almost any perspective by reprojecting or reformatting the original three-dimensional voxel data. These images can be used for diagnostic imaging (Kawamata et al,. 2000). A patient's slice data from CT scan images is analyzed via automatic contouring algorithms to provide a representation of the surface of the studied structures (Woolsen et al,. 1986). These structures can be displayed on the screen, compared against normative references for surgical planning, and modified to represent a simulated surgical operation. Implant design and bony augmentation can be simulated on-screen as well (Benjamin, 2002).

Computer tomography (CT) assisted implant planning systems can considerably enhance the quality of implant therapy by improving the transfer from planning to surgery and the ability to convey the treatment plan to the patient. The significance of proper prosthetically driven treatment planning was reorganized first with the aim of the optimal crown position used as a guide to implant position. CT is considered a valuable tool towards achieving this goal and enables the use of a three-dimensional image for the diagnosis of osseous features, including its density, volume and architecture, and the identification of vital anatomic structures (such as the maxillary sinus and the mandibular canal) in the radiographic image. Prosthetic and radiographic implant planning can be further enhanced with computer software, using template-guided surgery enabling the clinician to optimize implant position, angle, diameter and length (Horwitz et al,. 2009).

In 1986, Fellingham first demonstrated the use of interactive graphics and 3D modeling for surgical planning, prosthesis, and implant design. 3D images were transmitted to a computer-controlled milling machine for reproduction of the anatomical structure. This technology was used to reproduce atrophic mandibular and maxillary jawbones for full arch subperiosteal implants (Fellingham et al,. 1986). After that, multiplanar reformatted CT had become the most comprehensive and accurate aid for endosseous implant treatment planning. Advancement in diagnostic technology, namely helical or spiral CT and stereolithography, have allowed the development of a CAD-CAM processed surgical guide to be placed directly on the bony site. The surgical guide facilitates the predictable transfer of the analysis of the bony morphology and accurate positioning of the endosseous implant (Cucchiara et al,. 2001).

Limitation of this technique includes the determination of bone quality by use of the imaging computer; hard copy images that only include a limited range of the diagnostic gray scale of the study; and the tilt of the patient's head during the examination, which is critical because all the cross-sectional images are perpendicular to the axial imaging plane. CT examinations are expensive and deliver a relatively high radiation dose to the patient. During dental radiographic procedures, organs most susceptible to the side effects of radiation are the hyoid gland, brain, active bone marrow, lymphatics, and salivary glands. However, although the biologic effects of radiation are known, the risk associated with CT is assumed to be low (Iplikcioglu et al,. 2002). Usually a diagnostic template is necessary to take full advantage of the technique. The diagnostic template enables the dentist to incorporate the three-dimensional treatment plan of the final prosthetic result into the imaging examination; evaluate the patient's anatomy relative to the proposed implant sites; esthetics; and occlusion; and record and transfer these finding to the patient at the time of surgery. CT enables identification of disease, determination of bone quantity, determination of bone quality, identification of critical structures at the proposed regions, and determination of the position and orientation of the dental implants (Misch, 2005).

4.2.4 Cone beam computed tomography

Cone beam volumetric tomography was pioneered at the Nihon University School of Dentistry during the 1990s, and the first machines became commercially available in 2000 (Terakado et al,. 2000; Ito et al,. 2001). Since then, numerous machines have been commercialized and much research on the usefulness of the technology in dentistry have been performed. Cone-beam technology is progressing rapidly and scanners are constantly being refined and upgraded. A reasonable number of scanners have already been installed in dental practices and radiology practices, and this number is sure to grow in the future. While CBCT permits three-dimensional visualization of the dental hard tissues in a similar manner to multislice CT, there are some fundamental differences. With the majority of cone-beam machines, the patient is seated or standing rather than being supine (Vannier, 2003; Monsour &Dudhia, 2008). This imaging modality is very promising with regard to pre-implant imaging. CBCT generally delivers a lower dose to the patient compared to CT and provides reasonably sharp images with three-dimensional information. While CBVT permits three-dimensional visualization of dental hard tissues in a similar manner to multi-slice CT (Vannier, 2003), there are some fundamental differences. Image acquisition times vary and are specific to particular models, but typically range between 10 to 70 seconds (Scarfe et al,. 2006; Pinsky, 2006). Acquisition time with a 16-slice CT scanner is shorter than the fastest CBCT scan, and newer 64-slice CT units reduce the scan time even further. This effectively minimizes the risk of patient movement. The theoretical resolution of CBCT is higher than CT (Sato et al,. 2004), but the difference may not be as significant as once through due to the impact of patient movement resulting from the increased scan times. Longer scanning times utilizing an increased number of images permits increased resolution or a decrease in image noise but with a significantly higher radiation dose and an increased risk of patient movement (Scarfe et al,. 2006). As cone-beam technology was built on the platform of complex-motion tomography, the radiation dose is typically lower than a multi-slice CT scan of the jaws (Terakado et al,. 2000; Hashimoto, 2003).

Recent studies indicate that CBCT images are of sufficient accuracy for use in pre-implant assessments (Pinsky, 2006; Ludlow et al,. 2007). It has been demonstrated that the error in measurements obtained from CBCT scans is less than 0.5 mm (Marmulla et al,. 2005). Volume-rendered images obtained from CT data have been found to be superior to those from CBVT. The low exposure parameters of CBVT result in poor soft-tissue contrast compared with CT, (Scarfe et al,. 2006; Katsumata et al,. 2006) and the inability to alter the exposure parameters in most machines means that image quality is compromised in larger patients. Furthermore, CBVT suffers from the same beam-hardening artifact that CT does, limiting the usefulness of the exam in patients with metallic restorations, posts or surgical plates (Guerrero et al, 2006).

While it is recognized that multi-slice CT is a higher dose examination way compared to CBVT, some reports indicate that low-dose CT protocols result in significantly less exposure than previously thought, without compromising image quality significantly (Ekestubbe, 1999). A consequence of the lower dose of CBVT is the reduced contrast and subsequent image quality. It is important to note that while the radiation dose from a CBVT scan may be less than that from low-dose CT, the dose is still significantly higher than that from other forms of dental radiographic examinations (Scarfe et al,. 2006).

4.2.5 Magnetic resonance imaging

Magnetic resonance imaging (MRI) has become a powerful imaging tool in medicine. This technique was announced first by Lauterbur in 1972.Useful medical images were produced in the early 1980s (Lauterbur, 1973).Using the magnetic properties of the hydrogen atom, MRI units are capable of producing images of the human body. As the technology is dependent upon the presence of hydrogen atoms, MRI is particularly suitable to imaging soft tissues. Using various radiofrequency pulse sequences and relaxation times, images may be produced to better demonstrate anatomy or pathology in the body. Since MRI relies on the use of a strong magnetic field, MRI examinations are contraindicated in patients with metal foreign bodies in the eyes, ferromagnetic intracranial aneurysm clips, cardiac pacemakers, cochlear implants and patients in the first trimester of pregnancy. The presence of certain metals such as amalgam and non-precious alloys will result in considerable artifact on the images and often render the examination useless (Hubalkova et al,. 2002; Hubalkova et al,. 2006). Pure titanium implants show no artifact with MRI, but if there are any impurities in the titanium artifact will appear. Other considerations include the significant cost to the patient for MRI examinations and claustrophobia is a real concern as the examinations are generally performed with the patient in a very confining tunnel. MRI is used in implant imaging as a secondary imaging technique when primary imaging techniques fail (Monsour &Dudhia, 2008).

Most studies using MRI for pre-implant imaging have focused on the ability of MRI units to locate the inferior dental canal (Eggers, 2005). With MRI the inferior dental canal appears as a black void within the high-signal cancellous bone. If the inferior dental canal is surrounded by sclerotic bone, visualization of the canal is more difficult with MRI as the presence of sclerotic bone results in a low bone marrow signal. The contrary is true for CT, as the presence of sclerotic bone in the mandibular body makes the inferior dental canal more obvious. Magnetic resonance imaging has a significant potential for pre-implant imaging due to the lack of ionizing radiation, but acquisition times can be as long as 30 minutes and there is limited bone information available (Monsour &Dudhia, 2008).

5. Surgical guides

In spite of significant advances in devices and techniques, placement of dental implants in correct position still remains a challenge. Diagnostic casts, probing depths and panoramic radiography can lead to unpredictable results as they do not give three-dimensional (3-D) radiographic information required for correct positioning and orientation of implant (Almong et al,. 2001). Moreover, predictable implant supported prosthesis also requires a determination of final prosthesis in treatment planning stage. Thus for a successful implant supported prosthesis, the prosthodontist should plan the implant positioning in accordance with accurate mesiodistal and buccolingual location, angulation with residual bone and correct implant orientation. To achieve these objectives, surgical guide (stent) with radiopaque marker in conjunction with dental CT scan imaging should be used.

The purpose of stent is to purview the definitive restoration and its relationship to adjacent structures, to communicate the restoration planned by the prosthodontist to the surgeon, to reduce osteotomy and to locate healing screws at the time of second stage surgery (Garber, 1995). For a successful implant supported definitive restoration the implant must be placed at a correct and pre-planned position and angulation. The mesiodistal placement of the implant should aid in preservation of papilla and provide an esthetic implant restoration profile (Lazzara, 1993). The implant should be placed at least 1.5 mm from the adjacent teeth with a minimum 3 mm interimplant distance. The distance of implant from buccal and lingual cortical plates should be greater than 0.5 mm. In the buccolingual plane the angle between the implant trajectory and residual bone trajectory should be less than 20 degrees to prevent unfavorable bending moment (Horiuchi et al,. 1995; Almong et al,. 1995). In multiple implant situations, non parallel implant placement is the primary cause of non axial loading and subsequent failure (Taylor et al,. 2000). It has been suggested to use stents to achieve the above mentioned objectives. Information present in the literature implies when the implants are placed using stents, the outcome of the positioning is more accurate than those placed without stent (Talwar et al,. 2011).

5.1 Diagnostic template

Evaluation of bone for implant placement may be provided through the use of radiographic or dual-purpose stents. Since the ultimate objective of implant placement is a functional, aesthetic, and durable restoration, the imaging of potential recipient sites should provide accurate information that facilitates precise placement of implants in a correct three-dimensional position (Cehreli & Sahin, 2000). Placement of implants in the anterior maxillary region requires special attention. localized soft tissue and bone contour may affect the emergence profile and the final appearance of the prosthesis. Implants over-angulated toward the labial can lead to aesthetic disharmony. For extremely malaligned implants, an opening for screw access on the facial surface of the prosthesis or its complete removal may be indicated. Implants placed in the inter-proximally areas of a prosthesis may cause aesthetic and hygiene problems, and implants placed too lingually generally result in a bulky prosthesis with an unfavorable lingual contour that may also interfere with speech (Iplikcioglu, 2002).

The goals of presurgical prosthodontics that converts to a radiographic stent include: (i) establishment of vertical dimension of occlusion and adjustment of sufficient interocclusal gap space, (ii) determination of centric occlusion at centric relation position (centric occlusion position is used to mount the casts of patients who are only partially edentulous and have enough remaining teeth), (iii) creation of a harmonious plane of occlusion, (iv) achievement of optimum esthetics, phonetics, and (v) incisal guidance so as not to alter the patient's speech patterns, and (vi) definition of the end result of treatment and its appearance.

Prior to the CT scan, a scan prosthesis that plays several critical roles in obtaining accurate roles in obtaining accurate input data is developed. The scan prosthesis stabilizes the opposing jawbones to prevent jaw movement during the CT scan. Movement is minimized with the helical CT, even slight jaw movement needs to be prevented. Second, occlusion and future tooth set-up can be simulated and represented in 2D and 3D reconstruction. The base of the scan prosthesis should be constructed to represent a radiolucent appearance on the transaxial images. Porous maxillary bone and knife-edge ridges on the mandibular bone must be distinguished from the CT scan prosthesis. Prosthetic teeth are represented as radio-opaque images clearly distinguishable in form and shape. Simulation of the prosthetic tooth position can be accomplished using opaque dental teeth, or coating acrylic teeth with barium sulfate, or using gutta percha markers or a similar radio-opaque material. In addition, the drilling hole must represent the drilling direction for implant insertion (Benjamin, 2002).

There are different surgical templates. Clear vaccuform stents are simple and quick to fabricate but the stents bear too much flexibility in the positioning of implant and are less accurate. Self cure acrylic stents with channels filled with gutta percha provide acceptable accuracy and are easy to fabricate and inexpensive. Self cure acrylic stents with metal sleeves are the most accurate tools in this respect.

Templates are usually fabricated in the laboratory with heat-cured acrylic resin. To indicate screw-access channels, 2-mm-diameter holes should be drilled in the cingulum area of the anterior teeth and the central fossa of the posterior area so that the channels do not interfere with the interproximal papillae or the opposing dentition. After fabrication of the surgical template, it will be drilled by the clinician forming pilot holes or grooves as indicators to implant positions or planned osteotomies, respectively (Zinner et al,. 2004). Figure 1 illustrates an image of milling machine used for the preparation of the access holes in the surgical template. During the surgery, these stents dictate the implant's position and angle. The stents can combine with CT scan to increase accuracy of the stent. Tomography and CT have been used to provide a three-dimensional picture of the region to be implanted (Ames et al,. 1980; Hollender &Rockler, 1980). Reformatted computed tomography (CT) has been proven to be an effective technique in planning complex cases in oral implantology (Besimo et al,. 2000). Pre -surgical imaging can provide important information in osseointegrated dental implant treatment. The use of cross-sectional images in the bucco-lingual direction, which can be delivered by computed tomography (CT), allows us to plan a more accurate design of implant placement before surgery (Naitoh et al,. 2000).

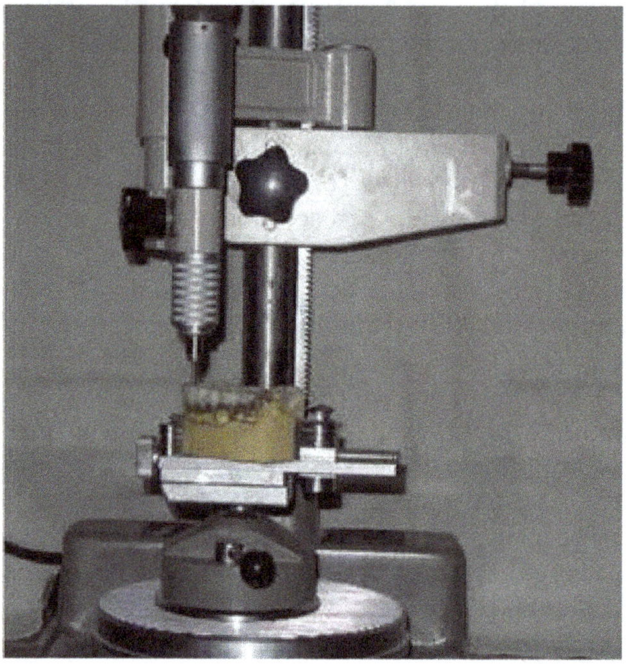

Fig. 1. A scheme of the preparation of implant access holes along the long axis of teeth using milling machine.

This template is the key to the system, since it allows the transfer of the predetermined prosthetic setup to the actual implant planning. The template is an exact replica of the desired prosthetic end result. Incorporation of the scanning template into the computerized tomography (CT) scanning data allows the surgeon to base implant planning on the desired prosthetic outcome. The treatment plan is thus driven by the prosthetic final result, not vice versa (Tardieu & Philippe, 2001). According to the literature, scannographic template can be made of 15wt% of barium sulfate in resin powder, or by means of other radiopaque substances (Wouteres et al,. 2000; Tardieu & Philippe, 2001). However, a variety of mixtures of barium sulfate ranging between 5 and 35wt% have been used. It has been experimentally revealed that the percentage should vary with respect to the surrounding elements (metal crowns or natural teeth) and also as a function of the opacity gradient that one wants to obtain within the same template containing several different radiopaque layers (Tardieu et al,. 2003). In figure 2, radiopaque templates are shown.

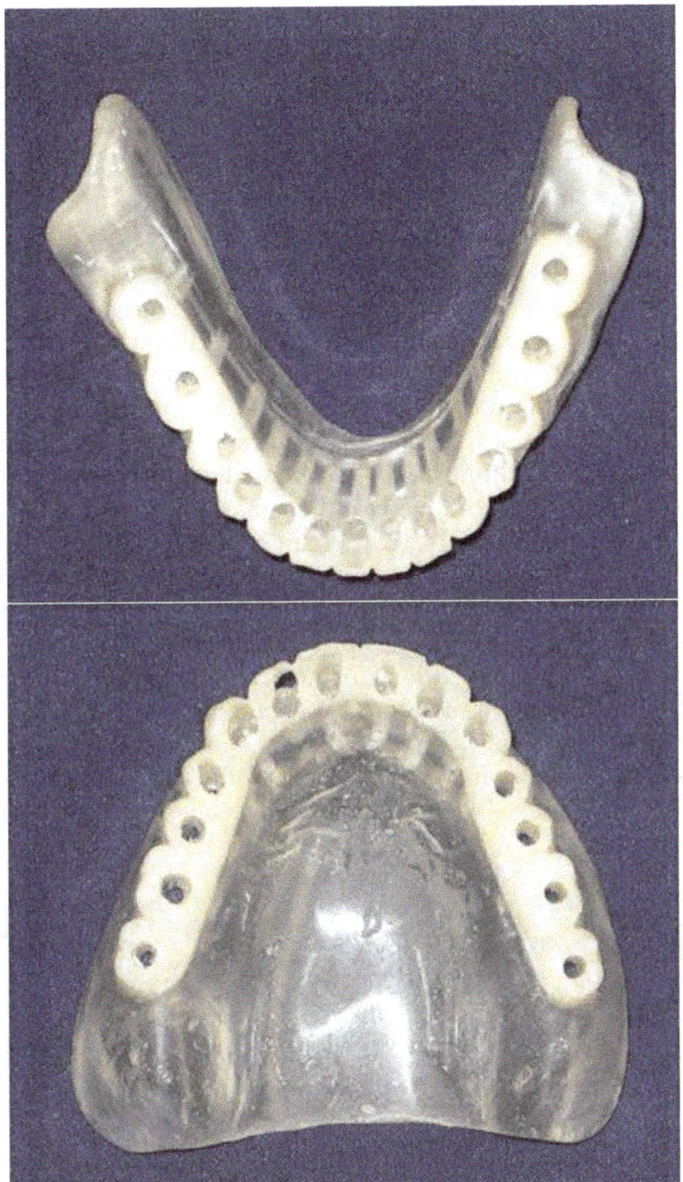

Fig. 2. Radiopaque templates.

In comparison to conventional radiographic stents, radiographic or dual-purpose stents with radiopaque markers offer the advantage of transferring the CT data onto the same stent for surgery. However, since errors which appear in the conversion of the stent may lead to malalignment of the implants, the angle of the radiopaque markers should facilitate reorientating the surveying table if guide channel preparation must be performed in a different angle.

The incorporation of treatment planning modified by CAD-CAM offers significant advantages, including the evaluation of the 3-D anatomy and the fabrication of anatomic site models and osseous-supported surgical templates. Other advantages include shorter surgery durations, shorter treatment times, minimizing of intraoperative radiographs during implant placement, less invasive surgical technique (flapless surgery, with less change of swelling, less pain, and faster initial healing times), prefabricated definitive prosthesis and immediate use of a fixed prosthesis (Saement et al,. 2003; Machrack, 2005). Furthermore, the surgical guides are useful to determine and insert the dental implant in appropriate position and length (Nokar et al,. 2011).

5.2 Scanning

The patient must be instructed on how to position the guide in the mouth and how to stabilize the guide by biting on two cotton rolls or on a bite template during CT scan (Fig. 3). The radiographic template can be visualized in both the 2D and 3D reformatted CT images. The concentration of barium sulfate used in creation of the ScannoGuide determines the level of visibility. It is crucial to remember that very low concentrations may result in a lack of visibility of the template in the CT images. And, concentrations of barium which are too high can cause artifacts and minimize proper visualization. It is possible to vary the concentration of barium between the teeth and the base plate of the ScannoGuide, so that both parts can be visualized separately. A hole can be drilled along the longitudinal axis of the tooth. This hole will appear black in the CT images and is clearly visible in 2D cross-sectional reconstructions. The following pictures illustrate what can be seen using a proper ScannoGuide in 2D and in 3D. Having the patient bite on cotton rolls has several advantages, it allows arches stabilization during CT scan, it gives a better comfort to the patient who can bite on something solid and it separates jaws avoiding artifacts from the opposite arch. The axial view clearly shows the image of teeth with open hole through. 3D images of the ScannoGuide can be combined with the bone information. The 3D reconstruction of the CT images of a ScannoGuide can show the teeth set-up for this partially edentulous case.

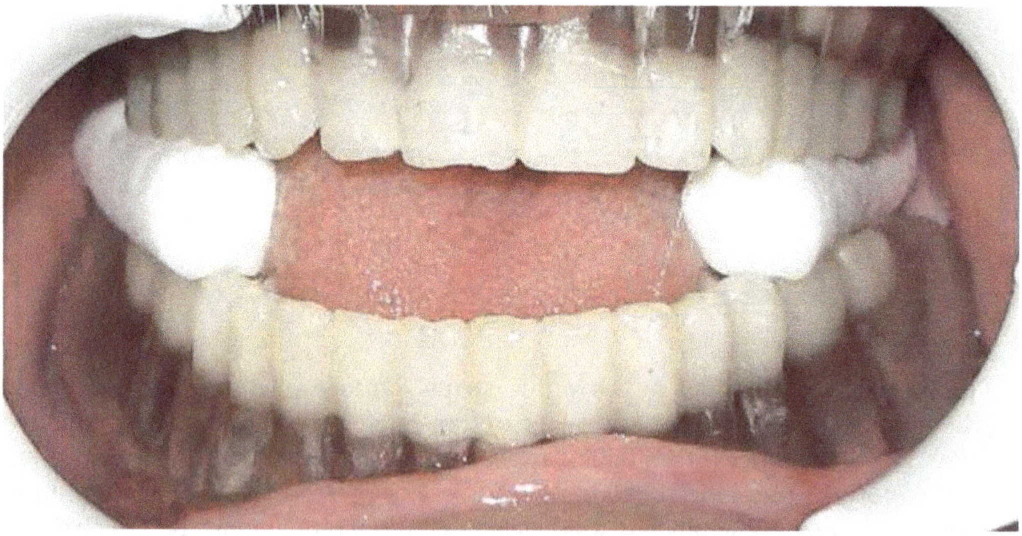

Fig. 3. Stabilizing the templates during CT scan

5.3 Process of the images and conversion of imaging data

The CT scan image data must be produced according to a specific scan protocol to obtain the data compatible with the imaging software. The imaging software (Mimics,

Materialise/Columbia Scientific, Glen Burnie, Md) converts slice image data into 2D and 3D computer models for analysis. The imaging software performs 2D image processing by reformatting the data along planes and/or curves. The simplest reformatting is the construction of images that show slices oriented orthogonally to the original plane of section. These are called planar reconstruction: sagittal if they pass through the midline and are oriented front to rear; coronal if they pass through the midline and are oriented left to right; parasagittal or pericoronal if they are parallel to the sagittal or coronal plane and do not pass through the midline; and paraxial if they are obliquely oriented (Herman &Liu, 1977) (Fig 4).

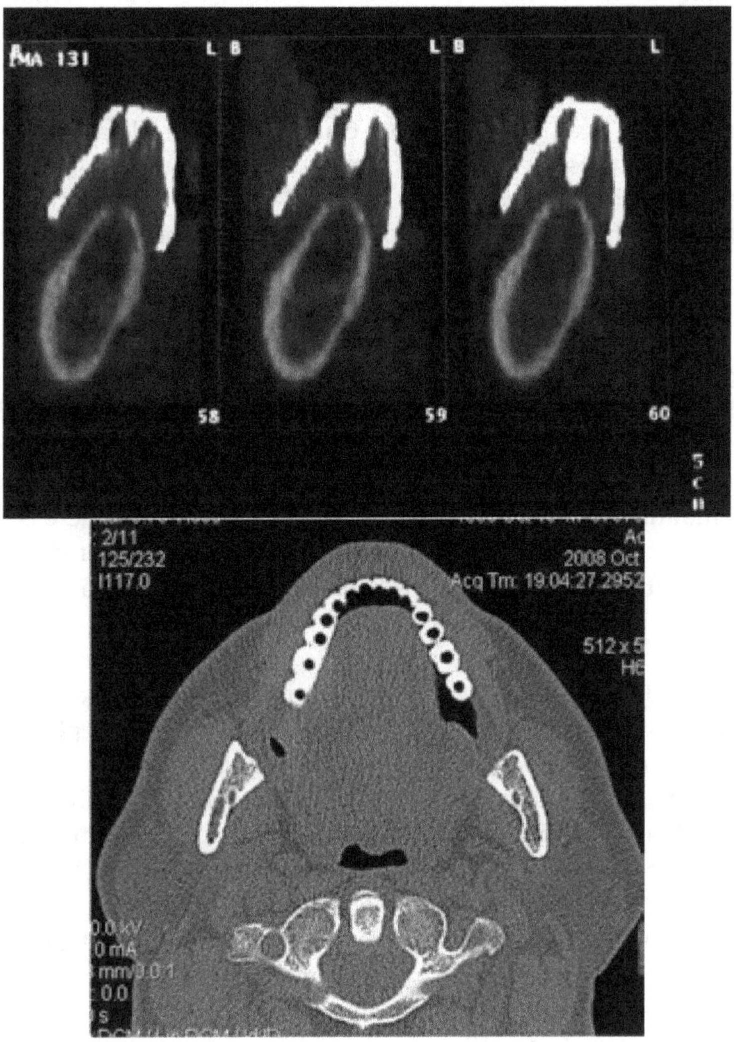

Fig. 4. CT scan images in two views, representing the access holes of radiographic template

In order to make 3D images of the anatomy, a 3D coordinate system must be established. Each slice of data has a location relative to the other slices given by the extent of the table indexed between acquisitions. The distance between slices develops the third dimension rather than the other 2 dimensions including right/left and up/down on each slice (Woolson et al,. 1986). The imaging software can interpret slices taken in a sequence in form of a "volume" of data, while the overlap of slices must be inhibited. In order to create a 3D image of bone, for example, the slices are individually processed to extract only the tissue of bone density range. Where necessary, slices are interpolated between the original slices to give a more realistic 3D image. The edges (or contours) of the anatomy of interest, i.e. bone, are stored for the entire set of slices (including the interpolated ones) as a "contour file". The processed contour file is used to create the 3D images (Herman & Liu, 1977; Liu, 1977). In addition, the imaging software provides the capacity to alter or to edit the contour files themselves. This is useful for editing out obvious metal artifacts, doing disarticulation, or for designing implants. Since the contour file itself is being modified, subsequent 3D images generated from that file will show the results of the editing operation (Woolson et al, 1986).

After completion of the scan, the data are sent for data processing. A computer engineer edits the images by removing the scattered and useless parasite images including spinal column, antagonist teeth, and projection of the upper extremities of the mandible for maxillary analysis). The scanning template can be easily identified in axial sections. Different anatomic structures such as maxilla and mandible and the template are separated in different masks. Each of these masks can be toggled on or off to allow separate visualization and interpretation. After calculation of the corresponding 3D models, the patient data were sent back to the surgeon and prosthodontist so that the implant treatment plan could be started (Tardiue et al,. 2003).

5.4 Treatment planning

Advances in implant dentistry over the past 40 years facilitate the predictable replacement of missing teeth. It is now common to treat edentulous areas in the mouth partially and fully with implant-supported restorations. In the standard planning for a dental implant case, the doctor procures mounted dental models and designs a surgical guide based on the model. Conventional dental radiographs and CT scans help the practitioner determine where the underlying bone relates to the final prosthesis. But in surgery, a crestal incision with subperiosteal reflection of the gingival, a method that can inadvertently displace the model-based surgical guide, is in most cases required to determine the anatomy of the alveolar ridge. Implants can only be placed in a flapless manner in cases associated with excess amounts of alveolar bone. Even with a model-based surgical guide, placing the implant in the preplanned position depends on the skill of the operator. The use of model-based guides to position dental implants becomes even more demanding especially in placing multiple implants, as in an edentulous arch with limited bone available (Spector L, 2008).

The incorporation of treatment planning modified by CAD-CAM offers significant advantages, including the evaluation of the 3-D anatomy and the fabrication of anatomic site models and osseous-supported surgical templates. Other advantages include: shorter surgery times, shorter treatment times, minimizing of intraoperative radiographs during implant placement, less invasive surgical technique (flapless surgery, with less change of swelling, less pain, and faster initial healing times), prefabricated definitive prosthesis and immediate use of a fixed prosthesis (Sarment et al,. 2003). Furthermore, the surgical guides are useful to determine and insert the dental implant in appropriate position and length.

The software allows the practitioner to view the axial images and also the 3D image. In this stage the length, diameter and position of the implant body can be determined. Using the method, the flapless surgical technique for oral implant placement may be promoted and the invasiveness of surgical techniques may be reduced. The system under test was observed to be reliable for the preoperative assessment of both the number and location of implants and implant size(s) needed, as well as potential anatomic complications. These procedures can be done using specialized software and also can be made using simple software. This method is very useful for fabrication of template in dentistry science field because it can eliminate rigid dependency on commercial companies and it can be used widely in clinical situation.

5.5 CAD/CAM surgical guide

CAD/CAM (computed-aided design/computed aided manufacturing) systems have evolved over the last two decades and have been used by dental health professionals for over twenty years. In 1971, Francois Duret introduced CAD/CAM in restorative dentistry and, in 1983; the first dental CAD/CAM restoration was manufactured (Priest, 2005). This system can be used in an intraoperative use for dental restoration and fabrication of surgical guides (Fuster-Torres et al,. 2009). Treatment planning decisions made with computer-aided design (CAD) can be easily transferred to the surgical treatment phase, be performed, in turn, with computer-aided manufacturing (CAM). It has been mentioned that CAD can be conducted through reading and interpreting multiplanar computerized tomography (CT) scans, performing measurements, and evaluating anatomic relationship by placing virtual images on the screen. In the CAM process, stereolithography method can be used for the fabrication of three dimensional surgical templates. The method includes a laser beam travelling above the photosensitive liquid acrylic, allowing the surgical template to be polymerized in the layers according to the design. Then, stainless steel tubes are inserted in the spaces that represent implant location. After insertion the tubes, the surgical template is ready for use. Thus, CAD/CAM surgical templates allow the software based planning to transfer to the surgical field. Template-guided implant surgery requires preoperative steps, starting with the fabrication of a radiographic template, CT acquisition with the template in position, computer-assisted implant planning and ending in fabrication and use of a surgical guide for drilling and implants insertion. Template-guided implant surgery requires pre-operative steps, starting with fabrication of a radiographic template, CT acquisition with the template in position, computer assisted implant planning and ending in fabrication and use of a surgical guide for drilling and implant insertion (Horwitz et al,. 2009).

5.6 Custom-made surgical guide

CT scans, when properly utilized, will help remove the limitations associated with two-dimensional imaging modalities for planning implants, and will empower clinicians with more diagnostic information to make informed decisions for their patients, especially when considering immediate-load protocols. The ability to visualize root, tooth-to-implant and implant-to-implant proximity through 3D technologies is an important step in the advancement of the science of dental implantology. Incorporating the restorative goal with interactive 3D planning tools for the creation of CT-derived surgical templates allows for the highest degree of accuracy and consistency in transferring the treatment plan to the patient at the time of surgical intervention. High-speed spiral CT image files can now be transferred to personal computers for further analysis and being used as reference, and computer programs are available to provide 3D jaw reconstruction and virtual surgical planning. With the advent of rapid prototyping techniques, virtual computer planning can be linked to the physical production of stereo models and surgical drill guides, which can then ensure an accurate transfer of data from the planning phase to the clinical setting. Van Steenberghe et al developed a procedure for immediate implant loading in the maxilla using 3D planning and a custom drill template (Van steenberghe et al, 2002). Their preliminary results indicated that this procedure is effective, precise, and safe (Chow, 2005). Furthermore, horizontal stabilization pins (a minimum of one in partially edentulous cases and up to four in edentulous cases) are virtually placed through the labial denture flange to anchor the surgical template during surgery. After the restorative dentist and surgeon approve the virtual treatment plan, the three-dimensional computer planning files are digitally sent through for fabrication of the stereolithically constructed surgical template (Spector L, 2008).

5.6.1 Computer simulation and virtual implant planning

Computer simulation and virtual implant surgery are valuable tools developed for treatment planning. Three dimensional images allow clinicians a direct visualization of the jawbone morphology, bone volume, level of the maxillary sinus floor, and the location and course of the inferior dental nerve. Computer simulation also allows clinicians to place dental implants according to the future prosthetic tooth position. Furthermore, clinicians can study their cases alternatively and modify the virtual surgical implant placement until they are fully satisfied with the plan. Such surgical rehearsal is a kind of mental navigation system allowing further improvement of clinical performance. Computer simulation and virtual planning are, however, associated with some disadvantages including radiation hazards, and greater requirements for resources and time.

Originally, surgical drill guides were used only for the preparation of implant osteotomy. In 2003, Tardieu and Vrielinck introduced the SAFE System for dental implant placement using a single surgical guide for both the drilling and implant placement. When it is possible to control the position, angulation, and the depth needed for drilling and implant placement, this kind of template-navigated procedure can be safe and accurate (Tardieu & Vrielinck, 2003). Although the precision of the surgical drill guides is high, the accuracy of actual implant placement can be affected by the following factors: (1) correct positioning of the guide; (2) fitting the guide to the underlying structures (bone, mucosa, or tooth); (3) stabilization mechanisms (bony irregularities, pins, or screws); and (4) discrepancies between the diameter of the implant drill and the corresponding metal drill sleeve (Chow, 2005).

SurgiCase software allows for the regeneration of 3-dimensional images of the jaw anatomy, which can simulate the insertion of the fixtures. Even bone density in the area of the future implant location can be taken into account. This system contains cylindrical representations of oral implants, and their lengths and diameters can be modified according to the available product sizes of the implant manufacturer so as to obtain the best use of the available bone, and when possible, the contact with the cortical parts of the jaw bone (Sarment et al,. 2003). The magnitude of bone density allows developing a bone map, where it is possible to identify the sites that could assure the fixtures' major primary stability and offer better resistance to the biting forces (Vrielinck et al,. 2003).

The effectiveness of CAD/CAM surgical guides has been studied. For instance, Van Steenberghe et al (Van Steenberghe et al,. 2003) examined the accuracy of a CAD/CAM surgical guide in cadavers or Vrielinck et al (Vrielinck et al,. 2003) performed a similar study in human subjects. Vercruyssen (Vercruyssen & Quirynen, 2010) has discussed possible errors of CAD/CAM surgical guides, which may occur at any of the following stages: CT-scan data collection, positioning of the radiographic guide, segmentation of bone, teeth, and/or tissue from the complete image, stereolithographic or CAD/CAM modeling, fixation of the surgical guide to the jaw bone, and use of precision sleeves. This type of precise surgical guide has also presented some challenges to clinicians. Yong and Moy studied early complications using CAD/CAM-guided implant placement with the NobelGuide system (Nobel Biocare AB, Goteborg, Sweden) claiming that the most common early surgical complication includes incomplete seating of the prosthesis due to bony interferences (Yong &Moy, 2008).

6. Stereolithography

Once CT scan data are segmented, the software interpolates the data on all 3 planes to form a smooth 3D model. A computer file of this model can be alternatively transferred to stereolithography equipment where a physical model of the patient's bone structure is created. The finalized treatment plan is thus used for fabrication of a surgical template using this technique.

The stereolithography process is a rapid prototyping method that produces physical models by selectively solidifying an ultraviolet sensitive liquid resin using a laser beam. It represents a relatively new technology in the diagnostic area. The status of this new methodology in clinical and surgical medicine is still at the prototype stage. It can be used for surgical simulation to assure predictable results and to diminish operation time (Choy JY, 2002). In oral implantology, this technology develops a precise evaluation of anatomic points such as the size of the maxillary sinus in the upper jaw and the location of the alveolar nerve in the lower jaw. It also provides information about size, direction, and bone location for accurate positioning of implants. In one study, the possible benefits in planning implant surgery using stereolithographic models and surgical guides relating to clinical guidance methodology have been indicated in detail (Sammartino G et al,. 2004).

From a detailed technical point of view, as point out earlier, stereolithography is a computer-driven process that creates precise models using laser and epoxy resin. A computer controlled HeCd laser generates an ultraviolet beam, which travels across the surface of a vat of photocurable liquid polymer. The laser draws each cross section of the anatomy one layer at a time. The photovoltaic energy from the laser polymerizes the epoxy immediately. The cured cross-sectional layer is lowered into the vat of resin and the next layer is processed. Successive layers of the anatomy are built in 0.15 mm increments until the model is completed (Herman GT& Liu HK, 1977).

Using this technique, surgical procedure would be simplified, reliable, and easily reproducible. Wound size and bone surface exposure would be minimal and no soft tissue trauma would be derived by use of burrs during bone drilling. Furthermore, during the operative procedure, there will no major problems of bleeding or nerve lesion. The postoperative time would be without complications.

This technique offers many advantages which include: correct management of the tissues with minimal trauma and a superior planned treatment. In cases of severe atrophy, this methodology allows fixture measurements by the indication of exact surgical limitations, and prevents complications related to poor stability of a denture. This technologic improvement can simplify oral management in implant dentistry and avoid complications related to the surgery (Sammartino G et al,. 2004).

The accuracy of anatomical models generated by this method depends on the quality of the CT scanners and the thresholding method (the computer process that determines what is soft tissue), but studies have shown a dimensional stability in general in the range of 0.6 mm (Choi et al,. 2002). The accuracy of steriolithographically made surgical guides have been studied by different groups. Sarment (Sarment et al,. 2003) used SIMplant software for fabricating template. A significant statistical improvement was found in all measurements when stereolithographic surgical guide was used compared to conventional guides. The average distance between the planned implant and the actual osteotomy was 1.5±0.7mm in conventional group and 0.9± 0.5 in stereolithographic group. Measurement of the angle formed in conventional group was 8± 4.5 degrees with an accuracy of 4.5±2 degrees in the stereolithographic group. In the other in-vitro study reported by Van steenbergehe and coworkers (Van Steenberghe et al,. 2002), LITORIM software was used for the fabrication of the guide and the match between planned implant and actual implants in the maxilla was on average within 0.8± 0.3mm and the match between planned and actual implant axis was on average within 1.8±1 degrees. Naitoh and colleagues (Naitoh et al,. 2000) suggested that angulation diverges by 5 degrees on average when utilizing a template based on the CT images. Application of stereolithographic surgical guides presented by Giacomo (Giacomo et al,. 2005) gave rise the match between the planned and the placed implant axis within 7.25±2.67 degrees. The differences in distance between the planned and placed position at the implant shoulder were 1.45±1.42mm. Besimo and associates (Besimo et al,. 2000) utilized a modified scannographic template for surgical guidance. Placement was evaluated by measurement on the casts of more than 70 clinical cases. They found 1.5mm differences at entrance point when used control guide and 0.9mm when the stereolithographic surgical guide was used. Van sttenberghe (Van Steenberghe et al,.2002) evaluated placement of 45mm long zygoma implants on human cadavers. They reported less than 3 degrees of deviation. Fortin (Fortin et al,. 2003) found that transfer error was less than 0.2 mm and 1.1 degrees.

Tardieu (Tardieu et al,. 2003) presented a case of implant placement using a drill guide created by stereolithography. They suggested that the scannographic template could be designed for proper transfer into a temporary fixed prosthesis which can be used in immediate loading. Mesiodistal accuracy influences implants from esthetic point of view especially in anterior region because the proper embrasures and golden proportional are not established yet. Length difference may also cause complication. A maximum length of 2 mm above the mandibular canal is generally recommended. If the length exceeds this limitation, it may cause parasthesia and pain leading finally to the removal of implant. Otherwise, if the length is very short, crown to implant ratio may be improper and biomechanical factors compromise the implant integrity. The accuracy of angle causes the forces directed towards the implant long axis.

The main drawback of the surgical template can be seen in the possible movement of the template during surgery and reproducibility of the splint position between the CT exam and surgical procedure. The template is supported on the remaining dentition or stabilized by a specific form of either the hard palate or the mandible. Sicilia (Sicilia et al,. 2000) reached a considerably higher precision using a fixed surgical template in the placement of implants in patients with edentulous maxilla. In a large edentulous area or completely edentulous jaw, the stereolithographic guide is advantageous since it is osseous-supported. The degree of the difference between the proposed and actual implant direction may be influenced by various factors, such as the construction accuracy of the template, the surgical accuracy using these templates, the accuracy of the study model, the accuracy of the stereolithographic machines and the measurement accuracy. The CT scan involves a higher dose/higher cost method. But the CT scan is less time consuming when multiple implants are required, and it allows imaging of the entire jaw, making it possible to use software for virtual implant placement (Nokar et al,. 2012). As long as radiographic imaging has been enhanced by the development of various techniques , multi-slice and spiral CT are being replaced by cone beam CT systems (CBCT) for oral and maxillofacial imaging, enabling a significant reduction dose (Loubele et al,. 2008).

7. Simplified CAD/CAM technique

This method has been recently developed to generate surgical guide by a much simpler method based on CAD/CAM. For making CAD/ CAM template, anatomic guide was digitized by ATOSII camera (optical measuring technique).The ATOS system was used to digitize the objects and process the data into an STL data set. Some reference points were applied onto the model. By using the photogrammetry camera and its supplied software, coordinates of the points were measured with high accuracy. Three reference markers were applied to each part added. At this stage, a second series of images were taken and the visible reference point coordinates were measured on these images. Using the points on the model, obtained with two sets of measurements, the second set of the points was transformed into the coordinate system that was previously defined after the first measurement. In the next step, all the measurement points were changed to IGES format with Rapid form software and consequently the IGES format was changed to SLD format using Solid work software. This model was assembled on the jaw model. The implant access holes were evaluated and the implant path and length in each tooth were determined. The length of implants was considered 2 mm above the mandibular canal and the diameter of implant holes was increased up to 4mm (Fig 5).

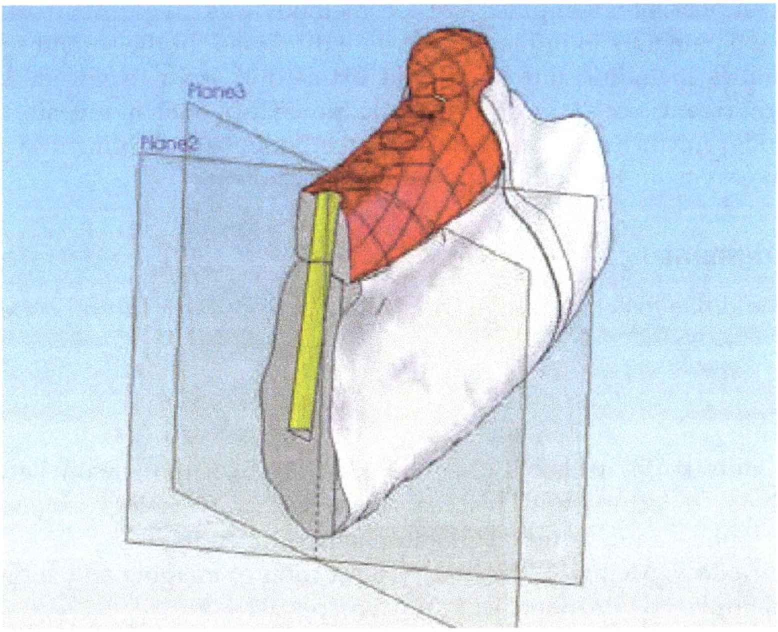

Fig. 5. Drilling direction and implant length determined in Solid work software.

This model, named gold standard model, was filed and applied for evaluating the results. After designing the implant path and length, the CAD-CAM surgical template was fabricated using stereolithographic rapid prototyping machine. Then, the stainless steel sleeves were fabricated to be used as drills of implants in two different sizes. The sleeves were, then, inserted in the CAD-CAM template. The sleeves kept the planned implants length and diameter as designed. In the first group, concerning the anatomical surgical template, implant path was modified via measuring CT scan file. For the second group, there was stereolithographic template with incremental guiding tube diameters, fabricated by CAD-CAM techniques (Fig 6).

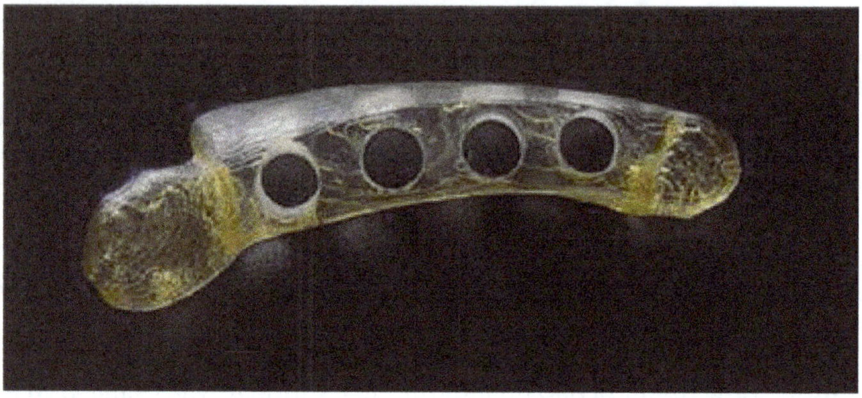

Fig. 6. Fabrication of the guide by stereolithography machine.

8. Conclusion

In this chapter an overview to different techniques of pre-surgical diagnosis and treatment planning with emphasis on computer assisted methods was given. At first the importance and all effective parameters in implantology were discussed. In the second section different imaging modalities including intra- oral and extra- oral were reviewed. The next parts described more recent pre-surgical diagnostic procedure which reveals that computer assisted methods enhance the capability of prosthodontists to diagnose and choose a convenient and easy to apply methods for implant placement.

9. Acknowledgment

The Author would like to acknowledge Dr Farzad Nasirpouri for careful review and edition of the text.

10. References

Almog DM, Onufrak JM, Hebel K, Meinter SW. (1995). Comparison between planned prosthetic trajectory and residual bone trajectory using surgical guides and tomography—a pilot study. J Oral Implantol 21:275–280

Almog DM, Torrado E, Meitner SW .(2001). Fabrication of imaging and surgical guides for dental implants. J Prosthet Dent , Vol (85), pp.504–508

Abarca M, van Steenberghe D, Malevez C, De Ridder J, Jacobs R. (2006). Neurosensory disturbances after immediate loading of implants in the anterior mandible: an initial questionnaire approach followed by a psychophysical assessment. Clin Oral Investig, Vol(10),No.4,pp.77

Ames JR, Johnson RP, Steven EA. (1980). Computerized tomography in oral and maxillofacial surgery, J Oral Surgery, Vol (38), pp.145-9

Bavitz JB, Harn SD, Hansen CA, Lang M. (1993). An anatomical study of mental neurovascular bundle-implant relationships. Int J Oral Maxillofac Implants, Vol (8), No.5, pp.563-7

Bavitz JB, Harn SD, Homze EJ. (1994). Arterial supply to the floor of the mouth and lingual gingivae. Oral Surg Oral Med Oral Pathol, Vol (77), pp.232-5

Benjamin L. (2002).The evolution of multiplanar diagnostic imaging: predictable transfe of preoperative analysis to the surgical site. J Oral Implantol, Vol (28), pp.135-143

Besimo CE, Lambrecht JT, Guindy JS. (2000). Accuracy of implant treatment planning utilizing template-guided reformatted computed tomography. Dentomaxillofacial Radiology, Vol (29), pp.46-51

Cehreli MC, Sahin S. (2000).Fabrication of a dual purpose surgical template for correct labiopalatal positioning of dental implants. INT J oral Maxillofac Implants, Vol (152), pp. 278-282

Chow JK. (2005).Computer-guided implantology:an overview with a case presentation. Hong Kong Dental Journal, Vol (2), pp.7-11

Choy JY, Choy JH, Kim NK, Kim Y, Lee JK, Kim MK, Lee JH, et al. (2002). Analysis of errors in medical rapid prototyping models. Int J Oral Maxillofac Surg, Vol (31), pp.23–32

Cucchiara R, Franchini F, Lamma A. (2001). Enhancing implant surgery planning via computerized image processing. Int j comput dent , Vol (4), pp.9-24

Dove SB, McDavid WD. (1993).Digital panoramic and extraoral imaging. Dent Clin North Am, Vol (37), No.4, pp.541-51

Eggers G, Rieker M, Fiebach J, Kress B, Dickhaus H, Hassfeld S. (2005).Geometric accuracy of magnetic resonance imaging of the mandibular nerve. Dentomaxillofac Radiol, Vol (34), pp.285–291

Ekestubbe A. (1999). Conventional spiral and low-dose computed mandibular tomography for dental implant planning. Swed Dent J Suppl, Vol (138), pp.1–82

Fellingham LL, Vogel J, Lau C, et al. Interactive graphics and 3D modeling for surgical planning and prosthetics and implant design. Presented at: National computer graphic association conference and exposition. Anaheim, CA, USA, May 11-15, 1986.

Fortin T, Bosson J, Coudert JL, Isidori M. (2003). Reliability of preoperative planning of an image guided system for oral implant placement based on 3D images: An In vivo study. INT J Oral Maxillofac Implants, Vol (18), pp.886-893

Fortin T, champleboux G, Lormee J, coudert J. (2000). Precise dental implant placement using surgical guides in conjuction with medical imaging techniques. Journal of Oral Implatology, Vol (264), pp.300-303

Fuster-Torres MA, Albalat-Estela S, Alcañiz-Raya M, Peñarrocha-Diago M. (2009).CAD / CAM dental systems in implant dentistry: update.Med Oral Patol Oral Cir Bucal, Vol (14), No.3, pp.E141-5

Garber DA. (1995). The esthetic dental implant: letting restoration be the guide. J Am Dent Assoc, Vol (126), pp.319–325

Giacomo DG, Cury P, Araujo N, Sendyk W, Sendyk C. (2005). Clinical application of stereolithographic surgical guides for implant placement: preliminary Results. J Periodontol, Vol (76), pp.503-507

Givol N, Chaushu G, Halamish-Shani T, Taicher S. (2000). Emergency tracheostomy following life-threatening hemorrhage in the floor of the mouth during immediate implant placement in the mandibular canine region. J Periodontol, Vol (71), pp.1893–1895

Goaz PW, White SC. (1992).Oral radiology:principles and interpretation, Mosby, ST Louis

Grandahl K, Ekestubbe A, Grondahl HG. (1996).Technical consideration for intraoral radiography in postoperative wxamination, Nobel Biocare Global Forum. Vol (10), pp. 10-11

Greenstein G, Tarnow D. (2006).The mental foramen and nerve: clinical and anatomical factors related to dental implant placement: a literature review. J Periodontol, Vol(77), No,12, pp. 1933-43

Guerrero ME, Jacobs R, Loubele M, Schutyser F, Suetens P, van Steenberghe D. (2006). State-of-the-art on cone beam CT imaging for preoperative planning of implant placement. Clin Oral Investig, Vol (10), pp.1–7

Hashimoto K, Arai Y, Iwai K, Araki M, Kawashima S, Terakado M. (2003). A comparison of a new limited cone beam computed tomography machine for dental use with a multidetector row helical CT machine. Oral Surg Oral Med Oral Pathol Oral Radiol Endod, Vol (95), pp.371–377

Herman GT,Liu HK. (1977).Display of three-dimensional information in computed tomography. Jconput assist tomogr, Vol (1), pp.155-160

Hofschneider U, Tepper G, GahleitnerA, Ulm C. (1999). Assessment of the blood supply to the mental region for reduction of bleeding complications during implant surgery in the interforaminal region. International Journal of Oral and Maxillofacial Implants, Vol (14), pp.379–383

Hollender L, Rockler B. (1980). Radiographic evaluation of osseointegrated implants of the jaws. Dento-maxillofacial Radiol, Vol (9), pp.91-5

Horiuchi M, Ichikawa T, Kanitani HWigianto R, Kawamoto N, Matsumoto N. (1995). Pilot-hole preparation for proper implant positioning and the enhancement of bone formation. J Oral Implantol , Vol (21), No.4, pp.318–324

Horwitz J, Zuabi O, Machtei EE. (2009).Accuracy of a computerized tomography- guided template-assisted implant placement system;an in vitro dtudy. Clin Oral Impl Res, Vol (20), pp.1156-1162

Hounsfield GN. (1995). Computerized transverse axial scanning (tomography): Part I. Description of system.Br J Radiol, Vol (68), No.815, pp.166-72

Hubálková H, Hora K, Seidl Z, Krásenský J. (2002). Dental materials and magnetic resonance imaging.Eur J Prosthodont Restor Dent, Vol (10), No.3, pp.125-30

Hubálková H, La Serna P, Linetskiy I, Dostálová T. (2006). Dental alloys and magnetic resonance imaging.Int Dent J, Vol (56), No.3, pp.135-41

Iplikcioglu H, Akca K, Cehreli MC. (2002). The use of computerized tomography for diagnosis and treatment planning in implant dentistry. Journal of Oral Implantology, Vol (28), pp.29-35

Jacobs R, Mraiwa N, vanSteenberghe D, Gijbels F, Quirynen M. (2002). Appearance, location, course, and morphology of the mandibular incisive canal: an assessment on spiral CT scan. Dentomaxillofac Radiol, Vol (31), No.5, pp.322-7

Katsumata A, Hirukawa A, Noujeim M, Okumura S, Naitoh M, Fujishita M, Ariji E, Langlais RP. (2006). Image artefact in dental cone-beam CT. Oral Surg Oral Med Oral Pathol Oral Radiol Endod, Vol (101), No. 5, pp.652–657

Kawamata A, Ariji Y, Langlais RP. (2000).Three-dimensional computed tomography imaging in dentistry. Dent Clin North Am, Vol (44), No.2, pp.395-410.

Kawamata A,Ariji Y,Langlais RP. (2000).Three-dimentional computed tomography imaging in dentistry.Dental Clinic of North America, Vol (44), pp.395-410

Klinge B, Petersson A, Maly P. (1989). Location of the mandibular canal: comparison of macroscopic findings, conventional radiography, and computed tomography. Int J Oral Maxillofac Implants, Vol (4), No.4, pp.327-332

Kohavi D, Bar-ziv J. (1996). Atypical incisive nerve: clinical report. Implant Dent, Vol (5), No.4, pp.281-283

Kopp KC, Koslow AH, Abdo OS. (2003). Predictable implant place ment with diagnostic surgical template and advanced radiographic imaging. J Prosthet Dent 2003, Vol (89), No.6, pp. 611-

Lauterbur PC. (1973). Imaging formation by induced local interactions: example employing nuclear magnetic resonanc. Nature , Vol (242), pp. 190

Lazzara RJ. (1993). Effect of implant position on implant restoration design. J Esthet Dent , Vol (5), pp.265–269

Liu HK. (1977).Two and three-dimensional boundary detection.Comput graph image proc, Vol (6), pp.123-134

Loubele M, Bogaerts R,Van Dijck E, Pauwels R, Vanheusden S, Suetens P, Marchal G, et al. (2009).Comparison between effective radiation dose of CBCT and MSCT scanners for dentomaxillofacial applications. European Journal of Radiology, Vol (71), pp.461-8

Ludlow JB, Laster WS, See M, Bailey LJ, Hershey HG. (2007). Accuracy of measurements of mandibular anatomy in cone beam computed tomography images. Oral Surg Oral Med Oral Pathol Oral Radiol Endod, Vol (103), pp.534–542

Makris N, Stamatakis H, Syriopoulos K, Tsiklakis K, van der Stelt PF. (2010). Evaluation of the visibility and the course of the mandibular incisive canal and the lingual foramen using cone-beam computed tomography. Clin Oral Implants Res, Vol (21), No.7, pp.766-71

Marchack CB. (2005).An immediately loaded CAD/ CAM-guided definitive prosthesis: A clinical report. J Prosthet Dent, Vol (93), pp. 8-12

Marmulla R, Wortche R, Muhling J, Hassfeld S. (2005). Geometric accuracy of the NewTom 9000 Cone Beam CT. Dentomaxillofac Radiol, Vol (34), pp.28–31

Mason M.E, Triplett R.G., Alfonso W.F. (1990). Life-threatening hemorrhage from placement of a dental implant. Journal of Oral and Maxillofacial Surgery, Vol (48), pp.201–204

McDonnell D, Reza Nouri M, Todd ME. (1994).The mandibular lingual foramen: a consistent arterial foramen in the middle of the mandible. J Anat, Vol (184), No.2, pp.363-9

Misch CE. (2005). Dental implant prosthetics, Elsevier, China

Monsour PA, Dudhia R. (2008). Implant radiography and radiology. Aust Dent J Suppl, Vol (53), pp.11-25

Moslehifard E, Nikzad S, Geramipanah F, Mahboub F. (2011). Full mouth rehabilitation of a patient with severely worn dentition and uneven occlusal plane: A Clinical Case Report. Journal of Prosthodontics. Accepted for publication

Naitoh M, Ariyi E, Okumura S, Ohsaki C, Kurita k, Ishigami T. (2000). Can implants be correctly angulated based on surgical templates used for osseointegrated dental implants, Clin Oral Impl Res, Vol (11), pp.409-414

Niamtu J, Richmond. (2001). Near Fatal airway obstruction after routine implant placement. Oral Surg Oral Med Oral Path Oral Radiol Endod, Vol (92), pp.597-600

Nokar S, Moslehifard E, Tootiaii B, Bayanzadeh M, Nasirpouri F.,Nokar A. (2011). Accuracy of implant placement using a CAD/CAM surgical guide: an in vitro study. Int J Oral Maxillofac Implants., Vol (26), PP.520-526

Parnia F, Moslehifard E, Mahboub F, Hafezeqoran A, Gavgani FE. (2010). Tomographic volume evaluation of submandibular fossa in patients requiring dental implants. Oral Surg Oral Med Oral Pathol Oral Radiol Endod, Vol (109), No.1, pp.e32-6

Pinsky HM, Dyda S, Pinsky RW, Misch KA, Sarment DP. (2006). Accuracy of three-dimensional measurements using cone-beam CT. Dentomaxillofac Radiol, Vol (35), pp.410–416

Priest G. (2005). Virtual-designed and computer-milled implant abutments. Oral Maxillofac Surg, Vol (63), No.9, pp.22-32

Richtert EJ. (1989). Basic biomechanical of dental implants in prosthetic dentistry.J Prosthet Dent, Vol (61), pp.602-609

Rosenquist B. (1996). Is there an anterior loop of the inferior alveolar nerve?. Int J Periodontics Restorative Dent, Vol (16), No.1, pp.40-5

Sakakura CE, Monteiro LC, Scaf G. (2004).Diagnostic agreement of conventional and inverted scanned panoramic radiographs in the detection of the mandibular canal and the mental foramen. Journal of Implantology, Vol (30), pp.2-6

Sammartino G, Della Valle A, Marenzi G, Gerbino S, Martorelli M, di Lauro AE, di Lauro F. (2004). Stereolithography in oral implantology: a comparison of surgical guides.Implant Dent, Vol (13), No.2, pp.133-9

Sarment DP, Al-shammari K, Kazor C. (2003). Stereolithographic surgical templates for placement of Dental Implants in complex cases. Int J Periodontics Restorative Dent, Vol (23), pp.287-295

Sato S, Arai Y, Shinoda K, Ito K. (2004). Clinical application of a new cone-beam computerized tomography system to assess multiple two-dimensional images for the preoperative treatment planning of maxillary implants: case reports. Quintessence Int, Vol (35), pp.525–528

Scarfe WC, Farman AG, Sukovic P. (2006). Clinical applications of conebeam computed tomography in dental practice. J Can Dent Assoc, Vol (72), pp.75–80

Schwarz MS, Rothman SL, Rhodes ML, Chafetz N. (1987).Computed tomography: Part II. Preoperative assessment of the maxilla for endosseous implant surgery. Int J Oral Maxillofac Implants, Vol (2), No.3, pp.143-8

Shenoy VK, Bhat SG, Rodrigues SJ. (2006).Iatrogenic complication of implant surgery. Journal of Indian Prosthodontic Society, Vol (6), 18, MYK19

Sicilia A, Enrile F, Buitrago P, Zubizarreta J. (2000). Evaluation of the precision obtained with a fixed surgical template in the placement of implants for rehabilitation of the completely edentulous Maxilla. INT J Oral Maxillofac Implants, Vol (15), pp.272-277

Spector L. (2008). Computer-Aided Dental Implant Planning. Dent Clin North Am, Vol (52), No.4, pp.761-75

Talwar N, Singh BP,Chand P.(2011).Use of Diagnostic and Surgical Stent: A Simplified Approach for Implant Placement. J Indian Prosthodont Soc, DOI 10.1007/s13191-010-0036-7

Tardieu PB, Vrielinck L, Escolano E. (2003). Computer-assisted implant placement. A case report: treatment of the mandible. Int J Oral Maxillofac Implants, Vol (18), pp.599-604

Taylor TD, Agar JR, Voigiatzi (2000) Implant prosthodontics:current perspective and future directions. Int J Maxillofac Implants 15:66–75

Terakado M, Hashimoto K, Arai Y, Honda M, Sekiwa T, Sato H. (2000). Diagnostic imaging with newly developed ortho cubic super-high resolution computed tomography (Ortho-CT). Oral Surg Oral Med Oral Pathol Oral Radiol Endod, Vol (89), pp.509–518

Truhlar RS, Morris HF, Ochi S. (1993). A review of panoramic radiography and its potential use in implant dentistry. Implant Dent, Vol (2), No.2, pp. 122-30

Tyndall DA, Brooks SL. (2000). Selection criteria for dental site imaging: a position paper of the American Academy of oral and maxillofacial radiology. Oral surg oral med oral pathol oral radiol endod, Vol (89), pp.630-637

van Steenberghe D, Naert I, Andersson M, Brajnovic I, Van Cleynenbreugel J, Suetens P. (2002). A custom template and definitive prosthesis allowing immediate implant loading in the maxilla: a clinical report. Int J Oral Maxillofac Implants, Vol (17), pp.663-70

Van Steenberghe D, Malevez C, Van Cleynenbreugel J, Bou Serhal C, Dhoore E, Schutyser F, Suetens P, Jacobs R. (2003). Accuracy of drilling guides for transfer from three-dimensional CT-based planning to placement of zygoma implants in human cadavers. Clin Oral Implants Res, Vol (14), No.1, pp.131-139

Vannier MW. (2003). Craniofacial computed tomography scanning:technology, applications and future trends. Orthod Craniofac Res, Vol (1), pp.23–30

Vercruyssen M, Quirynen M. (2010). Long-term, retrospective evaluation (implant and patient-centred outcome) of the two-implant-supported overdenture in the mandible. Part 2: marginal bone loss. Clin Oral Implants Res, Vol (2), No.5, pp.466-72

Vrielinck C, Politis S, Schepers M, Pauwels M, Naert I. (2003). Image-based planning and clinical validation of zygoma and pterygoid implant placement in patients with severe bone atrophy using customized drill guides. Preliminary results from a prospective clinical follow-up study. Int J Oral Maxillofac Surg, Vol (32),No.1, pp.7–14

Wismeijer D, van Waas MA, Vermeeren JI, Kalk W. (1997). Patients' perception of sensory disturbances of the mental nerve before and after implant surgery: a prospective study of 110 patients. Br J Oral Maxillofac Surg,Vol (35), No.4, pp.254-9

Woolson ST, Dev P, Fllingham LL, Vassiliadis A.(1986).Three-dimensional imaging of bone from computerized tomography. Clin Orthop Relat Res, Vol(202), pp.239-248

Worthington P, Rubenstein J, Hatcher DC. (2010).The role of cone-beam computed tomography in the planning and placement of implants. J Am Dent Assoc, Vol (141), No.3, pp.19-24

Wouters K, Vrielinck L, Wivell C, Dhoore E. (2000). Further development of drilling templates for the placement of regular dental implants and zygomatic fixtures, based on preoperative planning on CT images. In: Lemke HU, Vannier MW,

Inamura K, Farman A (eds). Computer-assisted radiology. Berlin:Elsevier Science,:945-949.

Yong LT, Moy PK. (2008). Complications of computer-aided-design/computer-aided-machining-guided (NobelGuide) surgical implant placement: an evaluation of early clinical results.Clin Implant Dent Relat Res, Vol (10), No. 3, PP. Epub 123-7.

Zahran MH, Fenton A. (2010). A radiopaque implant template for partially edentulous patients. J Prosthet Dent, Vol (103), No.6, pp.390-2

Zinner ID, Panno FV, Small SA, Landa LS. (2004). Implant Dentistry: From Failure to Success. Quintessence Publishing

4

Bone Substitutes and Validation

Christopher Ogunsalu
Human Anatomy and Forensic Dentistry
Department of Basic Medical Sciences
Faculty of Medical Sciences, University of the West Indies, Mona Jamaica
Caribbean Institute of Oral and Maxillofacial Implantology and Surgery
Jamaica

1. Introduction

This chapter will focus on the review of the various bone grafting materials in the market for implant dentistry with much emphasis on the fact that they are all second-hand bones (bone substitutes) when compared with the autogeneous bone graft which is the gold standard to which all bone substitutes are compared.

Bone grafting implies to the application of autogenous bone or other bone substitute obtained from natural or synthetic source to an area of with boney defect. Bone grafting is a procedure and should not be confused with bone regeneration which is the actual formation of new bone in the grafted defect. Bone grafting does not necessarily lead to bone regeneration. It is so important that the clinician and the patient are aware of the difference in terminology because of the clinical, scientific and medicolegal implications.

The use of bone substitutes or bone replacement source has increased tremendously in implant dentistry today and will continue to be so because of the unavailability of autogenous bone from the intra-oral site in most situation and patients are becoming more and more tolerant to clinicians harvesting bone from the extra-oral site such as the iliac crest or the tibial tuberosity.

The mechanisms available for bone regeneration will be fully described and classification of bone substitutes under these mechanisms will be attempted so as to assist the surgeon make a decision regarding which bone substitute to be used for pre-implant, intra-implant surgery and post-implant bone grafting and regeneration.

Theses previously mentioned bone regeneration mechanisms are actually positive mechanisms (osteogenesis, osteoinduction and osteoconduction). The author will introduce a newly discovered mechanism called the osteo-obstructive mechanism as a negative bone regeneration mechanism. This osteoobstructive mechanism was accidentally discovered by the author on single photon emission computerized tomography (SPECT) with histologic correlation during animal experiment to validate bone grafting technique and substitutes in the Ogunsalu sandwich bone regeneration technique. This osteoobstuctive mechanism has been histologically confirmed to be due to foreign body reaction.

In this chapter bone grafting will be mentioned distinctly from bone regeneration, similarly bone substitute (second -hand bone) will be distinctly separated from autogeneous bone graft.

The best GTR-membranes which will be preferably used with bone substitutes will be mentioned against the background of a new bone grafting technique called the Ogunsalu sandwich technique.
Finally the only available method for the qualitative and quantitative validation of bone substitutes and their comparism with one another will be described, in conjunction with histologic correlation. This method utilizes SPECT as a dynamic way for assessing osteoblastic activity after bone grafting and during bone regeneration.

1.1 Classification, types and source

This has been dealt with poorly in most standard textbook and as such I would attempt to adjust the existing classifications and sources. The source of bone graft could be autogenous or non autogenous with the autogenous bone source being the gold standard by which the non autogenous sources are to be compared for efficiency in effecting bone regeneration in the desired site. The autogenous bone can be derived from both intraoral or extra-oral sites. The intra-oral site includes the, chin, maxillary tuberosity, the body of the mandible , the ramus of the mandible, zygomatic buttress or even the exostosis including the oral tori (Fig. 1)

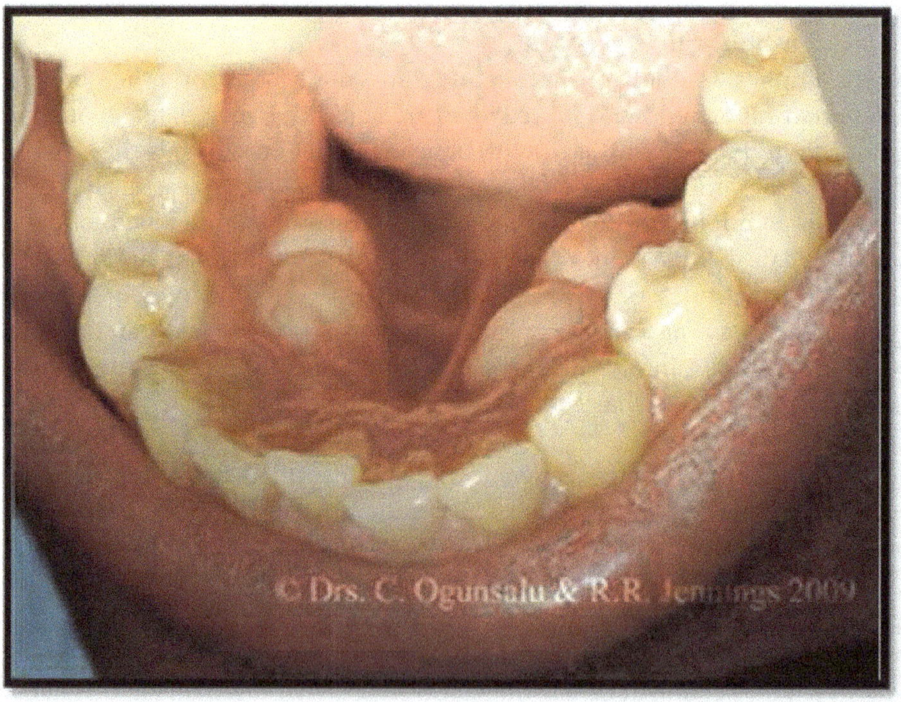

Fig. 1. Bilateral, multilobulated oral tori of the mandible.

The non-autogenous source are therefore second-hand in comparism to the autogenous source, for this reason I will call them the second-hand bones or bone grafting material(bone substitutes). Autogenous bone used for bone grafting should as such not be called bone grafting materials but rather a bone graft source.

The second hand bones are basically the allograft, alloplast of which the commercially available xenograft and the synthetic graft materials are generally considered a subgroup of the alloplastic bone grafting source.
The figure 2 shows the classification of bone grafting sources taken from the Glossary of implant dentistry II, published by the international congress of oral implantologists. I would however suggest that the classification shown in figure 3 be considered a reasonable variation of the former classification.
The origin of the bone graft will dictate the mechanism of its action with the understanding that none of them is osteogenic in action like the autogeneous bone graft source, which is an organic bone source harvested from the patient. This autogeneous bone also additionally forms bone by osteoinduction and osteoconduction, the two mechanisms ascribed to the second hand bones.

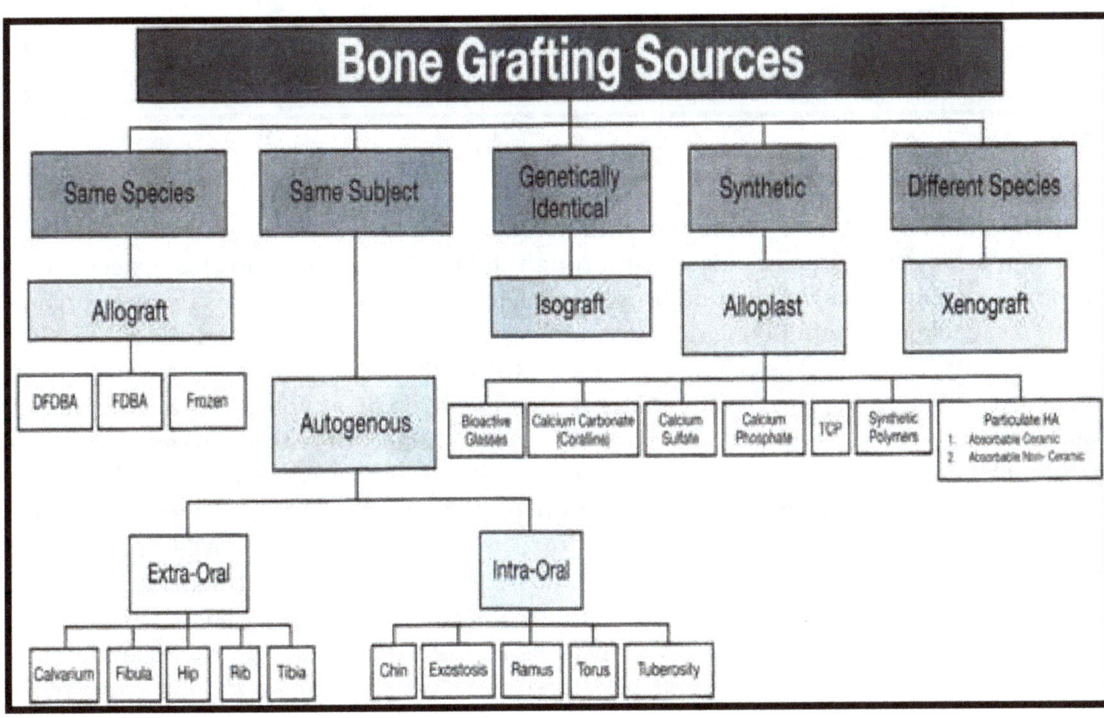

Fig. 2. Showing a reasonable classification of bone grafting source

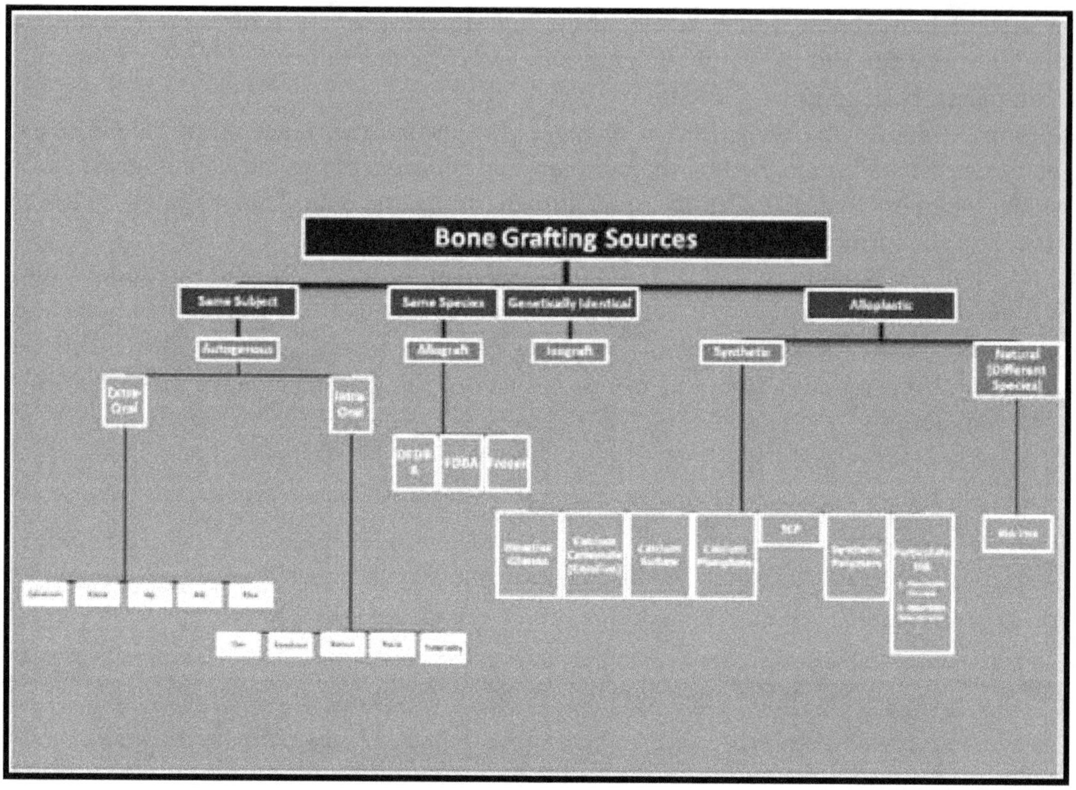

Fig. 3. Showing a much better classification of bone grafting source

1.2 Mechanism of action of bone substitutes

Bone grafts can effect bone replacement through three different mechanisms: osteogenesis, osteoinduction and osteoconduction (Misch and Dietsh 1993). Osteogenesis refers to organic material capable of forming bone directly from osteoblast (Misch and Dietsh 1993 and Marx and Saunders 1986). An osteogenic graft can therefore be said to be derived from or composed of tissues involved in the natural growth or repair of bone. It is for this reason that they can even encourage bone formation in soft tissues or activate more rapid bone growth in bone sites (Garg 2004, Wood and Moore 1988). Osteoinductive materials are capable of inducing the transformation of undifferentiated meseneymal cells into osteoblasts or chondroblast and enhance bone growth or even grow bone where it is not expected (Misch and Dietsh 1993). Urist (Urist 1980 and Urist 1965) recognized the mechanism as dependent upon many factors which includes specific proteins (e.g. bone morphogenic proteins [BMPs] located primarily in cortical bone. Osteoconduction is characteristic of a material (often organic) which permits bone apposition from existing bone and requires the presence of bone or differentiated mesenchymal cells (Rejda, Peelen and deGroot 1977 and Jarcho 1981). Osteoconduction provides a physical matrix or scaffolding suitable for the deposition of new bone. Osteoconductive graft are conductive to bone growth and allows bone apposition from existing bone, but do not produce bone formation themselves when placed within soft tissue (Garg 2004, Wood and Moore 1988). The healing of dental implants with a direct bone contact has been described as an osteoconductive process (Albrektsson 1985, 129-143).

Transplanted osteogenesis is another term for bone grafting. This term emphasizes that bone is dynamic and forms by cellular regeneration, which produces osteoid that becomes mineralized. A graft is not a solid bone block that heals into place (Garg 2004 and Marx and Garg 1998). Bone grafting is accomplished through osteogenesis, osteoinduction and osteoconduction (Lane 1995, Frame 1987, Pinholt, Bang and Haanaes 1991, and Lancet 1992). Osteogenesis refers to the formation and development of bone by osteocompetent cells. Osteogenic graft materials which are derived from or comprised of tissue involved in the natural growth and repair; it can encourage bone formation in soft tissues, and stimulates faster bone growth in bone implant site, whereas osteoinduction is the process of activating osteogenesis by recruiting cells from the surrounding natural bone that then differentiate into bone-forming cells. Osteoinductive grafts can enhance bone generation, sometimes even resulting in the extension or growth of bone where it is not normally found (Marx and Garg 1998). Osteoconductive grafts are those that act as nonviable scaffold on to and within which the patient's own natural bone grows. They are conductive to bone growth and allow apposition from existing bone but do not produce or trigger bone formation themselves when placed in soft tissue.
The table below shows the properties of the various types of bone graft sources in terms of mechanism of action with regards to bone regeneration.

Properties of various types of bone graft source.

	Osteoconductive	Osteoinductive	Osteogenic
Alloplast	+	-	-
Xenograft	+	-	-
Allograft	+	+/-	-
Autograft	+	+	+

Table 1. Showing the properties /mechanism of action for various bone source

It is important to note that all bone grafting materials have one or more of these three modes of action. Mixing of bone grafting substitutes can assist in bringing about a desired combination of modes of action for bone formation. For example Bio-Oss which is basically osteoconductive can be mixed with allograft as a deliberate or circumstantial cocktail to effect both osteoconductive and some osteoinductive properties. Because of making up the quantity of bone required in defects that definitely will benefit more from autogenous bone graft, any bone substitute can be mixed with autogenous bone graft to additionally effect all the mechanisms of action of bone regeneration attributed to autogenous bone graft.
Osteogenesis can form bone more rapidly and in conditions which have the least amount of bone. Autogenous bone is suggested even when additional operating time and surgical site preparation is required when limiting factors exist. Osteoconductive materials require the most ideal condition to grow bone, yet are the easiest material to obtain and manipulate. The amount of remaining host bone in the region and mode of action and physical characteristic of available graft materials must be considered prior to the selection of any one type or combination for use in implant dentistry (Misch and Dietsh 1993).
Osteogenesis, osteoinduction and osteoconduction are all positive mechanisms of bone regeneration with Osteogenesis being the fastest and most reliable. Bone substitute that regenerate bone via the osteoconductive mechanism are the least efficient.

In his classical experiment using animal model, Ogunsalu et al accidentally discovered the negative mechanism that will prevent bone regeneration (Ogunsalu 2009). This new mechanism called osteobstruction will be discussed in detail towards the end of the chapter.

2. Review of the literature on bone replacement source

The three primary types of bone graft material are autogenous bone, allograft and alloplast of which commercially available xenografts are generally considered a subgroup (Garg 2004). The mechanism by which these graft materials work normally depends on the origin and composition of the material (Misch and Dietsh 1993 and Lancet 1992). Autogenous bone, an organic material harvested from the patient, forms new bone by osteogenesis, osteoinduction and osteoconduction. Harvested from the cadavers, allografts which may be cortical or trabecular, have osteoconductive and possible osteoinductive properties (Garg 2004), but definitely they are not osteogenic. The alloplasts, which may be composed of natural or synthetic material, are typically only osteoconductive (Garg 2004).

In determining what type of graft material to use, the clinician must consider the characteristics of the bony defect to be restored (Misch and Dietsh 1993). In general, the larger the defect to be restored, the greater the amount of autogenous bone required. For small defects and for those with three to five bony walls still intact, alloplast may be used alone or with allografts. For relatively large defects or those with only one to three bony walls intact, autogenous bone must be added to any other type of graft material being considered. One of the complications during augmentation procedures with any grafting material is soft tissue ingrowths; it is for this reason that guided bone regeneration (GBR) using resorbable or non-resorbable membrane is to be employed (Schopper, Goriwoda, Moser, Spassova, Watzinger and Ewers 2001).

With regards to Maxillary sinus lift procedure, various materials including autogenous bone (Kent and Block1989, Jensen, Simonsen and Sindet- Pederson 1990, Reghoebar, Browne, Reintsena and Van Dort 1993, Adell R, Lekholm, Grondahl, Branemark, Lindstorm and Jacobsson 1990, Kahnberg, Nystrom and Bartholdsson 1989 and Nystrom, Kahnbourg and Gunne 1993), bone allograft (Misch and Dietsh 1993,Lane 1995, Lancet 1992, Wood and Moore 1988, Rummelhart, Mellonig, Gray and Towle 1989, Mellonig 1987, Tatum et al. 1993 and Tatum 1996) and alloplasts such as tricalcium phosphate (TCP), resorbable and non resorbable hydroxyapatite (Misch and Dietsh 1993, Rummelhart et al. 1989, Fetner, Hartigan and Low 1994, Schepers et al. 1993 and Smiler et al. 1992) bovine bone derivative (bovine-derived mineralized deprotinised bone) (McAllister et al. 1999) and bioactive glasses are used. It is important to note that an ideal graft is non-toxic, non-antigenic, non-carcinogenic, strong, resilient, easily fabricated, able to permit tissue attachment, resistant to infection, readily available and inexpensive (Wagner J 1989).

Autogenous bone which has long been considered the gold standards of grafting materials is currently the only osteogenic graft material available to clinical practitioners. When utilized_for bone grafting autogenous bone heals into growing bone through all these modes of bone formation; these stages are not separate and distinct, but rather, overlap_each other (Misch and Dietsh 1993). Autogenous bone can be harvested from extraoral sites such as the iliac crest or tibial plateau and intraoral sites sites such as the mandibular symphysis, maxillary tuberosity, ramus or exostosis (particularly the oral tori) (Misch and Dietsh 1993, Koole, Bosker, van der Dussen 1989 and Garg 1996).

It is well documented that less resorption is associated with the use of mandibular bone graft than with iliac crest grafts (Koole, Bosker, van der Dussen 1989). The use of expanded polytetrafluoroethylene (e-PTFE) membranes or slowly resorbable collagen membranes has been documented to enhance bone grafting (Buser, Dula, Hirt, Schenk et al.1996). Furthermore, bone graft obtained intraorally would generally result in less morbidity; however intraoral bone sites provides a significantly smaller volume of bones than do extraoral sites such as the iliac crest or tibeal plateau. The volume and type of regenerated bone needed for the site, will dictate the optimal donor site. The posterior iliac crest provides the greatest amount of bone (Koole, Bosker, van der Dussen 1989).

As previously stated, the autogenous bone graft is highly osteogenic and best fulfils the dental grafting requirement of providing a scaffold for bone regeneration (Hislop, Finlay and Moos 1993). Significant disadvantages associated with the use of autogenous bone include the need for a second operative site, resultant patient morbidity and in some cases the technical difficulties relating to obtaining a sufficient amount of graft material (this particular disadvantage relates to intraoral donor sites). In fact, it is these disadvantages and limitations that have lead to the development of less suitable alternatives such as allograft and alloplasts (Lane 1995, 36, Rummelhart, Mellonig, Gray and Towle 1989).

Autogenous bone graft forms the rigid scaffold which supports teeth and implants. It is composed of organic and inorganic structures. Resilience, toughness, and continuity are related to collagen, of the organic component. Stiffness, hardness and rigidity are characteristics of the inorganic aspect; a crystalline, ceramic-like material which is primarily hydroxyapatite (HA). This inorganic matrix contains organic components of osteocytes, osteoclasts, osteoblasts, osteogenic signaling proteins and various amount of mesenclymal tissue. Without any doubt, autogenous bone is the only osteogenic material (Misch and Dietsh 1993) and the various sites for harvesting autogeneous bone include intra-oral sites such as the chin, ramus, body of the mandible, maxillary tuberosity, oral tori and other exostosis, zygomatic buttress. The extra-oral sites are; tibial tuberosity, iliac crest (Misch and Dietsh 1993 and Garg 2004). Banked debris during implant osteotomy preparation is also another source of autogenous bone graft which is usually omitted by various authors (Misch and Dietsh 1993, Garg 2004, Koole, Bosker, van der Dussen 1989 and Garg 1996).

As shown in Figure. 4, grafted autogenous bone heals in three phases. During the first phase, the surviving cells are responsible for the formation of osteoid by osteogenesis. They are most active within the first four weeks after bone grafting (Marx and Saunders 1986, 347-428). The blood vessels from the host bone and the connecting tissue invade the graft. Bone cells from the host tissue follow the blood vessels and remodel the graft by a coupled resorption and formation phenomenon as reported by Roberts et al (Roberts et al. 1987). The BMP derived from the mineral matrix of the grafted bone through the resorbing action of osteoclast, acts as a mediator for the second phase (Urist 1980 and Urist 1965). The BMP and other proteins must be released prior to the osteoinduction cycle. Phase three occurs as the inorganic component of bone acts as a matrix and source of minerals during replacement of the matrix by the surrounding bone and resembles an osteoconductive mode of action. The three phases overlaps in the time sequence and are not separate phases of growing bone from the grafted autogenous material.

Grafted autogenous bone can be trabecular (cancellous), cortico-cancellous or cortical. The cancellous portion of grafts provides the cells for osteogenesis and survives best when a blood supply from the host bone is readily available. Cortico-cancellous block grafts permit

AUTOGENOUS BONE	
Phase 1	Osteogenesis
↓	Surviving cells - 4 weeks --> osteoid
Phase 2	Osteoinduction
↓	BMP release - 2 weeks --> 6 months
	Peaks at 6 weeks
Phase 3	Osteoconduction Inorganic Matrix - Space fillers Cortical plate - Guided Tissue Regeneration (GTR) since it acts as a barrier to soft tissue invasion.

Fig. 4. Grafted autogenous bone healing, depicting the three phases of bone healing.

contouring and adaptation of the graft to the recipient bed anatomy. It is important however to quickly point out at this stage that the Ogunsalu sandwich bone regeneration technique (Ogunsalu 2009) will permit the cancellous portion of the autogeneous bone graft to be contoured and adapted to the recipients bed anatomy also. The trabecular portion is placed on the host bone and the cortical aspect is positioned on the surface of the graft. The cancellous portion is primarily responsible for the living bone cells and osteogenesis and therefore placed closest to the new blood vessels which arrive from the host bone and enter the graft at a rate of 0.5mm/day (Marx and Saunders 1986, 347- 428). The cortical graft supports osteogenesis only from the surviving cells (fewer than trabecular bone) and also provides more of the BMP compared with trabecular bone for the second osteoinductive phase (Longacre, Converse and Knize 1977). The cortical aspect also provides a more resistant scaffold for the third osteoconductive phase. In addition, it may act as a barrier to soft tissue invasion (thus excluding the need for a GTR membrane) and provide an extended period for blood vessels to enter the graft from the host bone (Misch and Dietsh 1993).

Allografts are obtained from cadavers or from patients' living relatives or non-relatives. Basically these bone grafts are of the same species but different genotypes. After processing, they are stored in bone banks. The advantages of allografts are availability, elimination of the donor site in the patient, decreased anesthetics and surgery time, decreased blood loss, and fewer complications. However, it is associated with some disadvantages which relate to bone tissues coming from another individual. Consequently the medical history must be thoroughly checked to eliminate donors with history of infection, malignant neoplasm's, degenerative bone diseases, hepatitis B or C, sexually transmitted diseases, autoimmune disease and other problems which affects the quality of the bone and the health of the recipient (Fonseca et al. 1986).

There are four main types of bone allografts: frozen, freeze-dried (lyophilized), demineralized freezed dried bone (DFDB), mineralized deproteinized and irradiated allograft. Fresh allografts are the most antigenic; freezing or freeze-drying the bone significantly reduces its antigenicity (Lancet 1992). Allografts are not osteogenic and so, bone formation takes longer and results in less volume than can be achieved with autogenous grafts (Misch and Dietsh 1993). Allograft is said to form bone by osteoinductive effect on surrounding undifferentiated mesenclymal cells in the soft tissue over the graft as the blood vessels grow into the graft. It may also form bone by the osteoconduction phenomenon when the host bone resorbs the material and grows into its scaffold.

Freeze dried bone allograft (FDBA) can be used in either a mineralized or a demineralized (DFDBA) form. Demineralization removes the mineral phase of the graft material and possibly exposes the underlying bone collagen and growth factors such as the bone morphogenic proteins (BMPs) which has been implicated as a factor that increases the osteoconductive capabilities of allografts (Lane 1995, Acil et al. 2002 and Wikesjo et al. 2002). Freeze dried bone allograft hardens faster than DFBA because it is mineralized. Clinical studies have shown that grafting of the sinus with DFDBA alone results in the presence of dense connective tissue after six months whereas grafting with FDBA results in the presence of new bone formation (Meffert 1998). The clinical and histological study conducted by Feuille, Knapp, Brunsvold et al in 2003 showed that sites grafted with FDBA and subjected to GTR by coverage with an e-PTFE barrier can yield predictable result when augmenting alveolar ridges prior to placement of implants (Feuille et al 2003). MTFC (Dentsply friadent Ceramid, Lakewood Co.) and puros (Zimmer dental, Carlsbond, CA) are examples of manufacturers' allografts. The MTF is an allogenic freeze-dried bone that is available in both mineralized and demineralized forms. The FDBA is more effective than DFDBA in the following situations: repair and restoration of fenestrations, minor ridge augmentation, fresh extraction site filler, sinus lift, bone grafting and in the repair of dehiscence's and failing implants. The Puros is an allogenic graft material that has been subjected to a well-tested processing method to reduce antigenicity and to minimize any cross infection with HIV or Hepatitis virus (Masullo 1995). Puros which is solvent-preserved (in comparison with the freeze-drying) to extract the water component has been demonstrated to osseointegrate as effectively as cryopreserved material and to be equally biotolerable (Gunther et al 1996). This material has been very promising with regards to good bone formation and repair (Sener et al. 1998, Becker et al. 1996, Dalkyz et al. 2000 and Alexopoulau et al 1998).

Moreover, because the water component is removed by solvents rather than by cryo-dehydration, which can alter the mineral as a result of volume expansion that occurs during the transition from the liquid to the solid phase, the mineral matrix is said to remain intact (Gunther et al 1996). This mineral also has both the mineral and collagen phases of allogenic tissues.

The use of DFDBA as a graft material continues to be questioned because of various reports showing that it is unpredictable in regenerating new bone. In one study in humans, for example, the DFDBA particles were found to be surrounded by uninflammed connective tissue (Brugnami et al. 1996). However, a more recent study (Feuille et al 2003) showed positive result with the use of DFDBA and a cell occlusive membrane. Incorporation of the DFDBA particles was observed in new bone that contained lacunae with osteocytes (Brugnami et al. 1996). The use of FDBA in this study instead of DFDBA might have yielded a more favorable outcome in terms of new bone regeneration. It is believe that BMPs and other non-collagenous protein in the expressed matrix are responsible for the osteoconductivity of DFDBA (Garg 2004). The osteoconductivity however, depends on the quality and quantity of the bone matrix in the graft material (Zhang, Powers, and Wolfinbarger 1997). Furthermore, studies have shown that different samples from the same bone bank and also different samples from different bone banks of the DFDBA can display different osteoconductive activity (Schwartz et al 1996).

To date, there are no widely acceptable tests or guarantee to ensure that DFDBA materials meet any minimum standards for osteoinductive properties; it is for this reason that this graft material had been avoided by many surgeons when bone grafting is considered. Invitro and in vivo assays have been utilized to a limited extent to assess the osteoconductivity of DFDBA (Zhang, Powers, and Wolfinbarger 1997).

DFDBA can be combined with other materials that have the potential to enhance bone growth. For example, the use of tetracycline with a DFDBA allograft has been studied; however, no benefit was derived from reconstituting the DFDBA particles in tetracycline hydrochloride during grafting of osseous defects (Masters et al. 1996). Osteogenin, a bone-inductive protein isolated from human long bones has been combined with DFDBA and studied in the regeneration of intrabony periodontal defects. Although this combination generated new attachment apparatus and component tissues more positively, it did not have any additional positive effect on new bone regeneration (Bowers, Felton and Middleton 1991).In another study, which compared Osteofil (Regeneration Technologies, Alachula, FL) a DFDBA with Grafton (osteotech, Eatontown, NJ) another DFDBA which, forms bone via osteoconductivity, suggested that the graft processing methods could represent a greater source of variability than do differences among donors (Takikawa et al. 2003).

Irradiated cancellous bone (Rocky Mountain Tissue Bank, Denver, Co.) has also been used as a substitute graft material for autogenous bone (Tatum, Lebowitz, Tatum and Borgner 1993, Tatum 1996). This is trabecular allograft obtained from the spinal column and treated with between 2.5 and 3.8 megarads of radiation. It has been shown that among all available allograft, irradiated bone is most similar to autogenous bone in terms of demonstrating rapid replacement and consistent establishment of a reasonable ratio of new bone with less expense and morbidity than that associated with autogenous material (Tatum, Lebowitz, Tatum and Borgner 1993 and Tatum 1996). Unfortunately, because of lack of further work in this area, the use of this material is not recommended (Garg 2004).

Gendler (Gendler 1986) in 1986 demonstrated by experiments that perforated demineralized bone matrix was a new form of osteoinductive material. Osteoinduction which is defined as transformation of non osseous connective tissue cells into osteogenic and chondrogenic cell, is an important biological process whose contribution to the physiology of bone remodeling and fracture healing at that time had only began to be appreciated (Mckibbin 1978 and Peck 1981).

In his unique experiment, Gendler demonstrated that subcutaneous implantation of perforated decalcified bone matrix (PDBM) induced multiple centers of endochondral osteogenesis with subsequent resorption of bone matrix and replacement by new bone. He therefore suggested that PDBM should be a useful research model to study osteoinduction and in the clinical management of orthopedic and reconstructive surgery for the filling of bone defects and stimulation of fracture healing (Gendler 1986).

Alloplast, xenografts and tissue-engineered materials are another group of bone graft substitutes. These include the deorganified bovine bone, synthetic calcium phosphate ceramics (e.g. hydroxyapatite, TCP) and calcium carbonate (e.g. Coralline). These ceramics form the new bone strictly by osteoconduction (Misch and Dietsh 1993 and Meffert et al. 1985) with the new bone formation taking place along their surface.

Basically alloplastic materials for bone growth are synthetic or deorganified biocompatible materials developed to cover a broad range of clinical applications for bone growth or soft tissue support. They come in a variety of textures, sizes and shapes and readily available and are mostly ceramics (Misch and Dietsh 1993).

Ceramic alloplasts may be bioinert or bioactive. Inert ceramics do not bond with the host bone. The relationship consists of an intimate mechanical contact which permits force transfer. They are rarely used as bone augmentation materials, but often are used as endosteal implants (e.g. aluminum oxide [$Al_2 O_2$] and titanium oxide [TiO_2]) as previously mentioned; the mode of bone formation for these ceramics is osteoconduction. Sub categories of bioactive calcium phosphate ceramics includes synthetic TCP and dense HA and those derived of natural origin (corallin or deorganified bovine and human bone). A chemical contact between the host bone and grafted material may be developed as well as possible stimulus for bone activity (Le Geros 1988).These materials exhibit good compressive strength, but poor tensile strength (similar to bone) (Le Geros 1983). Additionally, particle size, porosity, chemical structure and composition of the bioactive ceramics greatly influence the resorption rate of the material and may be another method of describing bioactive materials (Misch and Dietsh 1993). The bioactive ceramics differ greatly in resorption properties. Although difference in the biologic response of implanted bone substitute occurs, all have been recommended for augmentation (Masters 1988 and Le Geros 1988). TCP can be used with osteogenic or osteoinductive materials to improve the handling characteristic of the graft during placement (Misch and Dietsh 1993). Both hydroxyapatite and TCP are safe and well tolerated.

Cerasorb (Curasan, Kleinostheinon, Germany) is a beta-tricalcium phosphate (beta-TCP) material that has been certified for use in bone defect regeneration in the entire skeletal system. It is also certified in Europe as a synthetic carrier of the patient's own platelet rich plasma. This material is resorbed completely and is a generally replace by natural bone in three to twenty four month period, depending on the type of bone.

Hydroxyapatite (HA) is the principal inorganic component of the calcified tissues in the human body and has calcium to phosperous ratio of 10:6. Its crystallographic similarity to the bone mineral apatite allows bone growth and contact when implanted in hard tissue (Misch and Dietsh 1993). Various types of HA can be distinguished according to physical or chemical characteristics. Physical properties are the surface area or form of the product (block, particle), porosity (dense, macroporous, microporous) and crystallinity (crystal or amorphous), chemical properties are related to the calcium-to- phosphorous ratio, elemental impurities (such as carbonate) ionic substitution in HA and the PH of the surrounding region (ToFe, Watson and Bowerman 1991). These properties all play a role in the rate of resorption and clinical application of HA material (ToFe, Watson and Bowerman 1991). The larger the particle size, the longer the material will remain at the augmentation size. Thus 75um particle will resorb more rapidly than 3000um particles. The porosity of the calcium phosphate also impacts on the resorption rate. Tofe et al (ToFe, Watson and Bowerman 1991) reported on the porosity of dense, macroporous and microporous HA. Dense HA may lack any macro or microporousity within the particles (Misch and Dietsh 1993). The longest resorption rate occurs with the dense HA type since osteoclasts may only attack the surface and cannot penetrate the dense material (Misch and Dietsh 1993). The greater the porosity, the more rapid the resorption of the graft material. The crystallinity of HA also affects the resorption rate of the material. The highly crystalline structure is harder for the body to alter and resorb. The crystalline form of HA has been found to be very stable over the long term under normal conditions while the amorphous structures are more likely to exhibit resorption, The less crystalline the material, the faster its resorption rate (Le Geros 1983).

The purity of HA bone substitute may also affect the resorption rate. The resorption of this bone substitution requires living cells, similar to the modeling/ remodeling process of living bone with the coupled resorption/ formation process. A solution-mediated resorption permits the dissolution of the material by a chemical process. Impurities in bioactive ceramics, such as calcium carbonate, permits solution-mediated resorption which then increases the porosity of the bone substitute. It is said that corallin HA does not demonstrate micropores around the larger holes, the HA has carbonates incorporated within the material, which hastens the resorption process (ToFe, Watson and Bowerman 1991).

The pH in the region in which the bone substitute is placed also affects the rate of resorption of HA. As the pH decreases (e.g. from the infection in the bone), the HA components of living bone and phosphates resorbs by the solution-mediated process. Bone, dense HA, macroporous HA, microporous HA, crystalline HA or amorphorous HA may all resorbs within a two week period.

Physical properties should determine the type of HA selected for residual ridge augmentation. Dense, crystalline, large particle size HA can be used for ridge augmentation. Dense HA particles may also act as space filler or modifier of soft tissue contours under pontics of a fixed partial denture or around implants (Jarcho 1981). Dense crystalline HA cannot be easily cut and should not be placed in bone defects when the insertion of endosteal implants is planned in the future, in addition when an implant is in contact with dense crystalline HA, the material cannot grow into or attach itself to the implant surface. As a result, less percentage of inert bone implant bone implant contact occurs and compressive forces cannot be transmitted as well to the HA particle-implant interface. This factor will increase the amount of force generated to the remaining bone contacting the implant.

As the resorption rate of macroporous HA is generally greater than thirty six months, it is used where a more long-term matrix is desired (e.g. ridge augmentation or subantral augmentation). The resorption rate of microporous HA (six to twelve months) is compatible with applications where scaffold is needed within bone during the first several months of healing, but where living bone is desired in the near future.

Tricalcium phosphate (TCP) has calcium to phosphorous ratio of 3:2, and is intended to provide a scaffold for initial bony proliferation. TCP has been reported to act as short-term biologic filler which is resorbed over time by osteoclasts and replaced by living bone cells which grow directly in contact with the material without any encapsulation process (ToFe, Watson and Bowerman 1991 and Heimke and Griss 1983). The resorption of TCP and its replacement by new bone occurs through various mechanisms. The process seems to be very dependent upon the material characteristics, primarily chemical structures, porosity and particle size. These characteristics are closely related to manufacturing processes (Swart, Rejda and de Groot 1979).

TCP is prepared by sintering processes. It is very sensitive to heat and sterilization, which may change its chemical structure and alter its properties, including resorption rate (Le Geros 1988). It can be used in combination with osteogenic and or osteoinductive materials because it provides improved handling characteristics to the graft during placement. In addition to Cerosorb®, which is mentioned above as β-TCP, other commercially available TCP products are; Calciresorb® (Ceraver Osteal, Paris, France), Synthograft (small size and dense) and Augmen (larger size and dense) (Miter, Warsaw).

Bovine-derived anorganic bone matrix materials (xenogenic alloplast) are utilized for bone grafting. An example of this is Bio-Oss (Osteohealth, Shirley, NY) which is anorganic bovine bone that has been chemically treated to remove its organic component.

After the Bio-Oss is sterilized, it can be used as a graft without causing a host immune response (Hislop, Finlay and Moos 1993). Bio-Oss is osteoconductive (Hislop, Finlay and Moos 1993 and Pinholt, Bang and Haanaes 1991) and over time, the graft undergoes physiologic remodeling and becomes incorporated into the surrounding bone. This type of bone graft can be used alone or in combination with barrier membrane in periodontal defects, dehiscences and fenestrations around implants and in small sinus osteotomies. In large alveolar ridge deficiencies, anorganic bone can be combined with autogenous bone for successful augmentation. Anorganic bone has been utilized in the treatment of intra bony defects, and for maxillary sinus augmentation and treatment of peri-implantitis (Garg 2004).

Bovine bone substitutes are widely used for treating osseous defects, however, there is a risk of transmitting bovine spongiform encephalopathy to human (Will 1999, Scott et al. 1999 and Vedrager 1999). As these materials are routinely and successfully utilized in surgical dentistry and orthopedic surgery, careful risk assessment has to be done. Bio-Oss and osteograft are bovine derived bone substitute which are processed from veterinary certified cows from the USA, a country that is known to be free of BSE-cases. Consequently it is unlikely that the starting material for the manufacturing of Bio-Oss or osteograft contains prions. However, it has recently been questioned whether the U.S.A. can still be considered as a BSE-Free country.

(http://europa.eu.int/com/dgs/healthconsumer/library/press/press66_en.html)

The issue has become more urgent as many biomaterial scientists, dental and orthopedic surgeons are getting more concerned about the bio-safety of biomaterials from bovine origin. There is an increasing interest in the analysis of the risk of transmitting BSE through grafting materials derived from the bovine bone. The theoretical risk assessment has been done according to a model proposed by the German Health Authority (Bundesgesundheitsamt 1994 and Bundesgesundheistamt 1996). This was done before for osteograft /N based on a model published in 1994 (Bundesgesundheitsamt 1994). Wenz *et al* in their publication of 2001 on the analysis of the risk of transmitting bovine spongiform encephalopathy (BSE) through bone grafts derived from bovine bone concluded that theoretical and experimental data indicate that the use of these materials does not carry a risk of transmitting BSE to patients (Wenz, Oesch and Horst 2001).

PepGen P-15 (Dentsply Friadent Ceramed) is another form of bovine-derived hydroxyapatie which is enhanced and contains an added synthetic short-chain peptide p-15. This component mimics the cell-binding domain of type I collagen which is responsible in natural bone for cell migration, differentiation and proliferation (Similer 2001). PepGen P-15 may provide the benefit of a synthetic graft containing an inorganic and an important organic component that together may mimic autogeneous bone in graft sites. This material has been reported to provide enhanced bone formation in a shorter time compared with the other bovine-derived hydroxyapatite plus DFDBA graft material traditionally used for sinus augmentation (Krauser, Rohrer and Wallace 2000). Another study indicated that enhanced bone formation and faster particle resorption can occur with Pep-Gen P-15 flow (PepGen p-15 particles suspended in biocompatible inert hydrogel consisting of sodium carboxymethyl-cellulose, glycerol and water) compared with the pep-Gen P-15 particles (Hahn, Rohrer and Tofe 2003).

Recently the bioactive glass ceramics have emerged as a bone grafting material. Bioglass (US Biomaterials, Jersey City, NJ) is composed of calcium salts and phosphate in a proportion similar to that found in bone and teeth, as well as sodium salts and silicon, which are essential for bone to mineralize. Bioglass is an amorphous material which is deliberately not manufactured in the crystalline form (to strengthen the material) because the developers foresaw that degradation of the material by tissue fluid and subsequent loss of the crystal could cause a loss of integrity. This material is not porous and as such, tissue and blood vessel in-growth is prevented. The biologic impact of this non-porous nature is not known, and only few studies support the use of this material in periodontal and maxillofacial procedures (Garg 2004).

Bioactive glass ceramics have two properties that contribute to the successful results observed with its use: (Misch and Dietsh 1993) a relatively quick rate of reaction with the host cell and (Marx and Saunders 1986, 347- 428) an ability to bond with the collagen found in connective tissue (Kirsh and Garg 1994). It has been documented that the high degree of bioactivity may stimulate the repair process and induces osteogenesis (Wilson 1993). Because the bioactivity index is high, reaction layers develop within minutes of implantation. As a result osteogenic cells in the implantation site may colonize the surface of the particles and produce collagen on these surfaces, osteoblast then lay down bone material on top of the collagen; an action which may supplement bone that grow by osteoconduction from the alveolus. In their seminal clinical trial and subsequent publication of 1993, Schepers *et al* (Schepers, Ducheyne, Barbier and Schepers 1993) reliably demonstrated that bioactive glass granules of narrow size range constitute a valuable material to aid in the repair of dental bone lesions.

The phenomenon of osteogenesis guided by bioactive glass particles with a narrow size range has been explained. The glass particles and the surrounding tissue fluids result in the formation of a silica gel, which is quickly covered by a calcium-phosphorous-rich layer. The particle size of the glass is such that the entire granule is transformed into silica gel (i.e. it is gelated). Phagocytosing cells penetrate the silica gel by means of small cracks in the outer calcium-phosphorous layer and partially resorbs the gel. This resorption leads to the formation of protective pouches in which primitive mesenchymal cells acquire phenotypic characteristics of osteoblasts. These osteoprogenitor cells adhere to the inner surface of the pouch. When the primitive cells are immobilized on this inner calcium-phosperous-rich layer (a bone-like surface), differentiation of these cells into osteoblasts occurs. In this way islands of new bone tissue are formed without the need for osteoblastic proliferation from the preexisting bone (i.e. the cavity walls (Schepers, de Clercq, Ducheyne and Kempeneers 1991 and Schepers, Ducheyne, Barbier and Schepers 1993). The size range of bioglass particles must be narrow (300 to 360 *u*m for the glass composition selected) due to several critical considerations (Schepers, de Clercq, Ducheyne and Kempeneers 1991 and Schepers, Ducheyne, Barbier and Schepers 1993), the phenomenon of preferential resorption of the gel is restricted to this size range. Particles with a size exceeding this range do not corrode throughout and therefore are not resorbed into their centers. Hence recruitment of primitive cells exhibiting osteoblastic differentiation throughout the bone defect does not occur and healing is slow since it must proceed from the pre existing bone tissue walls. Particles with smaller diameter are fully resorbed and cannot act as a substrate for enhancement of mesenchymal cells. Glass granules preparations that contain the critical 300 to 360mm size range and also smaller particles are not active as described. Another critical aspect related to small size range is the packing of the particles (Schepers, de Clercq, Ducheyne and Kempeneers 1991 and Schepers, Ducheyne, Barbier and Schepers 1993). When granules have uniform dimensions, dense packing will still leave space between the particles. With a wider size range, smaller particles fill up the spaces in between the larger particles. Such a granular mixture will extensively fill a defect space and leave very little room for tissue infiltration and regeneration (Fig. 5).

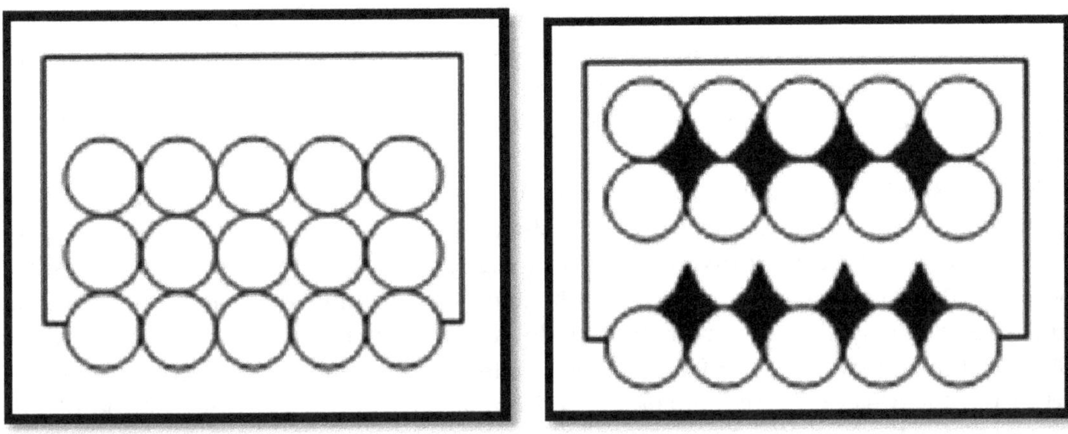

A B

Fig. 5. Difference in packing when a limited size range of particles is used (A) as opposed to a larger size range (B)

The endosseous ridge maintenance implant (ERMI, US Biomaterials) is another Bioactive glass bone substitute. It is a cone-shaped device made of bioglass that is placed in the extraction site (Kirsh and Garg 1994). This bone implant system can be used for maxillary and mandibular premolars and anterior teeth. It can also be used for preserving the contour of the alveolar ridge following tooth removal. This bone implant acts under a time-dependant kinetic modification of its surface after placement within one hour of implantation; a chemical bond appears to form within the bone tissue (Kirsh and Garg 1994). Based on a study (Kirsh and Garg 1994), denture wearers showed a retention rate of approximately 90% for up to seven years when the Bioglass implants were used for alveolar ridge maintenance (Kirsh and Garg 1994).

Perioglass (Mova Bone, Alachu, FL) is a synthetic particulate form of Bioglass that bond to both bone and certain soft connective tissues (Wilson 1993). Perioglass is composed of calcium, phosphorous, silicon and sodium (Fetner, Hartigan and Low 1994). The quality and quantity of new bone deposition may increase with the use of perioglass particles compared with hydroxyapatite crystals (Oonishi 1994). Perioglass is indicated for the treatment of intrabony defects and the criteria for successful perioglass use includes pre-treatment planning, debridement of the defect, preservation of soft tissue vascularity and infection control (Quinones and Lovelace 1997).

Perioglass has demonstrated two favorable characteristics: ease of compactability and ability to promote hemostasis (Fetner, Hartigan and Low 1994). When well packed into osseous defects, it becomes strongly adherent and hardens into a solid mass incapable of being disturbed by a suction tip or hand piece. Fetner, *et al* concluded that by bonding to both bone and connective tissue, perioglass achieved improved grafting results (Fetner, Hartigan and Low 1994).

Biogran (3i, Implant Innovations, Palm Beach Gardens Fl.) is another resorbable bioactive glass bone grafting material which have granules that are chemically identical to perioglass and are composed of calcium, phosphorous, silicon, and sodium. The difference between perioglass and biogran is the size range of the particles- 300 to 355 *u*m for biogran and 90 to 710 *u*m for perioglass. Biogran is hydrophilic and slightly homeostatic; it stays in place in the defect when bleeding occurs. Once in contact with the patient's blood, it forms a cohesive mass that is shaped into the defect (Garg 2004). Bone transformation and growth occurs within each granule. This osteogenesis which is guided by bioactive glass particles occurs at multiple sites, rapidly filling the osseous defects with new bone that continuously remodels in the normal physiologic manner (Rummelhart, Mellonig, Gray and Towle 1989, Schepers 1993 and Duchenyne et al 1992). This bioactivity permits material and bone transformation to occur simultaneously.

Bioplant HTR Polymer (Bioplant, Norwalk, CT) is a microporous composite with a calcium hydroxide graft surface (Ashman 1993 and Ashman 1984). This polymer resorbs slowly and is replaced by bone after approximately 4 to 5 years. This bone grafting material has been reported to be effective for ridge maintenance post extraction, ridge augmentation (immediate or delayed) and repair of periodontal and other bone defects. Boyne (Boyne 1995) concluded that in the HTR-implanted defects, bone tended to become lamellated (cortical) in the area of the particulate grafted implant particle over a long period of time. This lamellated bone structure suggests that such crestal regions should resist resorption in clinical areas. Porous bone material (Bio-Oss, Switzerland) that slowly resorbs and remodelled slowly also has been shown to confer a similar resistance to resorption on edentulous ridges in clinical situation (Boyne 1991). HTR is non-resorptive and may offer the same type of ridge support against resorption. The ability of HTR to produce an environment that resists resorption should be determined on a long-term basis by controlled clinical studies of conventional and root form implant supported prosthesis.

Garg (Garg 2004) argues that the use of autogenous bone, allografts and alloplasts or tissue engineered materials, alone or in combination should be based on the osteogenic potential of the recipient site. The decision should be based on the individual's systemic healing ability, considering among other things age, systemic illness affecting healing, (such as diabetes or autoimmune disorders like scleroderma and lupus), previous surgeries to the area, previous radiation treatment or chemotherapy, and irradiated tissue bed. Local osteogenic potential of the defects (e.g. defect size, ratio of host bone to graft material, number of walls of the defect, soft tissue bed, adjacent scar tissues, health of adjacent periostium, stability of the graft material, soft tissue closure, use of interim restorative device over and around grafted site should also be considered. The osteogenic potential of the graft, the surgeon's skill and the time available for graft maturation are also critical to the decision.

It is as such important at this stage to indicate that the membrane sandwich technique allows us to enhance, combine, and maintain osteogenic potential at the required site.

3. Application of bone grafting materials and selection criteria

The application of bone grafting materials and selection criteria should be done against the background of the understanding that autogenous bone graft is the gold standard for utilization in any peri-implant or periodontal bony defect, because it forms bone by osteogenesis and additionally by osteoinduction and osteoconduction.

For the predictable long-term success of dental implants it is important to appreciate the available bone (Misch 1990). When available bone is inadequate, bone substitute represent a viable treatment modality. The extraction sockets, ridge defects and sites where bone volume is inadequate may be filled to maintain or improve ridge anatomy, improve esthetics and function, and/ or prepare the site for endosteal implants. Bone graft substitutes can also be found beneficial in the treatment of peri-implant defects which may occur after or during implant placement. It is important that the composition of the graft used to fill defects correspond to the mode of action of the graft material, and the number of walls of host bone remaining in contact with the graft (Misch 1993).

With regards to defects in the oral cavity that may require bone grafting, we have; five-wall defects, four-wall defects, two or three-wall defects and one-wall defects; each defect requires a particular type or combination of bone grafting substitute for optimum healing. It is for this reason that in this Section; I have dealt with bone grafting requirements per defect.

3.1 Five-wall defect (with one wall missing)

An extraction socket can be compared with a five-walled pocket (Fig. 6), similarly a cystic cavity is comparable to a five-walled pocket. This pocket is expected to fill with new bone by appositional growth. In order to maintain the width of the extracting socket and to improve the chance of success of future dental implants placement, an extraction socket can be filled with inexpensive resorbable calcium phosphate material to prevent the usually documented percent to 60% of the width of the ridge resorption which primarily occurs from the facial dimension (Khan et al 1981).

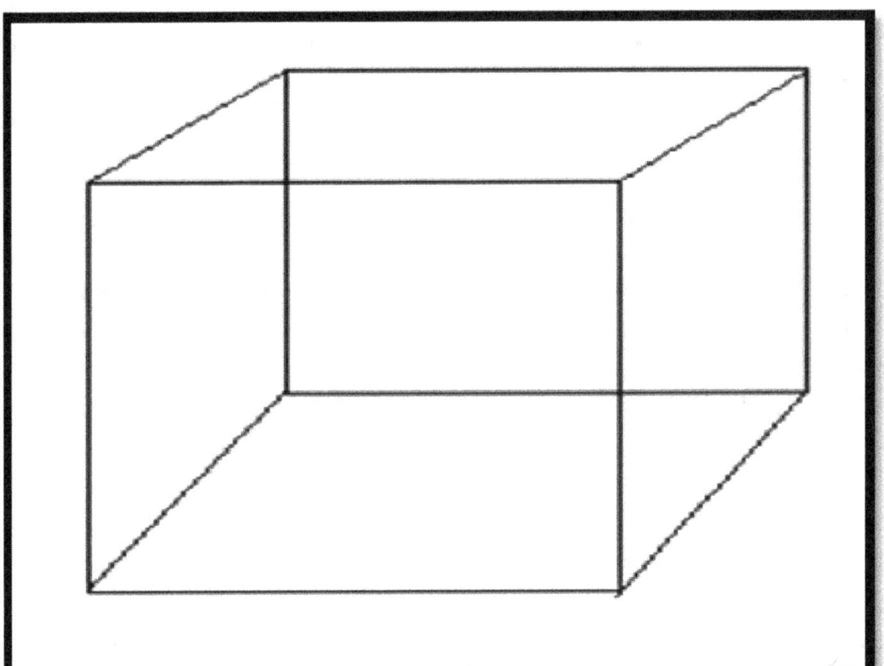

Fig. 6. Five-wall defects such as at tooth extraction socket or cystic cavities are filled with inexpensive resorbable calcium phosphate material to maintain ridge width. Autogenous bone is least indicated, but may always be used when readily available, since it is an osteogenic material and has no cost.

Autogenous bone may be used in any defect. It is often readily available without any cost to the clinician and forms bone by osteogenesis. When the harvesting site for bone is difficult to access, the five-wall defect may be grafted with any resorbable material, and then covered with a collagen or synthetic membrane to contain the resorbable material, particularly in situations where complete approximation of the soft tissue is not possible. With this procedure, it is advisable that 4 to 6 months elapse before re-entry and implant placement (Misch and Dietsh 1993).

3.2 Four-wall defect (defect with two walls missing)

If the host bone site has lost an additional wall of bone (usually the labial wall), it is called a four-wall defect. Additional active elements are beneficial in this graft since bone does not surround the defect. In such cases the addition of DFDB to the alloplastic calcium phosphate is recommended in order to compensate for the lack of labial bone and additional soft tissue in approximation to the graft (Roberts et al. 1987). It is suggested that the calcium phosphate be mixed with DFDB and over packed or contoured beyond the defect and this material is covered further with DFDB. This will allow the DFDB to be intact with the overlying soft tissue to modify the undifferentiated cells into osteoblast (Fig. 7).

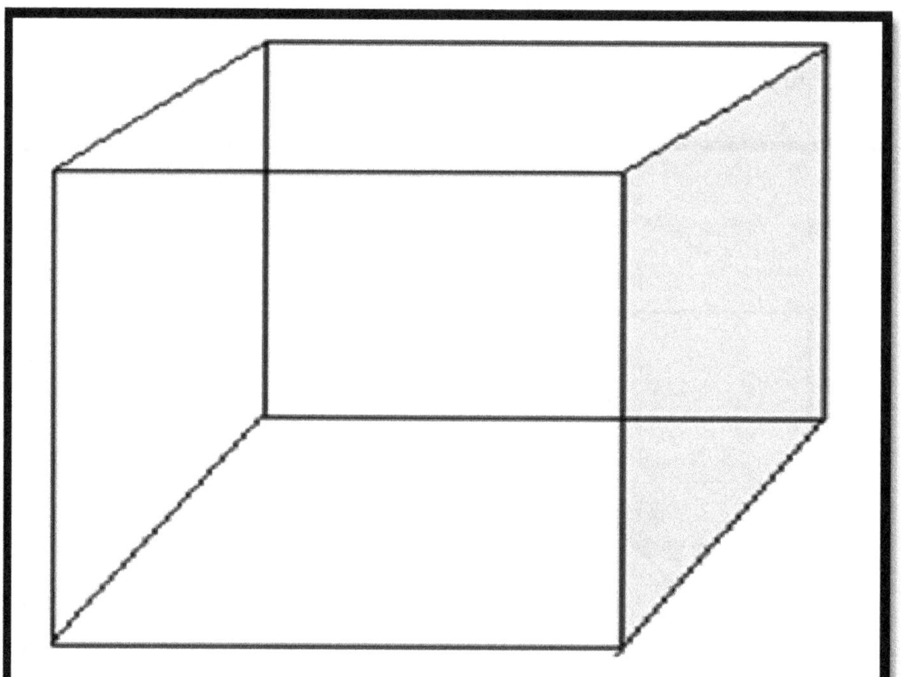

Fig. 7. With four remaining walls (usually labial and occlusal walls missing), calcium phosphate mixed with DFDB is placed over the host bone to retard soft tissue ingrowth. DFDB is placed on top of the calcium phosphate mixture so it is close to soft tissue for an osteoinductive effect.

The calcium phosphate acts similar to a barrier (due to its bulk) to retard the amount of soft tissue in growth within the graft and allows more bone formation in the region. DFDB when used alone in defects has not yielded much satisfactory results since it is eliminated too rapidly to permit a predictable volume of bone formation in the defect with the four- wall defect as such a healing period of at least 6 months should elapse before implant placement (Misch and Dietsh 1993).

3.3 Two or three-wall defect (defects with 3 or 4 walls missing

The loss of three or four bony walls will create a two or three wall defect. This type of defect requires the use of autogenous bone. The autogenous bone can be harvested intraorally from the maxillary tuberosity or with a trephine drill under the roots of the mandibular incisors and is positioned in the defect in contact with the host bone. Such placement allows for blood supply from bone to be established, to maintain trabecular cell survival. DFDB is laid over the autogenous bone chips to begin the osteoinduction process. Calcium phosphate and DFDB are added on top and the entire graft is covered with a membrane. A resorbable membrane is preferred to prevent the need for early re-entry and to reduce the risk of infection. Overall this approach allows guided tissue regeneration technique to impair epithelial in growth into the graft which would otherwise impair the healing process. Although the two-three wall defects are larger, the healing time is more rapid with the autogenous bone component. In approximately six months the implant can be inserted (Misch and Dietsh 1993) (Fig. 8).

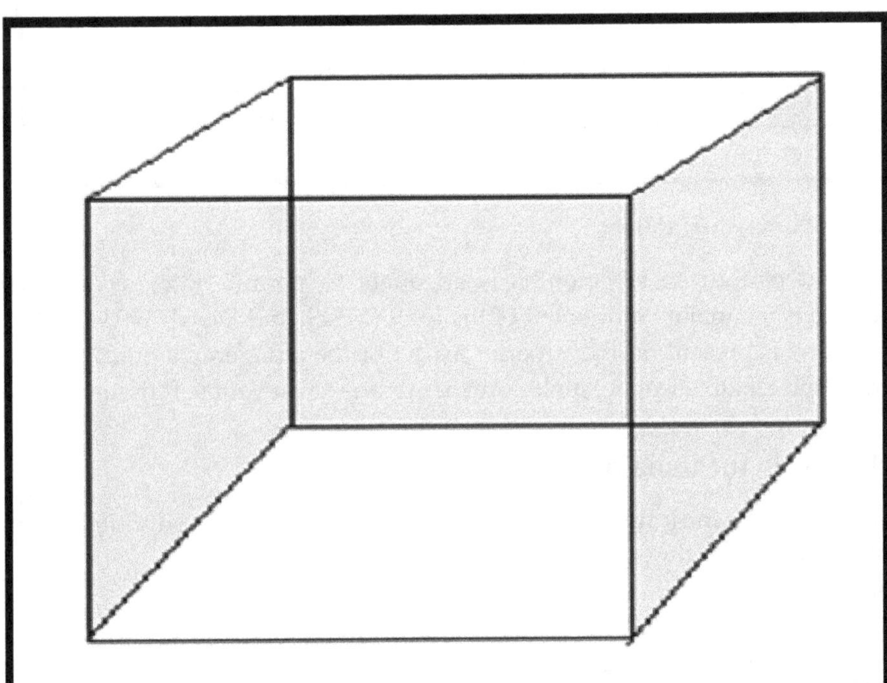

Fig. 8. The loss of three to four bony walls (a two or three wall defect) necessitates the use of autogenous bone

3.4 One-wall defect

Defects with five missing walls (one-wall defect) warrant the use of an autogenous corticotrabecular bone to regenerate a good volume of bone in the recipient site. A block graft is therefore the most preferable approach. The cortical aspect of the block is placed superiorly to act as a barrier to the invergination of the soft tissue within the graft. A mixture of chips of autogenous bone, then DFDB and then calcium phosphate and DFDB can be used to fill any defects around the block of the bone (Fig. 9).

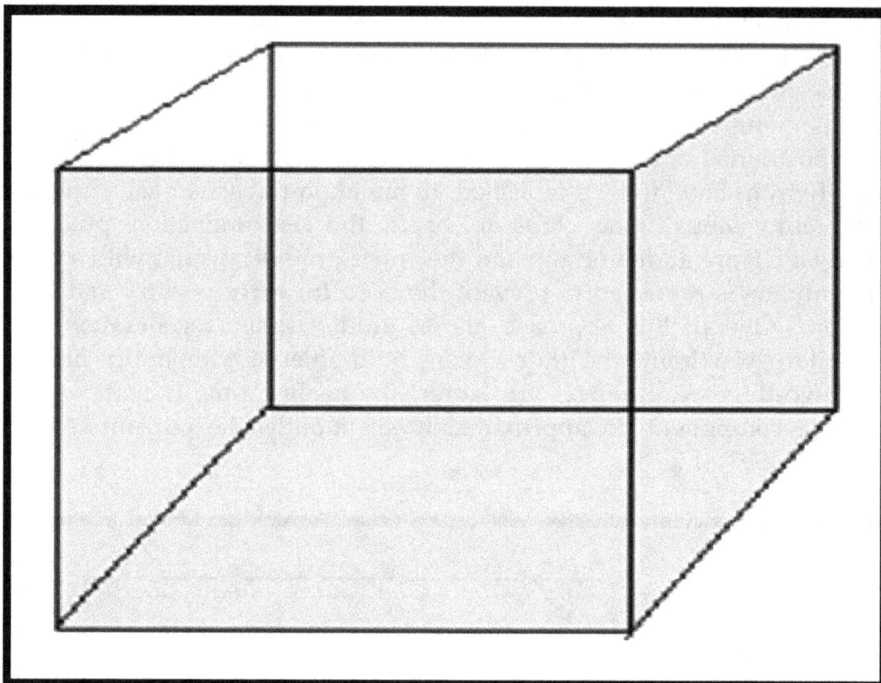

Fig. 9. Showing a one-wall defect

A healing period of four to six months is adequate to permit ridge reconstruction since autogenous bone is the major component of the graft (Misch and Dietsh 1993 and Misch 1993). If the cortical bone is present on the superior aspect of the autogenous graft, the area may be covered with a thin DFDB sheet or small pore membrane to prevent soft tissue ingrowth.

4. The indications for uses of bone substitutes

In implant dentistry the indications for use of bone substitutes can be divided into:

a. Pre-implant bone grafting needs such as:
   i. Ridge augmentation
   ii. Maxillary sinus lift procedure
   iii. Extraction socket for delayed implant placement
   iv. Extraction socket for ridge preservation
   v. Intrabony defect
   vi. Furcation involvement of teeth adjacent to implant site
   vii. Recession
   viii. Pneumatized sinus
b. Intra-implant surgery bone grafting needs such
   i. Intra-operative per-implant placement (precautionary of mandatory)
   ii. Extraction socket during immediate implant placement

iii. Repair of cortical bone plate dehiscence
iv. Alveolar or mental nerve protection
v. Conventional maxillary sinus lift procedure
vi. Osteotome technique for maxillary sinus lift and simultaneous implant placement
vii. Ballooning technique for maxillary sinus lift and simultaneous implant placement
viii. Intra-operative ridge preservation
ix. Furcation involvement, recession and intrabony defect of teeth adjacent to the implant site.

c. Post -implant bone grafting needs such as;
i. Implant failure
ii. Peri-implantitis

The repair of defects around previously inserted endosteal implants can also be performed with bone substitutes. At the time of uncovering, defects and bone resorption are best identified around the implant with a full-thickness reflection. The defect filled with soft tissue can be curetted and filled with autogenous bone. The defect is then covered with DFDB since such defects are similar to three or four wall defects (Misch and Dietsh 1993).

Subantral augmentation after sinus elevation in the posterior maxilla is the most predictable region of the oral cavity where the atrophic ridge can be augmented in height with the use of allografts and alloplastic material (Misch and Dietsh 1993). Autogenous bone is an excellent material for this procedure, but the quantity of bone necessary to fill the antrum often requires harvesting host bone from an extraoral site. The procedure has been further modified to permit the use of less autogenous bone and incorporation of both allografts and alloplastic materials. Results from structures show that the subantral region is similar to a three or four-wall defect and the graft should include autogenous bone, DFDB and TCP or microporous HA to combine osteogenic, osteoinductive and osteoconductive modes of bone regeneration (Misch and Dietsh 1993).

The fact that the last fifteen years have seen the introduction of several bone substitutes. Those materials can modify the bony structure of the patient prior to implant treatment, during implant treatment and after dental implant treatment. It is as such very important to understand the characteristics of the different materials in reference to crystallinity, porosity, particle size, chemical structure, and PH in order to be able to select the most appropriate type or combination to achieve a predictable result.

5. Validation of bone substitutes (second-hand bone)

Bone substitutes are best validated utilizing single photon emission computerized tomography (SPECT)TO disclose in a dynamic way the osteoblastic activity and calculated index around the bone grafting site over a period of time . It is the intention of this section to explain SPECT and its various applications and then to describe the SPECT experiment to be used to a compare second hand bone such as Bio-Oss with autogeneous bone (both of which are contained in the Ogunsalu sandwich unit).

5.1 Single Photon Emission Computerized Tomography (SPECT)

The literature is replete with the various applications of single photon emission computerized tomography (Khan et al. 1980, Ell et al. 1981, Flood and Russel 1998, Lima et al. 2004, Van der Wall and Fogelman 2007, Horger and Bares R. 2006, Schafers and Stegger 2008, Dasgeb Mulligan and Kim 2007, Sarikaya, Sarikaya and Holder 2001, Ozyurt et al.

2008, Kalita et al. 2008 Crespo et al. 2008, Massardo et al. 2008 and Ellis et al. 2008), however, there is a dearth of information on the applications of SPECT in relation to implant assessment and osseointegration .Reports in the medical literature on the radiologic evaluation of per-implant bone changes in the context of osseointegration are limited to one-dimensional quantitaions of heights of the defects. Despite the fact that digitized radiography and computerized tomography can facilitate quantification of bone changes, these methods generally reflect morphologic changes but may fail to detect the dynamics of osteoblastic activity (Massardo et al. 2008, Ellis et al. 2008, Alberto 1998 and Galasko 1975).

Bone scintigraphy which is a well established imaging technique that accurately reflects osteoblastic activity (Ogunsalu et al. 2008) can be utilized to radiographically assess osseointegration. In most clinical situations, the data from planar or conventional radiographic views are usually sufficient for diagnosis, but accurate quantitative analysis may not always be possible because of interference by superimposed structures. The single photon emission computerized tomography (SPECT) provides an additional refinement to planar imaging, it allows accurate quantitation common to most tomographic techniques by removing regions not of clinical interest.

Although the SPECT technique is well established and successful in clinical application for the study of many organ systems, (including skeletal system) (Khan et al. 1980, Ell et al. 1981, Flood and Russel 1998, Lima et al. 2004, Van der Wall and Fogelman 2007, Horger and Bares R. 2006, Schafers and Stegger 2008, Dasgeb Mulligan and Kim 2007, Sarikaya, Sarikaya and Holder 2001, Ozyurt et al. 2008, and Kalita et al. 2008), its application by clinicians and manufacturers alike have been very much non- existent in the clinical or experimental assessment of osseointegration of bone grafts and implant systems. Recently however, Ogunsalu and co-workers have utilized SPECT to successfully assess osseointegration of a new bone grafting/ regeneration technique (Ogunsalu et al. 2008 and Ogunsalu et al 2008) and also for comparative assessment of osseointegration relating to implant systems (Ogunsalu et al. 2008 and Ell et al. 1982).

The underlying principles of SPECT are common to most tomographic imaging techniques. When a radiopharmaceutical agent containing a single gamma-photon emitting radionuclide such as technetium 99m is injected intravenously it is possible to obtain a three-dimensional representation of the distribution of radioactivity within an organ or an area of interest in which the radiopharmaceutical agent is localized by using radiation detectors and rotating gamma cameras which detects the emitted radioactivity as the camera is rotated around the clinical or experimental area of interest. The acquired data can then be processed by a computer which will initially provide a cross-sectional (trans-axial) representation of the distribution of radioactivity. The transaxial data can additionally be used to reconstruct sagittal and coronal images.

It is the ability for multiplane image reconstruction with SPECT which confers greater diagnostic accuracy to SPECT. Additionally, SPECT permits accurate volumetric measurement and it is thus possible, for quantitation of the distribution of radioactivity in terms of Mc_i per unit volume of tissue (Khan et al. 2000). This unique ability to quantitate physiologic events, by using a bone-seeking radiopharmaceutical sets SPECT apart from other tomographic techniques such as computerized tomography (Khan et al 2000). CT Scans (computerized tomography) is able to provide excellent morphological details but unlike SPECT, it is unable to provide functional data.

In a highly significant publication, Khan et al (Khan et al 2007 and Ogunsalu 2007) described SPECT as capable of accurate quantitation of bone changes, before and after titanium dental implants in edentulous patients. "A novel approach that has the value in imaging bone changes dynamically and further offers an objective method for monitoring such dynamic changes before, during and after implantation" (Khan et al 2007).

6. Experiment

6.1 Materials and methods

Experimental Animals

Seven pigs 4 months old and weighing between 25 and 30 kg (Fig.10) were used. Pigs were used for this experiment because of the similar metabolism to human and the ease of ethical approval which should have been problem if dogs were used for obvious reasons. The pigs were all obtained from the same swineherd and, as far as possible, from the same litters. The pigs were housed at holding pens (Fig. 10) in the School of Veterinary Medicine for a of 2-3 week period of acclimatization prior to the surgery.

On the day of surgery, each pig was pre-anaesthetised with Azaperone (Stresnil,) and Butophanol at the dose rates of 6mg/kg and 0.2mg/kg respectively, induced with 5% Thiopentone at 10 mg/kg, intubated and maintained with isofluorane in oxygen. An Omicron Plus Multiparameter monitor was used to evaluate the vital parameters, including ECG, heart rate, pulse rate, invasive arterial blood pressure, respiratory rate, SpO_2, and end tidal CO_2. The anaesthetized pig was placed in dorsal recumbency and the mandibular area was prepared for surgery by clipping the hair, thorough washing with chlohexidine surgical scrub solution (Hibitane) followed by two alternating applications of povidone iodine and surgical (70%) alcohol.

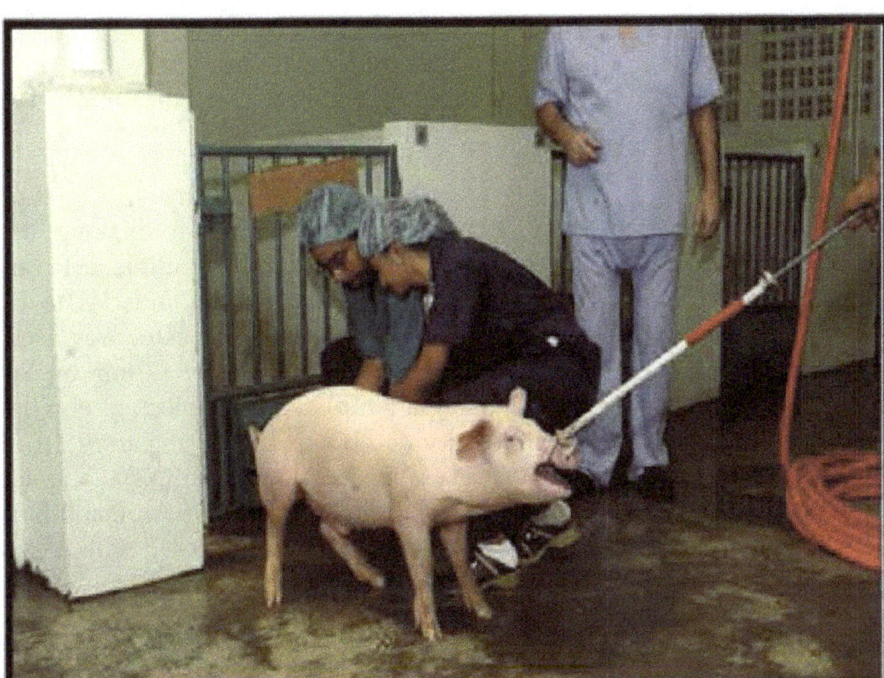

Fig. 10. Showing a 4 month old pig weighing approximately 30kg being cleaned and prepared for the operating room

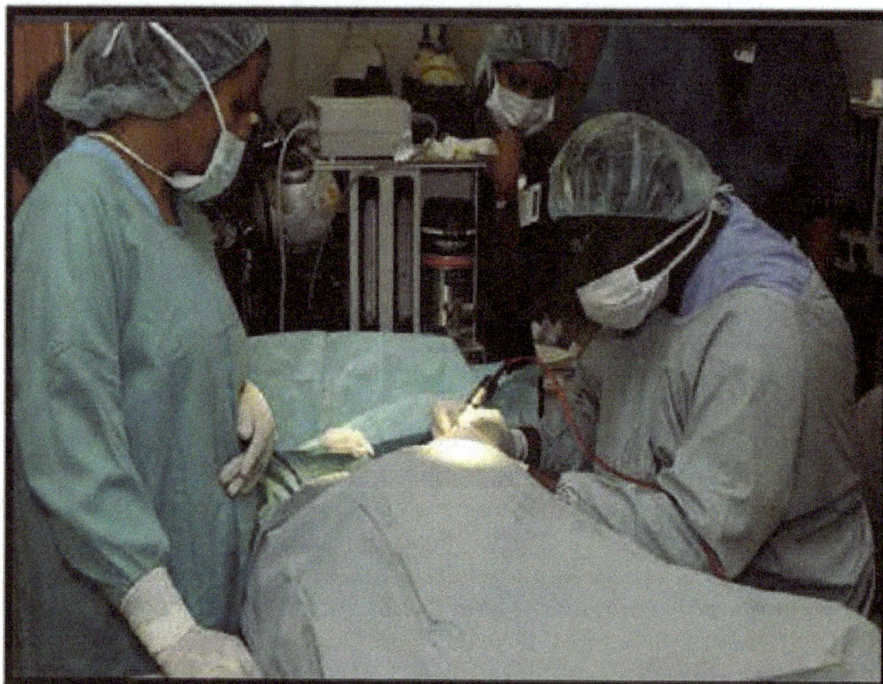

Fig. 11. Showing the operating room set-up and operator at work on the appropriately draped animal.

Surgical procedure

The animal was then drapped as shown in Figure 11 prior to making an incision (approximately 6 cm long) along the ventro-lateral aspect of the mandible just cranial to the masseter muscle. The incision was extended to the subcuticular muscles to expose the mandible without damaging the facial artery. A self-retaining retractor was used to allow adequate exposure of the bone. An area measuring approximately 17 mm by 16 mm was marked on each mandible (left and right) using a template, and a block of bone measuring approximately 17 x 16 x 4 mm was removed from each mandible using an Elcomed implant surgical motor and a surgical fissure burr at a speed of 18000rpm (NI). The appropriate graft (with or without the sandwich) were placed in the appropriate mandibular defect. Subcutaneous tissue was then closed with Vicryl (0), and the skin closed with #3 Vetafil.

The Sandwich

The sandwich is prepared as shown in Figure 12 below. Two sheaths of restorable membrane (Bio-Gide) are utilized and tailored with a restorable suture material into a pillowcase before the particulate bone grafting material (Bio-Oss) is placed in it. The tailoring was completed by suturing the fourth side with the same suture material to produce a closed sandwich unit ready to be implanted in the surgical site.

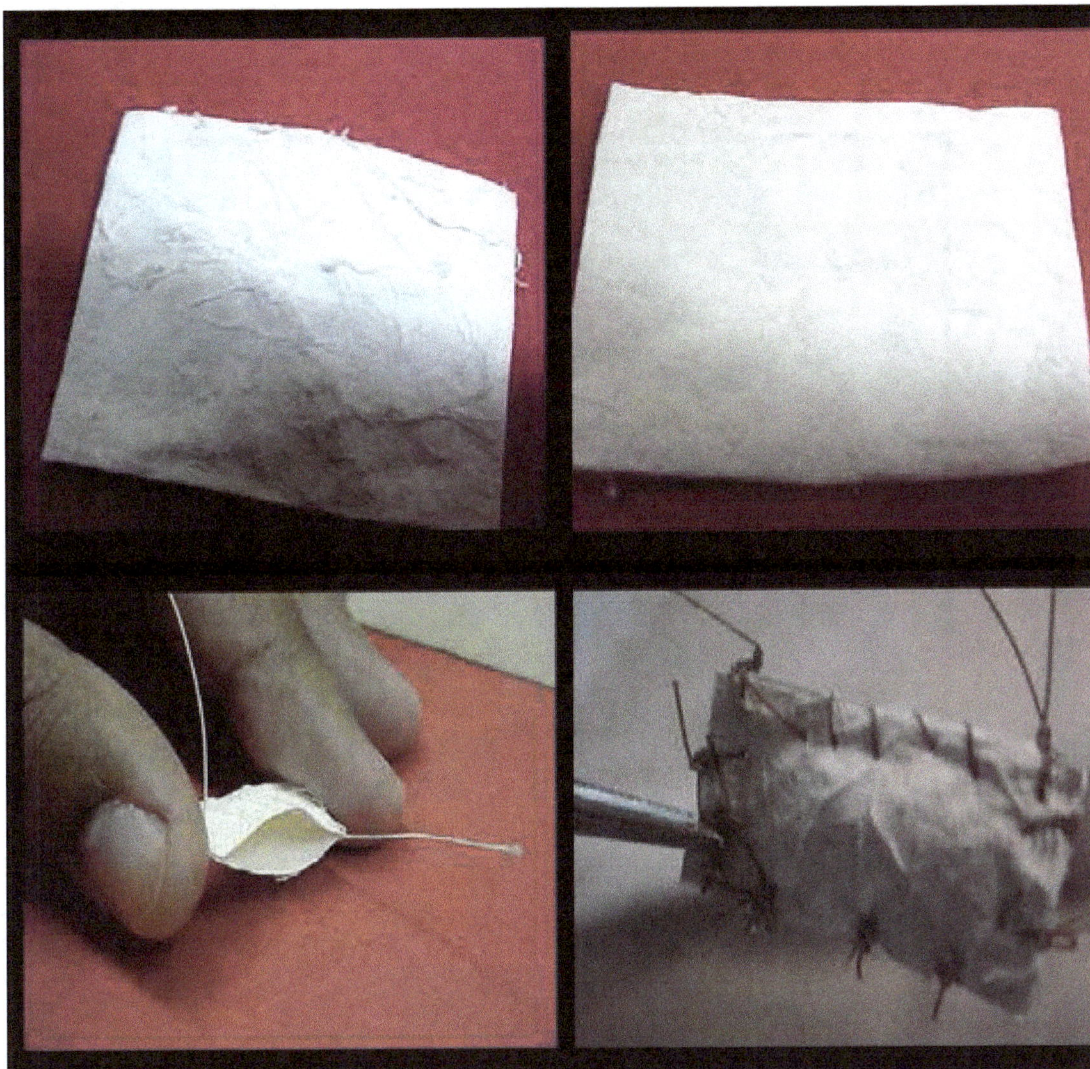

Fig. 12. The creation of the sandwich unit with Bio-Gide, Bio-Oss and resorbable sutures.

Evaluation of bone regeneration and ossification

Bone regeneration and osseointrgration were evaluated by (a) Computer Assisted Tomography scan (CT scan), (b) Single Photon Emission Computerized Tomography (SPECT), and (c) Histological and Histomorphometric techniques.

Single Photon Emission computerized tomography (SPECT):

SPECT studies focused primarily on evaluating the osteoblastic activities, especially the vascularization in and around the site of the graft or region of interest (ROI) At the end of each implantation period, the pig was anaesthetized and given an intravenous injection (into the ear vein) of 740MB_q (20 mci) technetium 99m-methylene diphosphate. The pig was subsequently euthanized two and half hours after the injection and then the mandible was removed. Tomographic images of the mandible in the region of interest (ROI) were acquired within 30 minutes of removal, using a Semens Orbiter II rotating large field-of-view gamma camera equipped with a low energy high resolution Collimater (Siemens Medical System

Inc, Erlangan, Germany). A total of 64 projections images (205/images) were acquired over 180 degrees in a 128 by 128 matrix with a dedicated nuclear medicine computer (Siemens ICON computer).

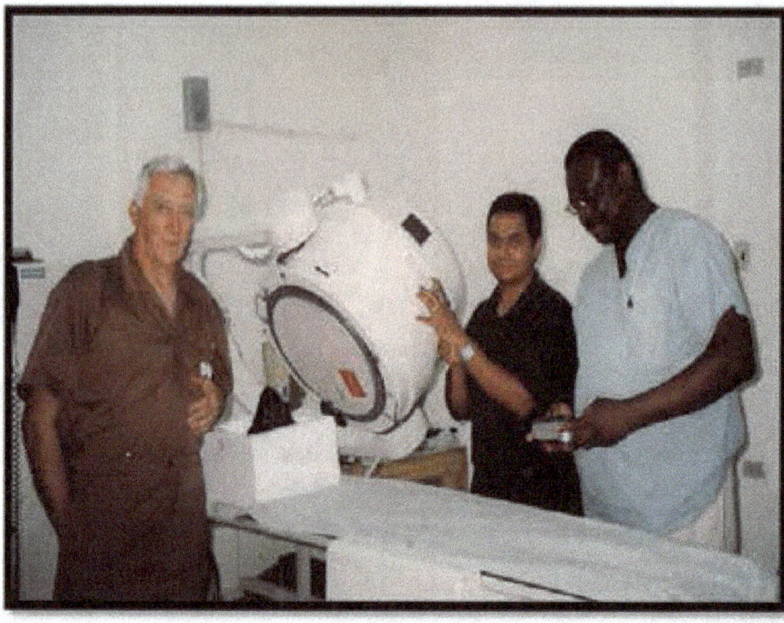

Fig. 13. The nuclear imaging team at work around the gamma camera and pigs mandible. From the left, Dr John Watkins, Mr Anthony Archibald and Dr Christopher Ogunsalu.

7. Results

7.1 Study I

SPECT Evaluation

The SPECT images demonstrated higher radioactivity on the right mandible compared to the left mandible, this indicates higher take-up of the radioactive material, which translate to higher osteoblastic activity. As such, on can conclude that the side with the autogenous graft (right side) has higher osteoblastic activity as shown in Figure 14. This result is presented graphically in Figure 15 which shows higher peak on the autogenous bone sandwich side compared with the xenograft sandwich side (left side). The average counts were 99.7 pixel and 78.1 pixels respectively (table 2) and a calculated relative activity ratio of 1:20.

SITE R	COMPONENT OF SANDWICH UNIT L	SIZE PIXEL	AVG COUNT	SUM
1. Right mandible	a. Membrane - Bio-Gide ® b. Bone substitute - autograft	112	99.7	11167
2. Left Mandible	a. Membrane - Bio-Gide ® b. Bone substitute - xenograft (Bio-OSS®)	129	73.1	9425

Table 2. Showing the comparasim of the osteoblastic activity between the xenograft and autograft sandwich

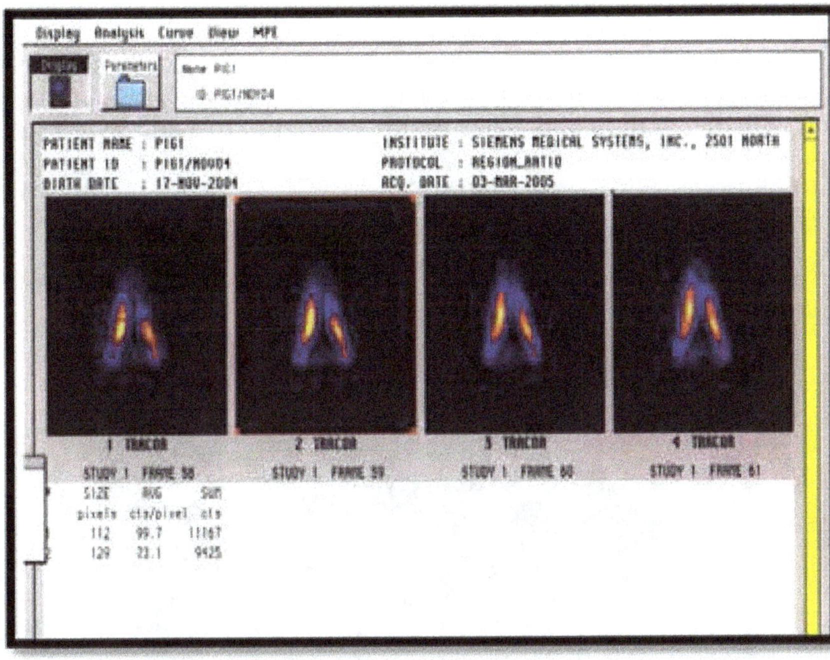

Fig. 14. Illistration of osteoblastic activity for Pig 1 at 14 weeks.

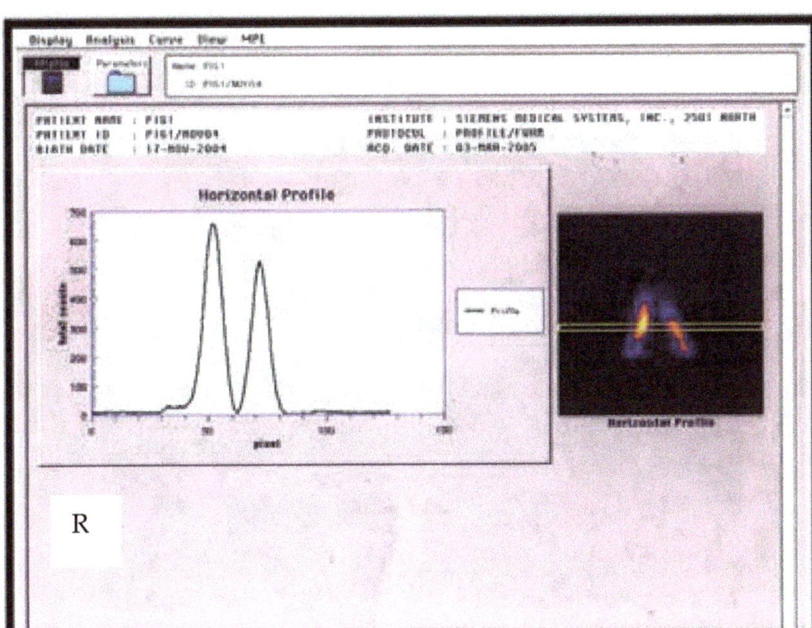

R = Right side

Fig. 15. Showing graphically the profile of osteoblastic activity of the autogeneous sandwich side (right side) versus the Bio-Oss sandwich side (left side), together with the activity ratio. The autogenous sandwich side obviously has more activity than the Bio-Oss sandwich side (note that the actual left side of the pigs jaw is represented by the right side of the profile).

CT–Scan evaluation

The CT-scan evaluation also depicted the morphological state of the bone regeneration site with the side which utilized the autogenous bone with the sandwich side having much more bone formation with obliteration of the marrow space (Figure 16 a and b)

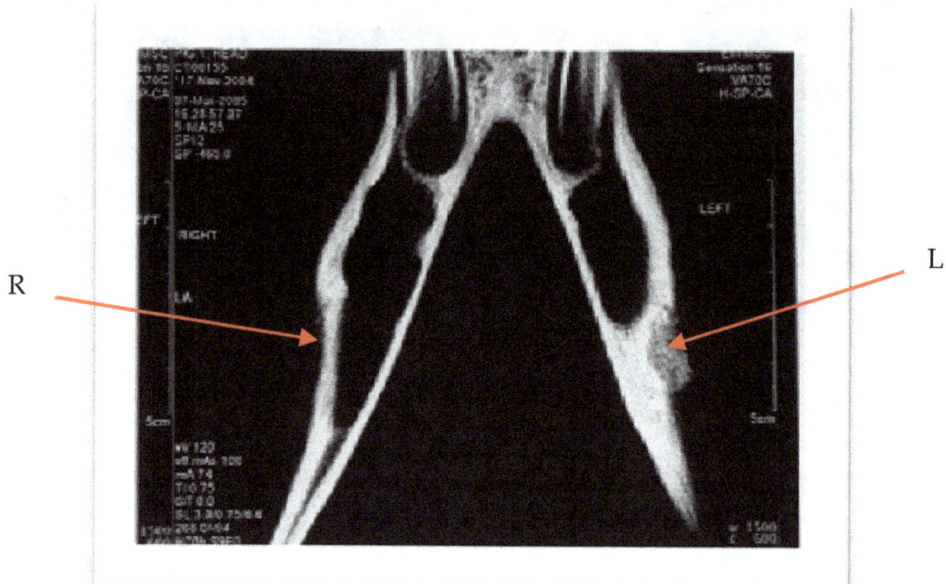

A

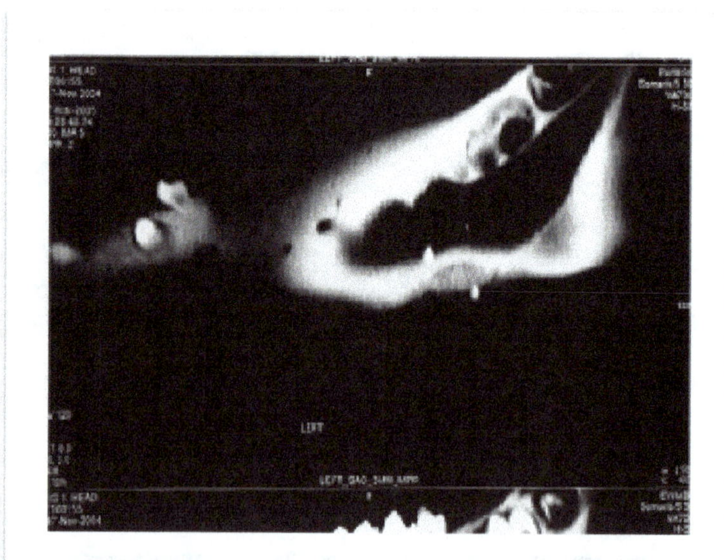

B

Fig. 16. (a- top and b- bottom): CT Scan showing the transverse saggital slices in the area of bone regeneration. Note the regular recortication on the side with autogenous sandwich (right side), compared with the side with Bio-Oss sandwich (left side), which shows less regular recortication with obliteration of the adjacent marrow space (see arrow).

8. The proper use of bone replacements

As mentioned earlier on in the chapter, bone replacement can be either autogenous in origin or non-autogenous and as such called second-hand bones or bone substitutes.
The proper use of the autogenous bone begins with its harvesting either as particulate, block or core graft to be placed in the site that requires bone to be regenerated. Recently the disposable bone scrappers became available in the market for the harvesting of particulate autogenous bone (Fig. 17). The attached CD will assist the clinician who is not knowledgeable with the use of the disposable bone scrapper to practice such utilizing a cadaver.

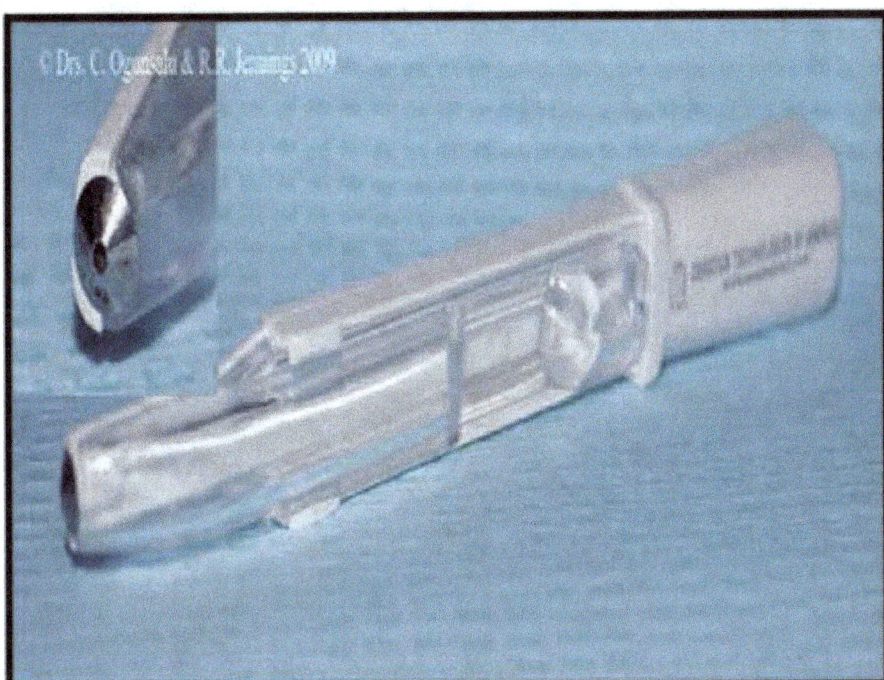

Fig. 17. Disposable bone scrapper for harvesting of particulate bone

Because of the technique sensitivity ascribed to the use of particulate bone substitute and the fact that it is the most common forms of bone substitute used in implant dentistry today, I will in stages describe the use of Bio-Oss (Osteohealth, Shirley, NY) particulate bone substitute in a furcation involvement in the mandibular molar region.
Bio-Oss (Fig. 18 and Fig. 19) is a xenogenic second hand bone obtained from bovine source and distributed in sterile packs and more important is the fact that it is sold only to practioners with current annual practicing license.

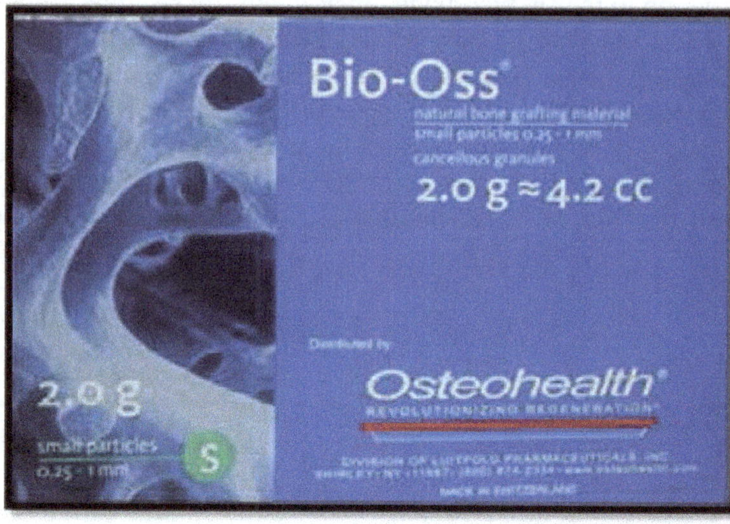

Fig. 18. Packing for Bio-Oss from Osteohealth

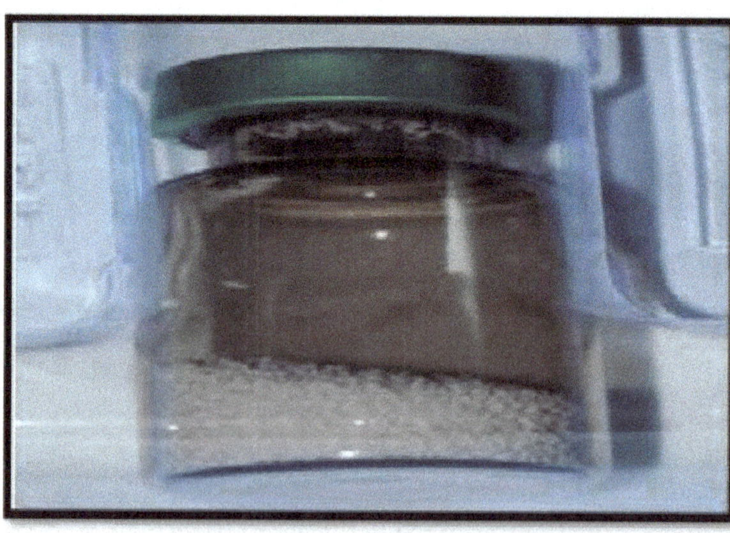

Fig. 19. Bottle of Bio-Oss particulate bone substitute(Xenograph)

In implant dentistry or in periodontal bone reconstruction or regeneration, it is best used with the resorbable membranes (Fig. 20 and 21)consistent with the guided tissue regeneration (GTR) technique.

Fig. 20. Bio-Gide resorbable membrane(smooth side)

Fig. 21. Bio-Gide resorbable membrane(rough side)

Once the surgical site has been exposed and all granulation tissue has been removed from the periodontal pathologic pockets and furcation area as shown in Figure 22 and 23.

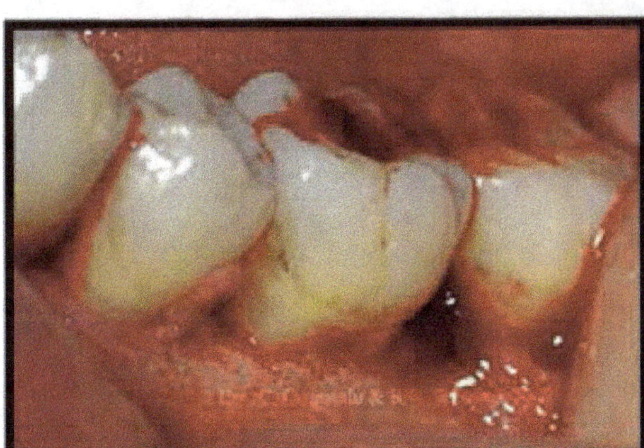

Fig. 22. Surgical site with some granulation tissue mesial to first molar tooth

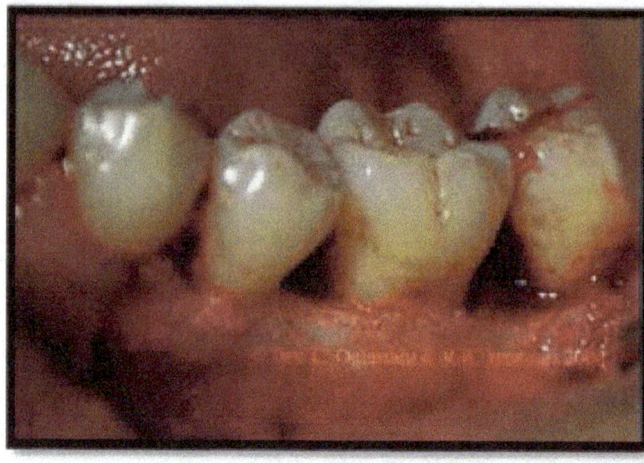

Fig. 23. Surgical site with all granulation tissue removed

The particulate bone which has been soaked with the patient's blood or sterile water is now condensed into the defect utilizing an amalgam plugger dedicated only for use in bone grafting (Fig. 24).

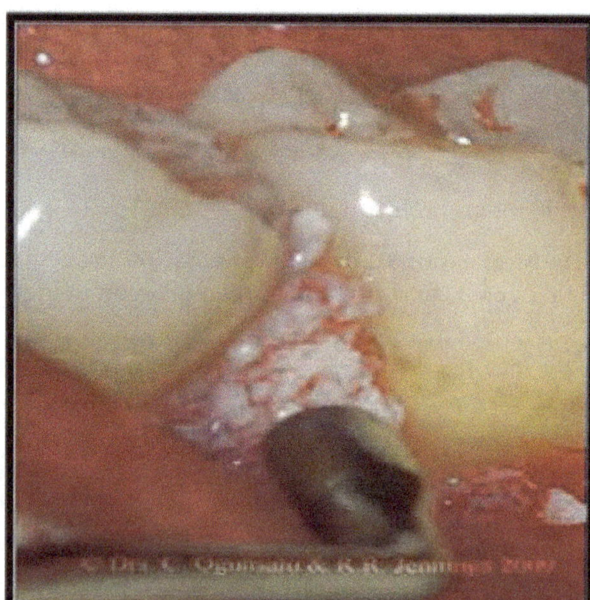

Fig. 24. Condensation of bone substitute with amalgam plugger

Once the particulate bone has been packed into the bony defect and appropriately condensed, the autotac pins and kit (Fig. 25) is now used to secure the GTR membrane which has been used to cover the grafted site (Fig. 26).

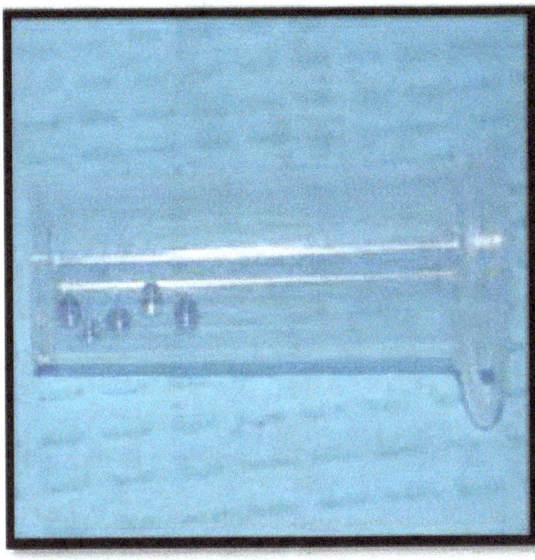

A

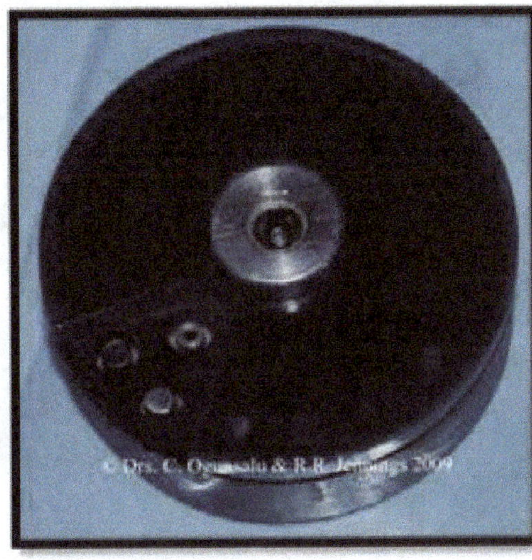

B

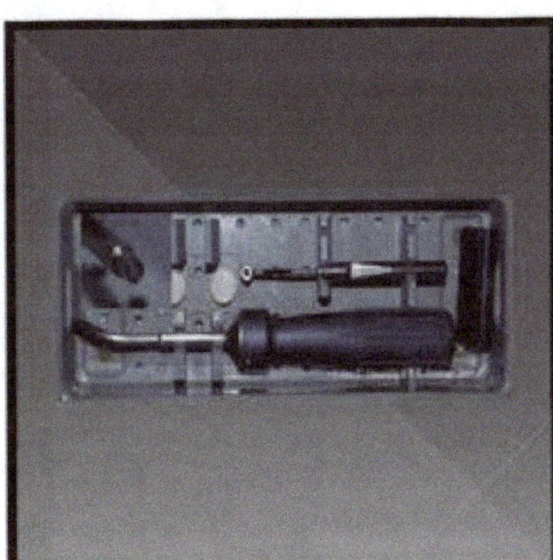

C

Fig. 25. Autotac kit with extra pins in sterile bottle

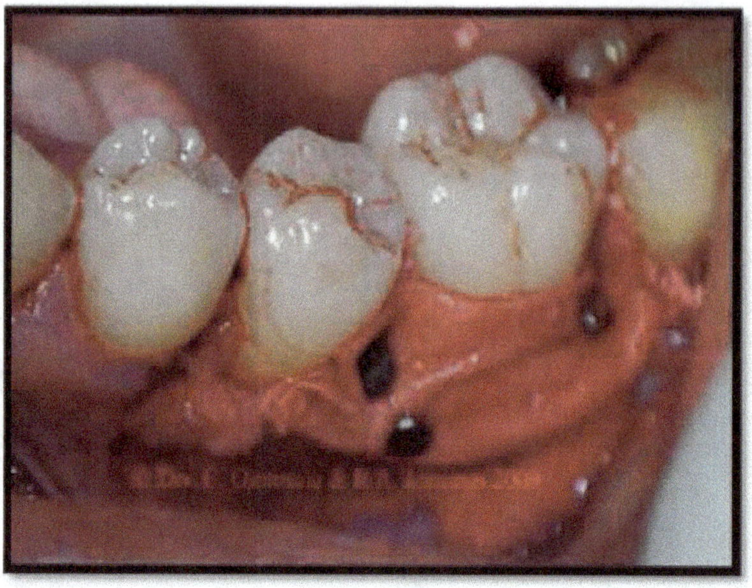

Fig. 26. Grafted site covered with resorbable membrane which is secured with stainless steel pins

The surgical procedure is then completed by suturing preferably with a non-resorbable suture material in such a manner that it is tension free (Fig. 27)

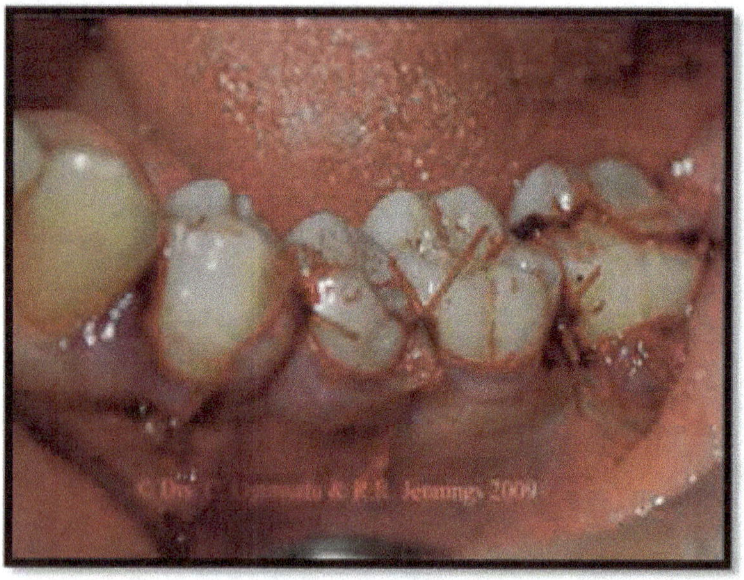

Fig. 27. Tension free suturing with resorbable suture

Most manufacturers of bone regenerative materials proudly explain the stage by stage use of their products in the appropriate section of their website. These information for use should be considered as very reliable and the clinician intending to use these products must adhere strictly to the suggested surgical sequence. For example Straumann, the manufacturers of a bone substitute, Emdogain proudly describe the use of this product which come in gel form variably by audiovisual on its website, *www.straumann.us.index/.../products-emdogain.htm*.

Additionally they also mention the functional advantage, cellular process involved in bone regeneration when Emdogain is used . The various scientific research to back-up this product is also mentioned.

9. Osteobstruction and bone substitutes

The osteobstruction mechanism in bone regeneration was coincidentally discovered during a sequential SPECT, histological and histomorphometric analysis on animal model in the validation of the Ogunsalu Sandwich Bone Regeneration Technique (Ogunsalu 2009).
This osteobstructive mechanism was demonstrated by episodes of overtaking and re-overtaking on SPECT following evaluation of osteoblastic activities in a sequential animal experiment to validate both the Ogunsalu Sandwich Bone Regeneration Technique (a double guided tissue technique; D-GTR) and the interceed membrane technique (a single guided tissue regeneration technique-;S-GTR) utilizing SPECT, histological and histomorphometric evaluation (Ogunsalu et al. 2008).
This new phenomenon of overtaking and re-overtaking and the newly discovered osteobstructive phenomenon, in bone regeneration are integral finding of my experiment, of which much discussion will follow in the next paragraph which will focus primarily on discussing the findings of sequential histological and histomorphometric findings, against the background of the SPECT findings at 8, 14,11,17,13 and 24 weeks. The implications of this sequential finding will also be discussed.
During the 8th week the total bone area was slightly more in the interceed side than the sandwich side and both side had vital bone with no non-vital bone. Also the marrow and fibrous tissue was more on the interceed side. This is in keeping with the superior osteoblastic activity on the interceed side on SPECT when compared with the sandwich side (Fig. 28)

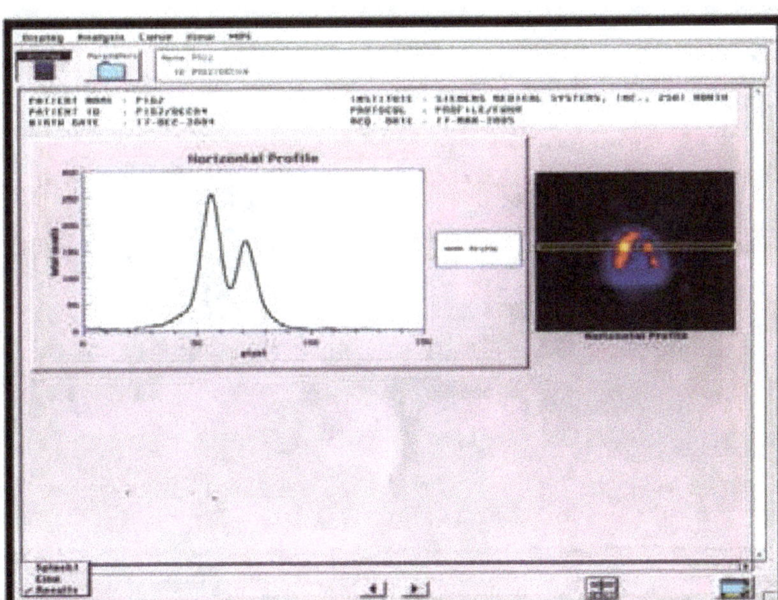

Fig. 28. Showing graphically the profile of osteoblastic activity of the sandwich side (SS) versus the interceed side (IS), together with the activity ratio. The IS obviously has more activity than the SS at 8 weeks. Note that the actual left side of the pig is represented by the right side of the profile.

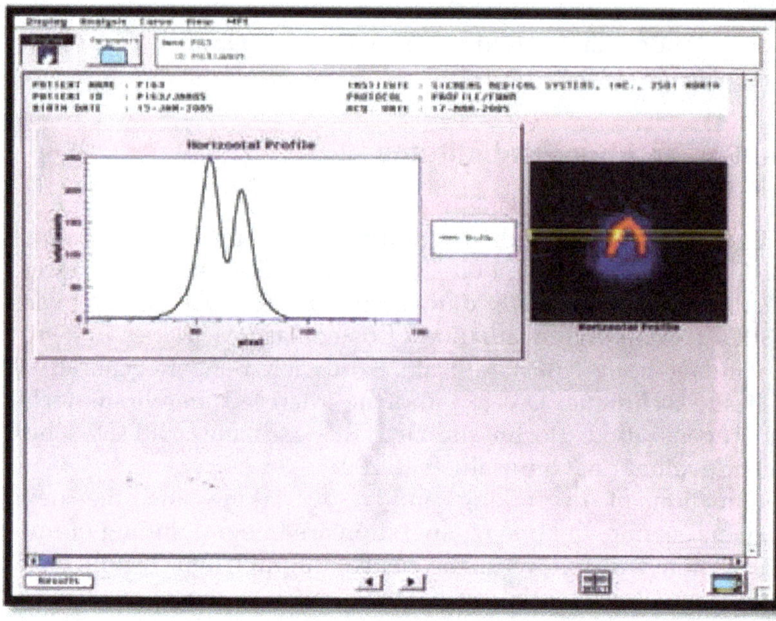

Fig. 29. Showing graphically the profile of osteoblastic activity of the sandwich side (SS) versus the interceed (IS) together with the activity ratio at 11 weeks. The interceed side still leads the SS at Fig 29: 11 weeks. Note that the actual left side of the pigs jaw is represented by the right side of the profile. The osteoblastic activity is still superior on the interceed side.

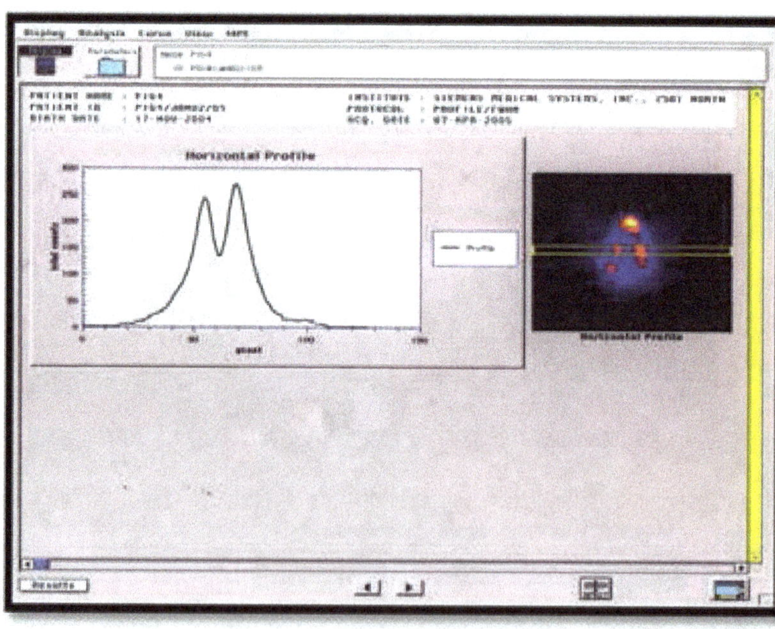

Fig. 30. Showing graphically the profile of osteoblastic activity of the sandwich side (SS) versus the interceed side (IS) together with the activity ratio at 13 weeks. The osteoblastic activity in the sandwich side has now overtaken the interceed side (slightly) at 13 weeks. Note that the actual left side of the pigs jaw is represented by the right side of the profile.

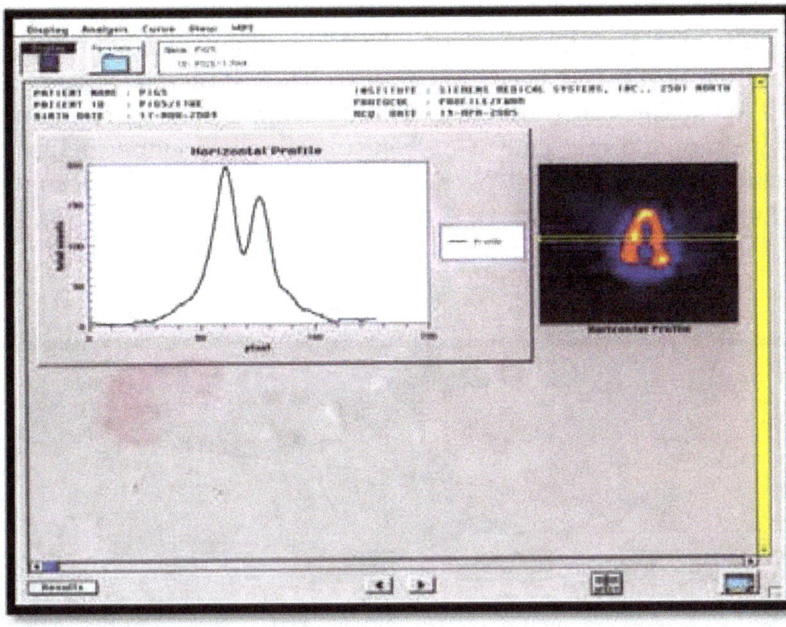

Fig. 31. Showing graphically the profile of osteoblastic activity of Sandwich side (SS) versus interceed side (IS) together with the activity ratio. The IS still leads the SS in terms of osteoblastic activity at 17 weeks as a result of an overtake. Note that the actual left side of the pigs jaw is represented by the right side of the profile

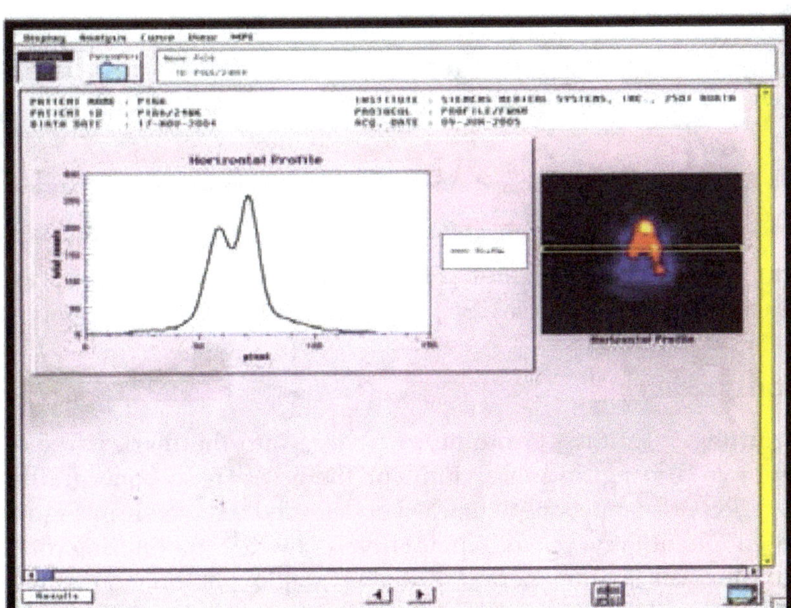

Fig. 32. Showing graphically the profile of osteoblastic activity of the sandwich side (SS) versus interceed side (IS), together with the activity ratio at 24 weeks. The sandwich side has finally exceeded the interceed side at 24 weeks.

The superiority of the interceed side was short lived at week 13 due to an overtake by the sandwich side (Fig. 29 to Fig. 32). This overtake as we found was due to the presence of foreign body reaction on the interceed side at week 11 as shown in Figure 33. The foreign body reaction is what can cause osteobstruction during bone regeneration. We as such include this as part of the mechanism of bone regeneration depite it being a negative mechanism when compared with osteogenesis, osteoinduction and osteoconduction which are all positive mechanisms.

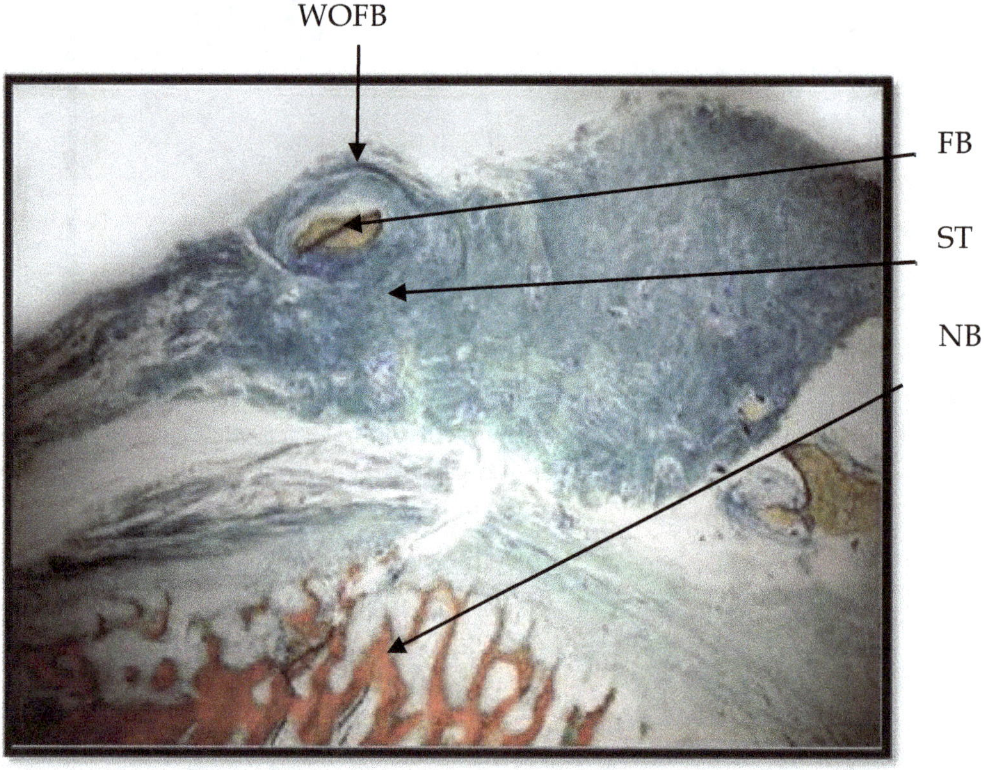

NB = New Bone, ST = Soft Tissue, FB = Foreign Body, WOFB = Walling off of foreign body

Fig. 33. Medium power photomicrograph showing Bio-Oss in soft tissue representative if foreign body reaction. (Slide 22-06-49M; Stevenel's blue and van Gieson's picro fuchsin)

10. Conclusion

Various bone grafting substitutes continue to emerge into the market to assist with bone regeneration prior to, during and after implant therapy. These bone grafting substitutes preferably called second hand bones should be classified as shown in Figure 3. They can only be validated quantitatively and qualitatively by the monitoring of the triggered osteoblastic activity over a time period utilizing single photon emission computerized tomography(SPECT) as demonstrated in the work of Ogunsalu and co-workers.It is this validation that will inform the clinician which bone substitute performs better in terms of bone regeneration and osteoblastic activity/ index. Further more, the osteo-obstructive phenomenon in bone regeneration discovered by the above mentioned workers is new and warrants more investigation.

11. References

Misch CE, Dietsh F. 1993. "Bone-grafting materials in implant dentistry." *Implant Dent.* 2(3):158-67.

Marx RE, Saunders TR. 1986. "Reconstruction and rehabilitation of cancer patients." In *Reconstructive preprosthetic oral and maxillofacial surgery* edited by Fonseca RJ and Davis WH, 347-28. Philadelphia: WB Saunders.

Garg AK. 2004. Bone: biology, harvesting, grafting for dental implants. Chicago, IL: Quintessence Publishing.

Urist MR. 1980. "Bone transplants and implants." In *Fundamental and clinical bone physiology,* edited by Urists MR. 331- 368. Philadelphia: JB Lippincott.

Urist MR. 1965. "Bone: formation by autoinduction." *Science*. 150: 893-99.

Rejda BV, Peelen JGJ, deGroot K. 1977. "Tricalcium phosphate as a bone substitute." *J. Bioeng*. 1: 93-97.

Jarcho M. 1981. "Calcium phosphate ceramics as hard tissue prosthetics." *Clinical Orthop*. 157: 259 -78.

Albrektsson T. 1985. "Bone tissue response." In *Tissue-integrated prostheses. Osseointegration in clinical dentistry* edited by Branemark P-I, Zarb GA, Albrektsson T. 129-143. Chicago, IL: Quintessence Publishing.

Garg AK, 2004, Bone: biology, harvesting, grafting for dental implants. Chicago, IL: Quintessence Publishing.

Marx RE, Garg AK. 1998. "Bone structure, metabolism and physiology; its impact on dental implantology." *Implant Dent*. 7: 267-76.

Lane JM. 1995 "Bone graft substitutes." *West J Med*. 163: 565-66.

Frame JW. 1987 "Hydoxyapatite as a biomaterial for alveolar ridge augmentation." *Int J Oral Maxillofac Surg*. 16: 642–55.

Pinholt EM, Bang G, Haanaes HR. 1991, "Alveolar ridge augmentation in rats by combined hydroxyapatite and osteoinductive material." *Scand J Dent Res*. 99: 64-74. Second-hand bones? Lancet 1992; 340: 1443.

Schopper C, Goriwoda W, Moser D, Spassova E, Watzinger F, Ewers R. 2001. "Long-term results after guided bone regeneration with resorbable and microporous titanium membranes." *Oral Maxillofac Clin North Am*. 13: 449-58.

Kent JN, Block MS. 1989. "Simultaneous maxillary floor bone grafting and placement of hydroxyapatite-coated implants." *J Oral Maxillofac Surg*. 47: 238-42.

Jensen J, Simonsen EK, Sindet- Pederson S. 1990. "Reconstruction of severely resorbed maxilla with bone grafting and osseointegrated implants: a preliminary report." *J Oral Maxillofac. Surg*. 48: 27-32.

Reghoebar GM, Browne TJ, Reintsena H, Van Dort RP. 1993, "Augmentation of the maxillary sinus floor with autogenous bone for placement of endosseous implants: a preliminary report." *J Oral Maxillofac Surg*.; 51: 1198-203.

Adell R, Lekholm U, Grondahl K, Branemark P-I, Lindstorm J, Jacobsson M. 1990. "Reconstruction of severly resorbed endentulous maxillae using osseointegrated fixtures in immediate autogenous bone grafts." *Int J Oral Maxillofac Implants*. 5: 233-46.

Kahnberg KE, Nystrom E, Bartholdsson L. 1989. "Combined use of bone grafts and Branemark fixtures in the treatment of severely resorbed maxillae." *Int J Oral Maxillofac Implants*. 4: 297-304.

Nystrom E, Kahnbourg KE, Gunne J. 1993. "Bone grafts and Branemark implant in the treatment of the severely resorbed maxilla." *Int J Oral Maxillofac Implants*. 8:45-53

Wood RM, Moore DL. 1988. "Grafting of the maxillary sinus with intraorally harvested autogenous bone prior to implant placement." *Int J Oral Maxillofac Implants.* 3: 209 – 14.

Rummelhart JM, Mellonig JT, Gray JL, Towle HJ. 1989. "A comparison of freeze-dried bone allograft and demineralized freeze-dried bone allograft in human periodontal osseous defects." *J Periodontol.* 60: 655-63.

Mellonig JT. 1984. "Decalcified freeze- dried bone allograft as an implant material in human periodontal defects." *Int J Periodontics Restorative Dent.* 4:40-55.

Tatum OH Jr, Lebowitz MS, Tatum CA, Borgner RA. 1993 "Sinus augmentation: rationale, development, long term results." *NY state Dent J.* 59: 43 -8.

Tatum OH Jr. 1996. "Osseous grafts in intraoral sites." *J Oral Implantol.* 22:51-2.

Fetner AE, Hartigan MS, Low SB. 1994. "Periodontal repair using Perioglass in nonhuman primates: clinical and histologic observations." *Compendium.* 15: 932, 935-38.

Schepers E, de Clercq M, Ducheyne P, Kempeneers R. 1991. "Bioactive glass particulate materials as filler for bone lesions." *J Oral Rehabil.* 18: 439-52.

Schepers E, Ducheyne P, Barbier H, Schepers S. 1993. "Bioactive glass particles of narrow size range: A new material for the repair of bone defects." *Implant Dent.* 2: 151-56.

Smiler DG, Johnson PW, Lozada JL, Misch C, Rosenlicht JL, Tatum OH Jr et al. Sinus lift grafts and endosseous implants. Treatment of the atrophic posterior maxilla. Dent Clin North Am. 1992; 36: 151-86.

McAllister BS, Margolin MD, Cogan AG, Buck D, Hollinger JO, Lynch SE. 1999. "Eighteen-month radiographic and histologic evaluation of sinus grafting with anorganic bone in the chimpanzee." *Int J Oral Maxillofac Implants.* 14: 361-68.

Wagner J. 1989. "Clinical and histological case study using resorbable hydoxylapatite for the repair of osseous defects prior to endosseous implant surgery." *J Oral Implantol.* 15: 186-92.

Koole R, Bosker H, van der Dussen FN. 1989. "Late secondary autogenous bone grafting in cleft patients comparing mandibular (ectomesenchymal) and iliac crest (mesenchymal) grafts." *J Craniomaxillofac Surg.* 17 Suppl 1: 28-30.

Garg AK. 1996. Practical implant dentistry. Houston, TX: Taylor Publishing Company. Buser D, Dula K, Hirt HP, Schenk RK. 1996. "Lateral ridge augmentation using autografts and barrier membranes. A clinical study with 40 partially edentulous patients." *J Oral Maxillofac Surg.* 54: 420-32.

Hislop WS, Finlay PM, Moos KF. 1993. "A preliminary study into the uses of anorganic bone in oral and maxillofac surgery." *Br J Oral Maxillofac Surg.* 31: 149-53.

Roberts WE, Turley PK, Brezniak N, Fielder PJ. 1987. "Implants. Bone physiology and metabolism." *Calif Dent Assoc J.* 15: 54-61.

Longacre JJ, Converse JM, Knize DM. 1977. "Transplantation of bone. In: Converse JM, editors. Reconstructive plastic surgery: principles and procedure in correction, reconstruction and transplantation. 2nd ed." Philadelphia: WB Saunders. 313-39.

Fonseca RJ, Frost D, Zeitler D, Stoelinga PJW. 1986. "Osseous reconstruction of edentulous bone loss." In *Reconstructive preprosthetic oral and maxillofacial surgery*, edited by Fonseca RJ, Davis WH. 117-65. Philadelphia: WB Saunders.

Acil Y, Springer IN, Broek V, Terheyden H, Jepsen S. 2002. "Effect of bone morphogenic proteins-7 stimulation on osteoblasts cultured on different biomaterials." *J Cell Biochem.* 86: 90-8.

Wikesjo UM, Sorensen RG, Kinoshita A, Wozney JM. 2002. "Rh BMP- 2/ alpha-BSM induce significant vertical alveolar ridge augmentation and dental implant osseointegration." *Clin Implant Dent Res.* 4: 173-81.

Meffert RA. 1998. "Current usage of bone fill as an adjunct in implant dentistry." *Dent Implantol Update*. 9:9-12.

Feuille F, Knapp CI, Brunsvold MA, Mellonig JT. 2003 "Clinical and histologic evaluation of bone-replacement grafts in the treatment of localized alveolar ridge defects. Part I: Mineralizied freeze- dried bone allograft." *Int J Periodontics Restorative Dent*. 23: 29-35.

Masullo C. 1995. "Estimate of the theoretical risk of transmission of Creutzfeldt Jakob disease by human dura mater grafts manufactured by the Tutoplast process: a commissioned report for Bio-dynamics International." Rowe, Italy: Institute of Neuorology, Catholic University.

Gunther KP, Scharf HP, Pesch HJ, Puhl W. 1996. "Osteointegration of solvent - preserved bone transplants in an animal model." *Osteology*. 5: 4-12.

Sener BC, Tasar F, Akkocaoglu M, Ozgen S, Kasapouglu O. 1998. "Use of allogenic bone grafts in onlay and sandwich augmentation technique." Paper presented at the XIV Congress of the European Association for Cranio- Maxillofacial Surgery in Helsinki, Finland, Sep 1-5.

Becker W, Urist M, Becker BE, Jackson W, Parry DA, Bartold M, et al. 1996. "Clinical and histologic observations of sites implanted with intraoral autologous bone grafts or allografts. 15 human case reports." *J Periodontol*. 67: 1025-33.

Dalkyz M, Ozcan A, Yapar M, Gokay N, Yuncu M. 2000. "Evaluation of the effects of different biomaterials on bone defects." *Implant Dent*. 9:226-35.

Alexopoulau M, Semergidis T, Sereti M. 1998. "Allogenic bone grafting of small and medium defects of the jaws." Paper presented at the XIV Congress of the European Association for Cranio- Maxillofacial Surgery in Helsinki, Finland, Sep 1-5.

Brugnami F, Then PR, Moroi H, Leone CW. 1996. "Histologic evaluation of human extraction sockets treated with deminerialized freeze-dried bone allograft (DFDBA) and cell occlusive membrane." *J Periodontol*. 67: 821-5.

Zhang M, Powers RM Jr, Wolfinbarger L Jr. 1997. "A Quantitative assessment of osteoinductivity of human demineralized bone matrix." *J Periodontol*. 68: 1076-84.

Schwartz Z, Mellonig JT, Carnes DL, de la Fontaine J. 1996. "Ability of Commercial demineralized freeze- dried bone allograft to induce new bone formation." *J Periodontol*. 67: 918-26.

Masters LB, Mellonig JT, Brunsvold MA, Nummikoski PV. 1996. "A Clinical evaluation of demineralized freeze-dried bone allograft in combination with tetracycline in the treatment of periodontal osseous defects." *J Periodontol*. 67:770-81.

Bowers G, Felton F, Middleton C. 1991. "Histologic comparison of regeneration in human intrabony defects when osteogenin is combined with demineralized freeze- dried bone allograft and with purified bone collagen." *J Periodontol*. 62: 690-702.

Takikawa S, Bauer TW, Kambic H. Togawa D. 2003. "Comparative evaluation of the osteoinductivity of two formulations of human demineralized bone matrix." *J Biomed Mater Res*. 65A: 37-42.

Gendler E. 1986. "Perforated demineralized bone matrix: a new form of osteoinductive biomaterial." *J Biomed Mater Research*. 20: 687-97.

Mckibbin B. 1978. "The biology of fracture healing in long bones." *J Bone Joint Surg Br*. 60B:150-62.

Peck WA. 1981. "Osteoporosis as a disturbance in the local regulation of bone cell activity." In *Osteoporosis*, edited by J Menczel, G.C. Robin, M. Makin and R Steinberg. 191-94. New York: John Wiley.

Meffert RM, Thomas JR, Hamilton KM, Brownstein CN. 1985. "Hydroxylapatite as an alloplastic graft in the treatment of human periodontal osseous defects." *J Periodontol*. 56: 63-73.

Le Geros RZ. 1988. "Calcium phosphate materials in restorative dentistry: a review." *Adv Dent Res*. 2: 164-80.

Le Geros RZ. 1983. "Properties of commercial bone grafts compared to human bone and new synthetic bone. Biomaterials." In *Program and abstracts of the 9th annual meeting of the Society for Biomaterials.* Abstract 86. Birmingham AL.

Masters DH. 1988. "Bone, bone substitute." *Calif Dent Assoc J*. 16: 56-65.

ToFe AJ, Watson BA, Bowerman MA. 1991. "Solution and cell mediated resorption of grafting materials." *J Oral Implantol*. 17: 345 abstract.

Jarcho M. 1981. "Calcium phosphate ceramics as hard tissue prosthetics." *Clin Orthop Relat Res*. 157: 259-78.

Heimke G, Griss P. 1983. "Tissue reactions to bone replacement materials." In *Bioceramics of calcium phosphate*, edited by de Groot K. 79-94. Boca Raton, FL: CRC Press.

Swart JGN, Rejda BV, de Groot K. 1979. "Porous calcium phosphate as alveolar bone implant." *J Dent Res*. 58 (Spec. Issue D): 2267, abstract 73.

Pinholt EM, Bang G, 1991. "Haanaes HR. Alveolar ridge augmentation in rats by Bio-Oss." *Scand J Dent Res*. 99: 154-61.

Will RG. 1999. "The transmission of prions to humans." *Acta Paediatr Suppl*. 88 (433):28-32.Review.

Scott MR, Will R, Ironside J, Nguyen H-OB, Tremblay P, De Armond SJ, Prusiner SB. 1999. "Compelling transgenetic evidence for transmission of bovine spongiform encephalopathy prions to humans." *Proc Natl Acad Sci USA*. 96:15137-42.

Vedrager J. 1999. "Risk of transmission of BSE via drugs of bovine origin." *Lancet* 354: 1304-5. Bundesgesundheitsamt. 1994. "Bekanntmachung der Sicherheits-anforderungen an Arzermittel aus Körperbestandteilan Von Rind, Schaf oder Ziege Zur Vemeidung des Risikos einer Ubertragung Von BSE bzw. Scrapis." *Bundesanzeiger*. 40: 1851-55.

Bundesgesundheistamt. 1996. "Bekanntmachung über die Zulassung and Registrierung Von Arzneimiffeln." *Bundesauzeiger*. 67: 4158-62.

Wenz B, Oesch B, Horst M. 2001. "Analysis of the risk of transmitting bovine spongiform encephalopthy through bone graft derived from bovine bone." *Biomaterials*. 22: 1599-606.

Similer DG. 2001. "Comparison of an organic bovine mineral with and without synthetic peptide in a sinus elevation: a case study." *Implant Dent*. 10: 139-42.

Krauser JT, Rohrer MD, Wallace SS. 2000. "Human histologic and histomorphometric analysis comparing OsteoGraft/N with Pep Gen P-15 in the maxillary sinus elevation procedures: a case report." *Implant Dent*. 9: 298-302.

Hahn J, Rohrer MD, Tofe AJ. 2003. "Clinical, radiographic, histologic and histomorphometic comparison of PepGen P-15 particulate and PepGen P-15 flow in extraction sockets: a same-month case study." *Implant Dent*. 12: 170-74.

Kirsh ER, Garg AK. 1994. "Postextraction ridge maintenance using the endosseous ridge maintenance implant (ERMI)." *Compendium*. 15: 234-38.

Wilson J, Clark AE, Hall M, Hench LL. 1993. "Tissue response to Bioglass endosseous ridge maintenance implants." *J Oral Implantol*. 19: 295-302.

Oonishi H, Kushitani S, Yasukawa E et al. 1994. "Bone growth into spaces between 45S5 bioglass granules." In Bioceramics, Vol 7: Proceedings of the 7th International Symposium on Ceramics in Medicine July 28-30, Turku, Finland, edited by Andersson OH, Yi-urpo A. 139-44. Oxford: Butterworth-Heinemann

Quinones CR, Lovelace TB. 1997. "Utilization of bio-active synthetic particulate for periodontal therapy and bone augmentation techniques." *Pract Periodont Aesthet Dent*. 9:1-7.

Duchenyne P, Bianco P, Radin S, Schepers E. 1992. "Bioactive materials: mechanisms and bioengineering considerations." In *Bone Bonding,* edited by Ducheyne P, Kokubo T, Van Blitterwijk CA. 1-12 Sutton: Reed Healthcare Publications.

Ashman A. 1993. "Clinical applications of synthetic bone in dentistry, Part II: Periodontal and bony defects in conjunction with dental implants." *Gen Dent*. 41: 37-44.

Ashman A. 1984. "The use of synthetic bone materials in dentistry." *Compendium Contin Educ Dent*. 13: 1020-34.

Boyne PJ. 1995. "Study of the use of HTR in tooth extraction socket to maintain alveolar ridge height and increase concentration of alveolar bone matrix." *Gen Dent*. 43: 470-3.

Boyne PJ. 1991. "Comparison of Bio-Oss and other implant materials in the maintenance of the alveolar ridge of mandible in man." In *International Symposium on Modern Trends in Bone Substitutes 1990 May Lucerne, Switzerland,* edited by Huggler AH, Kuner EH. 98-103. Hefte Zur Unfallheilkunde, Heft 216, Hrsg. Springer-Verlag.

Misch CE. 1990. "Divisions of available bone in implant dentistry." *Int J Oral Implantol*. 7: 9-17.

Misch CE. 1993. "Edentulous alveolar ridge augmentation and restorative grafting: residual ridge augmentation." In *Contemporary Implant Dentistry,* edited by Misch CE. 422-431. St. Louis: CV. Mosby.

Khan O, Ell PJ, Jarritt PH, Cullum ID, Williams ES. 1981. "Comparism between emission and transmission computed tomography of the liver." *Clin Res Ed*. 283: 1212-4.

Khan O, Ell PJ, Jarrit PH, Cullum ID. 1980. "Radio Iso-tope Section Scanning." *Cancer Res*. 40:3059-64.

Ell PJ, Khan O, Jarrit PH, Callum ID. 1981. "Radionuclide section scanning." *Semin Nucl Med*. 1: 50-60

Flood TR, Russel K. 1998. "Reconstruction of nasal defects with implant on retained nasal prosthesis." *Br J Oral Maxillofac Surg*. 36:341-5.

Lima RS, De Lorenzo A, Pantoja MR, Siqueira A. 2004. "Incremental prognostic value of myocardial perfusion 99m-technetium-sestamibi SPECT in the elderly." *Int J Cardiol*. 93:137-43.

Van der Wall H, Fogelman I. 2007. "Scintigraphy of benign bone disease." *Semin Musculoskelet Radiol*. 11: 281-300.

Horger M, Bares R. 2006. "The role of single-photon emission computerized tomography/ computed tomography in benign and malignant bone diseases." *Semin Nuci Med*. 36: 286-94.

Schafers KP, Stegger L. 2008. "Combined imaging of molecular function and morphology with PET/CT and SPECT/CT: image fusion and motion correction." *Basic Res Cardiol*. Mar 103: 191-9.

Dasgeb B, Mulligan MH, Kim CK. 2007. "The current status of bone scintigraphy in malignant disease." *Semin Musculoskelet Radiol*. 11: 301-11.

Sarikaya I, Sarikaya A, Holder LE. 2001. "The role of single photon emission computerized tomography in bone imaging." *Semin Nuci Med*. 31: 3-16.

Ozyurt G, Kaya FN, Kahveci F, Alper E. 2008. "Comparison of SPECT findings and neuropsychological sequele in carbon monoxide and organophosphate poisoning." *Clin Toxicol (Phila)*. 46: 218-21.

Kalita J, Misra UK, Ranjan P, Pradhar PK. 2008. "Pattern of cerebella perfusion on single emission computed tomography in sub cortical hematoma: a clinical and computed tomography correlation." *Neurol India*. 56: 17-21.

Crespo C, Gallego J, Cot A, Falcon C, Bullich S, Pareto D, Aguiar O et al. 2008. "Quantification of dopaminergic neurotransmission SPECT studies with 1231-labelled radioligands: a comparison between different imaging system and data acquisition protocol using Monte Carlo Simulation." *Eur J Nucl Med Imaging*. 35: 1334-42.

Massardo T, Lavados H, Jaimovich R, Herrera E, Quevedo L, Alfaro L et al. 2008. "Interobserver correlation in the interpretation of 99m Tc sestamibi SPECT in reperfused acute myocardial infarction." *Rev Esp Med Nuci*. 27: 83-9.

Ellis RJ, Zhon EH, Fu P, Kaminsky DA, Sodee DB, Faulhaber PF, et al. 2008. "Single photon emission computerized tomography with c apromab pendetide plus computed tomography image set co-registration independently predicts biochemical failure." *J Urol*. 179: 1768-73.

Alberto PL. 1998. "Implant reconstruction of the jaws and craniofacial skeleton." *Mt Sinai J Med*. 65: 316-21.

Galasko CS. 1975. "The pathologic basis for skeletal scintigraphy." *J Bone Joint Surg Br*. 57: 353-9.

Ogunsalu et al. 2008. "Single photon emission computerized tomography and histological evaluation in the validation of a new technique for the closure of oro-antral communication: an experimental study in pigs." *West Indian Med J*. Mar; 57(2):166-72.

Ogunsalu C, Ezeokoli C, Daisley H, Adogwa A, Watkins J, Archibald A et al. 2008. "Single photon emission computerized tomography in the evaluation of the osteoblastic activities of a new bone regeneration technique: analysis of 12 mandibular sites in six experimental pigs." *West Indian Med J*. 57(5): 500-7.

Ogunsalu C, Archibald A, Watkins J, Stoian C, Ezeokoli C, Daisley H, et al. 2008 . "Comparative study of the osteoblastic activity of two implant systems (Endopore versus Entegra) utilizing Single Photon Emission Computerized Tomography (SPECT): Experimental study in pigs model." Paper presented at the 16th General Meeting and Biennial Conference of the Caribbean Academy of Science, Grande Anse, Grenada, Oct 11-13.

C. Ogunsalu, C, Ezeokoli, A Archibald, J Watkins, C Stoian, H. Daisley et al. 2008. "Comparative study of osteoblastic activity of same implant (Endopore) in immediate extraction site utilizing single photon emission computerized tomography: Peri-implant autogenous bone grafting with GTR versus no peri-implant bone grafting- Experimental study in pig model" Paper presented at the 16th General Meeting and Biennial Conference of the Caribbean Academy of Science, Grande Anse, Grenada, Oct 11-13.

Ell PJ, Khan O, Jarrit PJ, Callum ID. Radionuclide section scanning; an atlas of clinical cases. Chapter 3, Clinical results. London: Chapman and Hall; 1982. p. 45-60.

Khan O, Archibald A, Thompson E, Maharaj P. 2000. "The role of quantitative single photon emission computerized tomography (SPECT) in the osseous integration process of dental implants." *Oral Surg Oral Med Oral Pathol Oral Radiol Endod*. 90: 228-30.

Ogunsalu C. 2009. "Double-Guided Bone Regeneration using the Ogunsalu sandwich regeneration technique: single photon emission computerized Tomography, Histology, and Histomorphometric analysis." PhD thesis, The University of the West Indies St. Augustine.

5

Ultrastructure of Dentogingival Border of Normal and Replanted Tooth and Dental Implant

Takashi Sawada[1] and Sadayuki Inoue[2]
[1]*Department of Ultrastructural Science, Tokyo Dental College,*
[2]*Department of Anatomy and Cell Biology, McGill University,*

1. Introduction

The interface between the gingiva and the tooth enamel is characterized by the presence of an attachment apparatus composed of well-developed hemidesmosomes at the basal surface of the junctional epithelium and internal basement membrane (Schroeder, 1986; Bosshardt & Lang, 2005). This apparatus plays an important role in the firm attachment of the epithelium to the tooth and in sealing the periodontal tissue from the oral environment. High resolution ultrastructural studies in our laboratory provided further evidence of this effective sealing (Sawada & Inoue, 1996, 2001a, 2003). In the first part of this review article, the ultrastructure of the dentogingival border in a normal tooth is described in detail.

The original attachment apparatus is mechanically broken down immediately after any surgical procedure such as tooth replantation or implantation. Whether the attachment apparatus is regenerated at the dento (implant)-gingival border in either case remains to be determined. In the latter half of this article, we will, therefore, describe the ultrastructure of the dentogingival border in replanted teeth and implants based upon our recent study (Shioya et al., 2009).

2. Materials and methods

The animals used in this study were as follows: Japanese monkeys (*Macaca fuscata*) and Rhesus monkeys (*Macaca mulatta*) provided by the Primate Research Institute of Kyoto University, Kyoto, Japan; a shark (*Cephaloscyllium umbratile*) freshly caught off the coast of Suruga, Shizuoka Prefecture, Japan; and Wistar rats purchased from CLEA JAPAN, Inc., Tokyo, Japan. All experiments were performed in accordance with the "Guidelines for the Use of Experimental Animals at Tokyo Dental College".

2.1 Monkeys

The head and neck regions of 3-5-year-old monkeys were perfused, under anesthesia, with a fixative containing 2.5% glutaraldehyde and 2% formaldehyde in 0.1M sodium cacodylate buffer, pH 7.4, through the carotid arteries for 60 min. Isolated upper and lower jaws were further fixed by immersing them in the same fresh fixative for 24 hr at 4°C. Molars with associated gingiva were isolated and washed with 0.1 M sodium cacodylate buffer containing 0.2 M sucrose. An aliquot of teeth was demineralized in 10% EDTA for 6-8 weeks at 4°C. Both demineralized and non-demineralized tissues were postfixed with 1% osmium tetroxide in 0.1 M sodium cacodylate buffer for 1.5 hr at 4°C, dehydrated in a graded series of ethanol, and embedded in epoxy resin. Semi-thin sections were stained with toluidine blue for light microscopy. Thin sections of tissue containing the internal basement membrane spanning from the cemento-enamel junction to the gingival groove were prepared for observation with either the H-7100 or H-7650 electron microscope (Hitachi Co., Tokyo, Japan), with or without counterstaining with uranyl acetate and lead citrate, and operating at 100 kV.

2.2 Shark

Tooth-bearing jaws of a shark were dissected out under anesthesia with MS222 and cut into small pieces. The pieces were fixed by placing them in a fixative containing 2.5% glutaraldehyde and 2% formaldehyde in 0.1 M sodium phosphate buffer, pH 7.4, for 24 hr at 4°C. An aliquot of the specimens was demineralized in 10% EDTA for 3-4 weeks at 4°C. Both demineralized and non-demineralized tissues were postfixed with 1% osmium tetroxide in 0.1 M sodium phosphate buffer for 1.5 hr at 4°C. They were further processed as described above for the observation of semi-thin and thin sections.

2.3 Rats

Experiment I: Tooth replantation was performed by a previously described method (Ihara et al., 2007). Briefly, under general anesthesia with ketamine hydrochloride, upper right molars were luxated with a dental excavator and carefully extracted with forceps in order to avoid damaging surrounding tissues. Then, they were immediately replaced in their original sockets. Gingiva around the maxillary left first molars was used as a control. All animals were allowed free access to water and a powdered diet. For ultrastructural examination as described below, the animals were sacrificed at 1, 2 or 4 weeks after the procedure.
Experiment II: After extraction of the tooth by the method described above, a screw-type implant was immediately placed in the socket. A custom-made pure titanium implant (Ti) (Fig. 1) 1.6 mm in diameter and 4 mm in length was used (Platon Japan Co., Tokyo, Japan). Sufficient space was left between the opposing lower first molar and the implant to avoid occlusal stimuli during mastication. After the operation, the animals were allowed access to water and a powdered diet *ad libitum*. They were sacrificed in groups at 1, 2, 4 or 8 weeks after the operation.
Under anesthesia with ketamine hydrochloride, the animals were perfused with a cold fixative containing 2.5% glutaraldehyde and 2% formaldehyde in 0.1 M sodium phosphate buffer, pH 7.4, for 20 min. Isolated upper jaws were further fixed by immersing them in the same fresh fixative for 5 hr at 4°C, after which they were washed with sodium phosphate buffer and demineralized in 10% EDTA for 4 weeks at 4°C. In experiment II, implants were mechanically separated from the surrounding tissue according to the method of Ikeda et al. (2000). Both replanted teeth with gingiva and peri-implant tissues were postfixed with 1% osmium tetroxide in 0.1 M sodium phosphate buffer for 1 hr, dehydrated in a graded series of ethanol, and embedded in epoxy resin. Thin sections were stained with uranyl acetate and lead citrate before observation by electron microscopy.

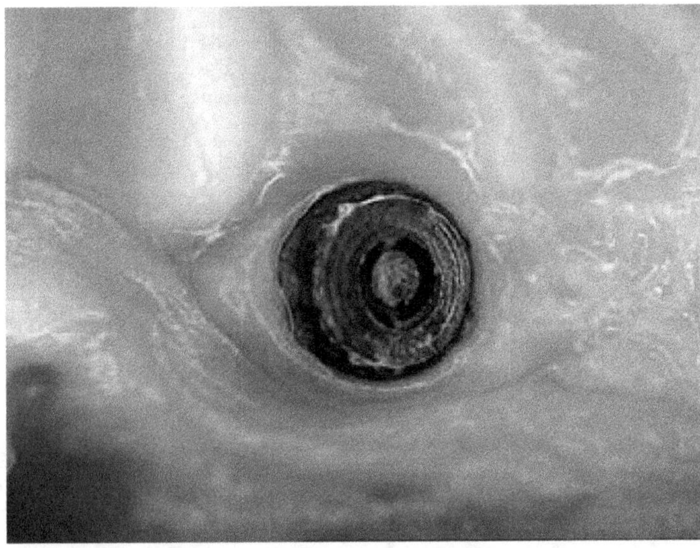

Fig. 1. Photograph showing rat upper jaw implanted with custom-made pure titanium implant

3. Ultrastructure of dentogingival border

3.1 Attachment apparatus in normal tooth

The surface (enamel) of the tooth is known to attach to the gingiva by means of an attachment apparatus. This attachment apparatus is composed of the hemidesmosomes of the junctional epithelium and the internal basement membrane (Listgarten, 1966, 1972; Schroeder, 1969; Schroeder & Listgarten, 1977; Stern, 1981). The internal basement membrane was initially described as an 80-120-nm wide homogeneous layer (Stern, 1981). It directly faced the enamel, and an intervening laminated or non-laminated layer of cuticles was found to be present in dog (Matsson et al., 1979), pig (Marks et al., 1994), monkey (Kobayashi et al., 1976; Sawada & Inoue, 2001b) and man (Listgarten, 1966; Schroeder & Listgarten, 1977). The internal basement membrane was either directly facing the surface of the enamel or doing so through intervening layers of cuticles (Kobayashi et al., 1976; Sawada & Inoue, 2001b) or afibrillar cementum in rhesus monkey (Kobayashi et al., 1976). The latter authors also reported that numerous fine strands crossed the lamina densa of the internal basement membrane at the hemidesmosomes. These strands may have been the anchoring filaments of hemidesmosomes, reported to be composed of kalinin and epiligrin (Eady, 1994; Garrod, 1993). In the cytoplasm of the cells of the junctional epithelium, the tonofibrils are associated with hemidesmosomes.

A more recent study investigated the internal basement membrane of the dentogingival border in monkey by transmission electron microscopy (Fig. 2) and found that it was uniquely specialized for mechanical strength, sealing off the periodontal tissues from the oral environment (Sawada & Inoue, 1996). Morphologically, basement membranes may be classified into three types: common, "thin" basement membranes; "double" basement membranes such as glomerular basement membrane; and often multilayered, "thick" basement membranes such as Reichert's membrane, the lens capsule, and the basement membrane matrix of mouse EHS tumor (Inoue, 1989).

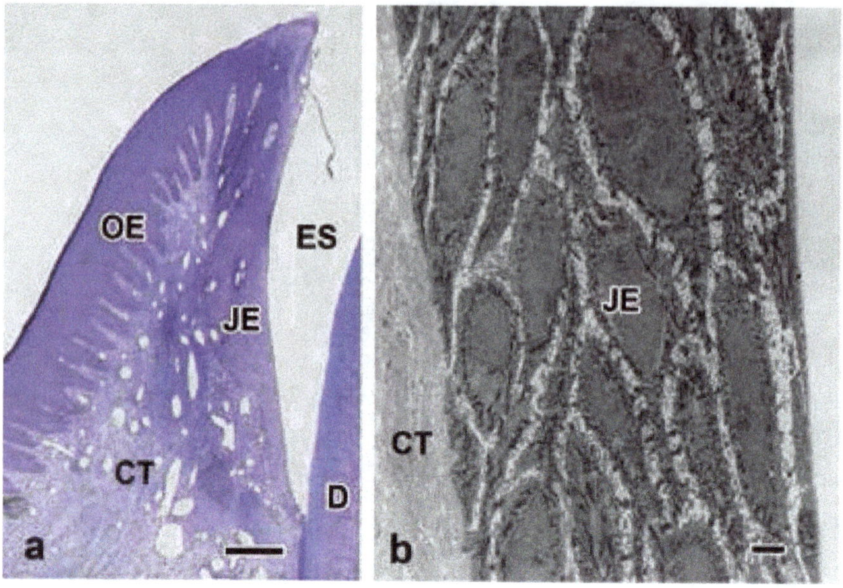

Junctional epithelium (JE) is bordered by enamel (enamel space, ES) and supporting gingival connective tissue (CT). OE, oral epithelium; D, dentin. Scale bars = 100 μm (a), 2 μm (b). Modified from Sawada & Inoue, 2003 © Calcified Tissue International.

Fig. 2. Light micrograph (a) of semi-thin section and electron micrograph (b) of thin section of an area of dentogingival border of monkey tooth

Firstly, in monkey, the internal basement membrane is unique in that it takes the form of both thin and multilayered thick basement membranes (Fig. 3). The thickening and multi-layering of the basement membrane may be directly related to the role of specific basement membranes such as the multilayered Reichert's membrane of the parietal yolk sac (Inoué et al., 1983). The capsular portion of Reichert's membrane provides reinforcement to the parietal wall of the embryonic yolk sac (Jollie, 1968). Similarly, multilayered internal basement membrane may provide mechanical strength for firm attachment of the tooth to the gingiva and the sealing off of the periodontal tissues from the oral environment. The monolayered, thin basement membrane portion of the internal basement membrane is also unique. This lamina densa, at 160 nm in width, is unusually thick compared with 30-80 nm in other types of basement membrane. Another example of unusually thick basement membrane is that of seminiferous tubules in rat (Inoue & Leblond, 1988). Again, the role of this particular basement membrane is mechanical strength to protect the integrity of the epithelium against the rhythmic contractions of the seminiferous tubules for the movement of sperm. Similarly, unusual thickening of the monolayered part of the internal basement membrane at the dentogingival border may provide mechanical strength for the tight sealing of this border.

Secondly, the finer level structure of the internal basement membrane, that is, the "cord" network, is also unique (Fig. 4). In basement membrane, in general, the basic texture of the lamina densa is made up of a 3-dimensional network formed by anastomosing, irregular, thread-like structures referred to as "cords" (Inoue, 1989, 1994; Sawada & Inoue, 2001a). In most types of basement membrane, the thickness of the cord is 3 nm-5 nm, and the average size of the openings in the network ("intercordal space diameter index") is 14 nm. The average thickness of the cords and the size of the openings in the internal basement membrane are 8.3 nm and 18.9 nm, respectively (Sawada & Inoue, 1996). These unusually wide cords and large openings are similar to those found in Reichert's membrane (5 nm and 15 nm, respectively) and the basement membrane of seminiferous tubules (4.5 nm and 14.1 nm, respectively). This indicates the role of the cord network in the mechanical strength of the internal basement membrane.

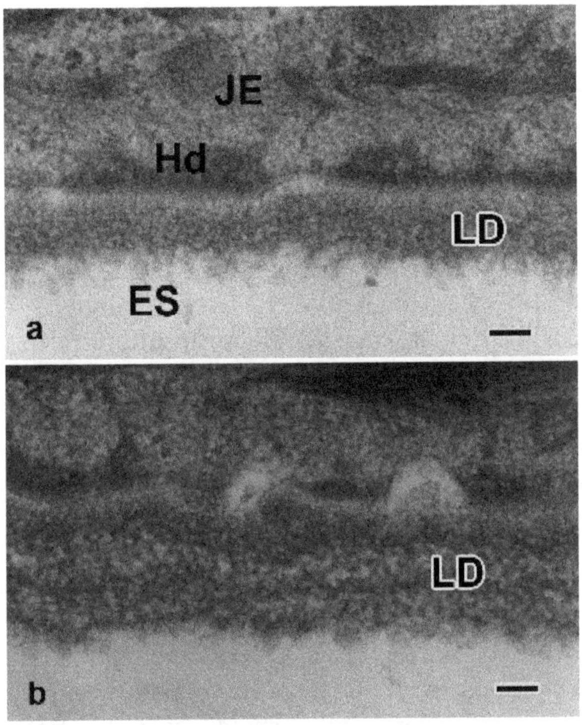

Internal basement membrane is composed of either single broad lamina densa (a) or multi-layers (b). JE, junctional epithelium; LD, lamina densa; Hd, hemidesmosomes; ES, enamel space. Scale bars = 0.1 μm. Modified from Sawada & Inoue, 1996 © The Anatomical Record.

Fig. 3. Electron micrograph of internal basement membrane of junctional epithelium

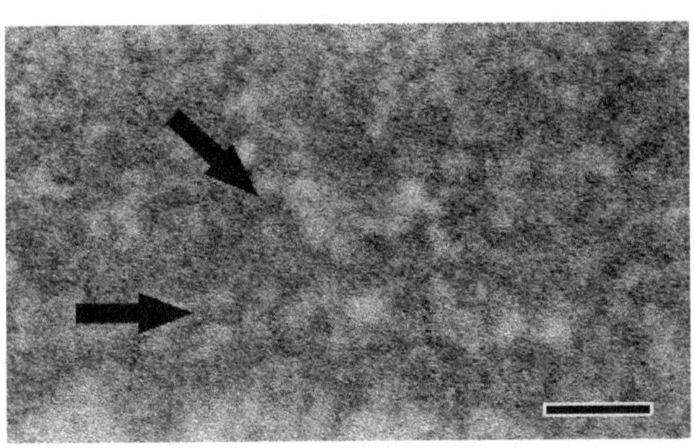

Lamina densa is composed of fine network of irregular anastomosing cords (indicated by arrows). Scale bar = 50 nm. Modified from Sawada & Inoue, 1996 © The Anatomical Record.

Fig. 4. High-magnification view of internal basement membrane of monkey tooth

3.2 Dental cuticle at dentogingival border

The dental cuticle is usually found at the dentogingival border in healthy teeth or at the surface of the roots of teeth with periodontal disease. Ultrastructurally, the dental cuticle has been described as an electron-dense, non-mineralized organic structure with an unlaminated amorphous appearance (Schroeder, 1986). In adult periodontitis, the dental cuticle covering the cementum showed a lobulated and layered structure with perforations (Friedman et al., 1993). Histochemical studies indicated that the structure may contain a protein-rich material (Kobayashi & Rose, 1978, 1979; López et al., 1990), or anionic polymers including glycoproteins (Friedman et al., 1993). Based on the results of morphological, as well as histochemical studies, the origin of the dental cuticle has been suggested to be a secretory product of the junctional epithelium (Ito et al., 1967; Listgarten, 1970; Nagatsuka, 1983; Sato, 1973; Schroeder & Listgarten, 1971), that is, either the accumulation of basement membrane components produced by the cells of the epithelium, or the formation of a layer of serum proteins originating from gingival exudates in the process of aging (Eide et al., 1983; Frank & Cimasoni, 1970; Friedman et al., 1993; Lie & Selvig, 1975; López et al., 1990); it has also been suggested to originate in hemoglobin resulting from the degradation of red blood cells (Hodson, 1966). Thus, its origin has yet to be conclusively determined.

In our previous study (Sawada & Inoue, 2001b), the detailed ultrastructural nature of the dental cuticle in monkey tooth was examined by high resolution electron microscopy. The dental cuticle, seen as a dense amorphous, usually unlaminated layer, was localized between the internal basement membrane and the enamel surface (Fig. 5a). High resolution electron microscopy showed that its basic structure was a fine network of irregular anastomosing strands identified as the cord network of the basement membrane of the junctional epithelium, as described above (Fig. 5b).

In the cuticle, openings of most of the network were filled with a dark amorphous material. Based upon the data, it was suggested that an additional layer of cord network formed from basement membrane components probably secreted by cells of the junctional epithelium during formation of the cuticle is added to the cord network of the lamina densa of the basement membrane. In addition, a dark amorphous material is deposited within the newly added cord network at the enamel side of the basement membrane. The origin of this dark material still remains to be clarified, but it possibly originates, as has previously been suggested, from either serum protein in gingival exudates or from hemoglobin produced by the degradation of red blood cells.

3.3 Mechanism of binding of normal tooth to gingiva

Detailed ultrastructural observation of the dentogingival border was carried out to elucidate how comparatively strong binding of the tooth to the gingiva is achieved in mammals (monkey) and non-mammalian vertebrates (shark) (Sawada & Inoue, 2003).

In monkey, this specialization of the lamina densa of the internal basement membrane is closely associated with an additional layer referred to as the supplementary lamina densa found on the enamel side of the tooth (Fig. 6a). Observation of non-demineralized tissue revealed that one part of the basement membrane, the supplementary lamina densa, was mineralized (Fig. 6b). This mineral deposit was continuous with that of the enamel of the tooth, and thus this deposit on the supplementary lamina densa formed an advancing edge of mineralization. Under this arrangement, two different phases, an organic and a mineral phase, overlap, with direct contact at this part of the basement membrane, ensuring intimate contact between and strong binding of these phases. Furthermore, detailed observation revealed that, in the mineralized portion of the lamina densa, mineral crystals were arranged in a network pattern which was comparable to the pattern of the cord network. This may facilitate more powerful gripping, and further demonstrates the elaborate mechanism by which firm binding of the mineral and organic phases is achieved.

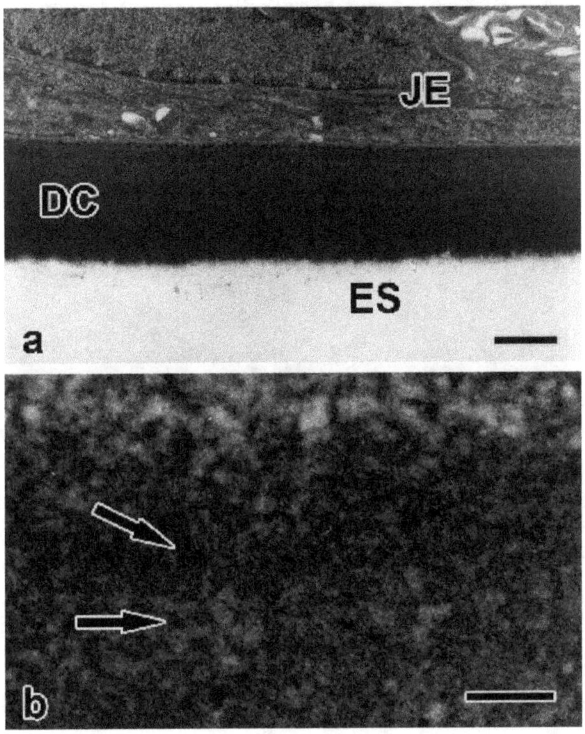

Cuticle contains network anastomosing structure (arrows) resembling cord network of internal basement membrane. Intercordal space is filled with dark amorphous material. JE, junctional epithelium; ES, enamel space. Scale bars = 1 μm (a), 0.1 μm (b). Modified from Sawada & Inoue, 2001b © Journal of Periodontal Research.

Fig. 5. (a) Dental cuticle (DC) found at dentogingival border in monkey (b) High magnification view of dental cuticle

The specialization of the lamina densa of the internal basement membrane in shark tooth was more complex (Fig. 7). Along the surface of the lamina densa of the internal basement membrane facing the oral epithelium (junctional epithelium), hemidesmosome-related, semicircular or rectangular bulges were intermittently present (Fig. 8a). In non-demineralized tissue, the entire lamina densa, apart from the specialized area of bulges, was mineralized, and this mineral deposit was continuous with that of enameloid/dentine (Fig. 8b). Furthermore, overlapping and binding of the organic and mineral phases was shown to occur throughout the internal basement membrane. Thus, in one comparative study (Sawada & Inoue, 2003), it was demonstrated that firm association of the tooth-gingiva occurs according to the same mechanism, that is, partial mineralization of the internal basement membrane, in both mammalian and non-mammalian vertebrates.

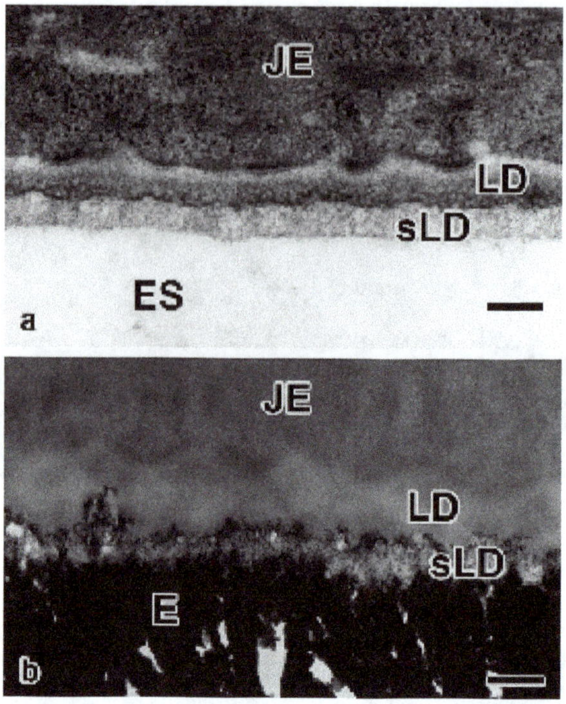

(a) Supplementary lamina densa (sLD) is well preserved after tissue demineralization with EDTA. It is composed of a network of cords similar to that of the internal basement membrane lamina densa (LD). (b) Supplementary lamina densa (sLD) is mineralized with deposit of fine mineral crystals which is continuous with mineral deposited in enamel (E). JE, junctional epithelium; ES, enamel space; LD, lamina densa. Scale bars = 0.2 μm. Modified from Sawada & Inoue, 2003 © Calcified Tissue International.

Fig. 6. Dentogingival border of monkey tooth from demineralized (a) and non-demineralized samples (b)

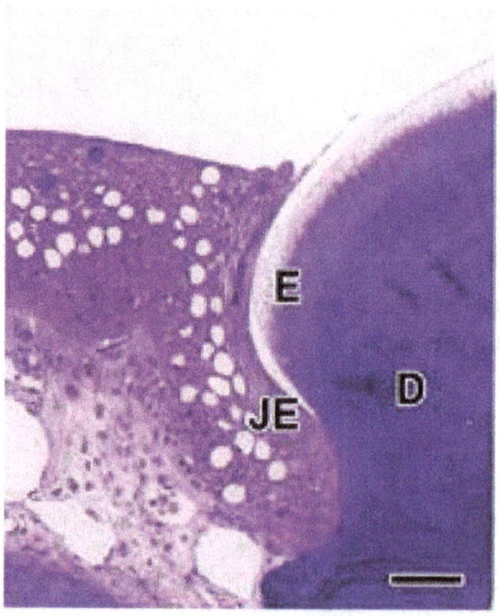

JE, junctional epithelium; E, enameloid; D, dentin. Scale bar = 100 μm. Modified from Sawada & Inoue, 2003 © Calcified Tissue International.

Fig. 7. Light micrograph of area of dentogingival border in shark tooth

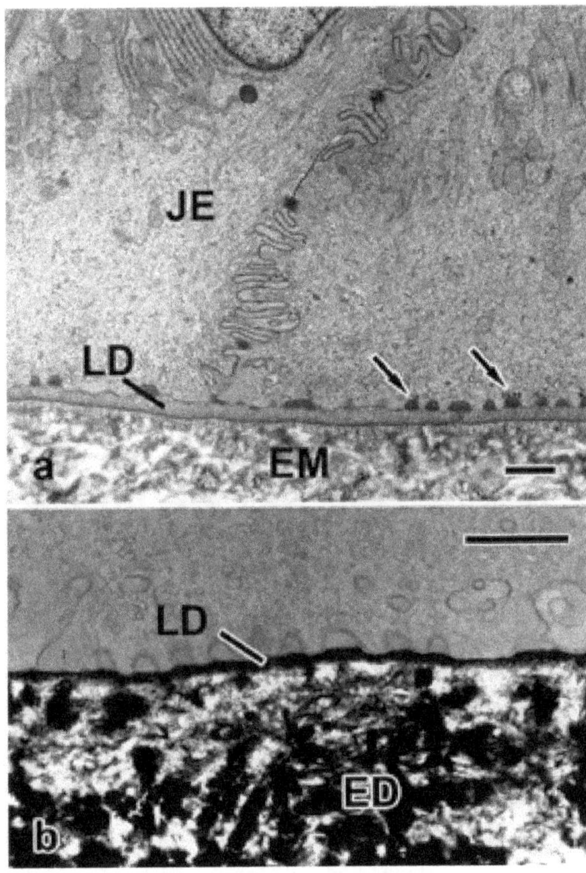

(a) Internal basement membrane of junctional epithelium (JE) is composed of lamina densa (LD) with extremely narrow lamina lucida to which semicircular or rectangular structures (arrows) are associated on its epithelial side. (b) Internal basement membrane at dentogingival border in shark tooth (non-demineralized sample). Lamina densa (LD) of internal basement membrane is mineralized by deposition of fine mineral crystals whose orientation is distinct from that of enameloid (ED). EM, matrix of enameloid/dentin. Scale bars = 1 μm. Modified from Sawada & Inoue, 2003 © Calcified Tissue International.

Fig. 8. Electron micrograph of dentogingival border in cervical region of shark tooth

Similarly, in the maturation stage of amelogenesis in monkey (Sawada & Inoue, 2000), mineralization of the lamina densa-like layer and part of the lamina densa was reported to proceed along the cords, ensuring firm attachment of the organic and mineral phases. The basement membrane of a layer of maturation-stage ameloblasts was specialized, showing an association between the lamina densa at its enamel side and a wider layer of what appeared to be an additional lamina densa (Fig. 9a). Observation of non-demineralized tissue revealed that almost the entire layer of combined lamina densa and its closely associated lamina densa-like structure were associated with enamel crystals, forming with advance in mineralization (Fig. 9b). Again, these grain-like crystals, unlike the larger needle-like crystals of enamel, were arranged along the individual cords of the cord network of the lamina densa or lamina densa-like layer (Sawada & Inoue, 2000).

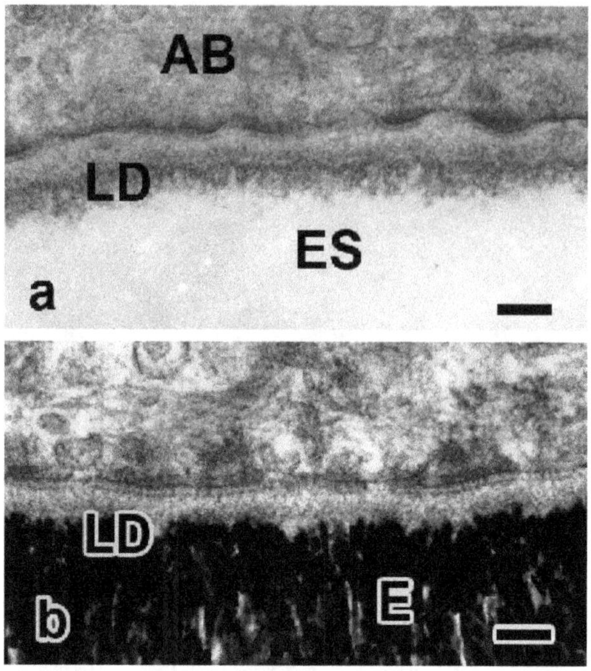

(a) Lamina densa (LD) is composed of cord network. (b) Part of lamina densa (LD) is mineralized and embedded in advancing edge of enamel (E). AB, maturation stage ameloblasts; ES, enamel space. Scale bars = 0.1 μm. Modified from Sawada & Inoue, 2000 © Calcified Tissue International.

Fig. 9. Electron micrograph of basement membrane of maturation stage ameloblasts

3.4 Dentogingival border of replanted tooth

The technique of tooth replantation has successfully been used in endodontic therapy. The original attachment apparatus is likely to be mechanically disrupted immediately following surgery. Regeneration of the attachment apparatus after gingival surgery has been reported (Listgarten, 1967; Maríková, 1983; Masaoka et al., 2009; Taylor & Campbell, 1972). However, whether or not regeneration of the attachment apparatus at the dentogingival border occurs following tooth replantation remains to be clarified. It is known that when replantation of avulsed teeth is delayed, conditions such as desiccation, bacterial infection and added inflammation cause damage to the periodontal ligament and may lead to unfavorable prognoses such as ankylosis. However, if avulsed teeth are immediately replanted with minimum extra-oral dry time, "favorable healing" results, with repair of damaged root surface by cementum (Andreasen, 1981; Line et al., 1974).

In a recent study, tissues around replanted teeth in rat were examined morphologically and ultrastructurally in detail in order to determine whether the attachment apparatus at the dentogingival border was regenerated following replantation (Shioya et al., 2009). Rat molars, luxated and extracted with care to keep damage to the surrounding tissues to a minimum, were immediately replanted into their original sockets. Most of the junctional epithelium at the dentogingival border was lost in one week. The coronal side of the enamel was covered with oral sulcular epithelium, from the tip of which a thin layer of epithelium formed and extended towards the apical side along the surface of the enamel. At the ultrastructural level, the cells composing this new epithelium closely resembled those of junctional epithelium. In addition, a basement membrane-like layer appeared along the surface of this new epithelium. Although many inflammatory cells were observed invading this area, two weeks later they had disappeared, and at this stage numerous hemidesmosomes appeared on the enamel side of the new epithelium closely attached to a newly formed internal basement membrane (Fig. 10a). Four weeks after replantation, the cells of the newly formed epithelium, which covered the enamel and extended towards the apical side, appeared almost identical to those of the junctional epithelium (Fig. 10b). No inflammation was present in the lamina propria at this stage.

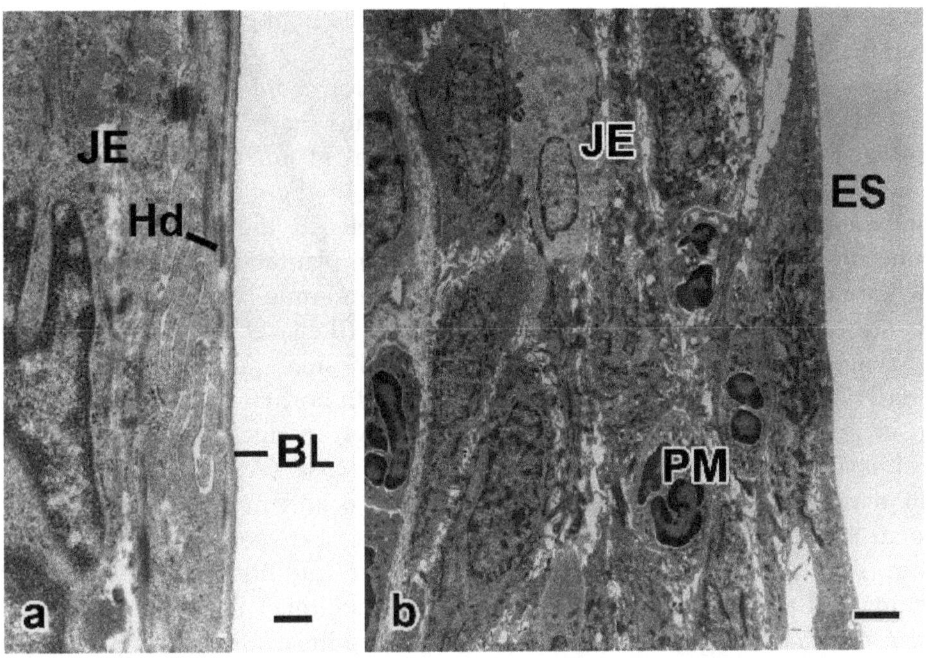

(a) Note occurrence of basal lamina-like structure (BL) at enamel surface. Well differentiated hemidesmosomes (Hd) are evident in regenerated junctional epithelium (JE). (b) Cells of regenerated junctional epithelium (JE) 4 weeks after replantation. Epithelial cells covering enamel were morphologically almost identical to cells of junctional epithelium in control animals. Polymorphonuclear leukocytes (PM) were observed between epithelial cells. ES, enamel space. Scale bars = 0.2 μm (a), 2 μm (b). Modified from Shioya et al., 2009 © Clinical Oral Implants Research.

Fig. 10. Electron micrograph showing interface at 2 (a) and 4 (b) weeks after replantation in rat

3.5 Tissues surrounding dental implants

In addition to tooth replantation, the technique of replacing teeth with dental implants has also been successfully applied (Weber & Fiorellini, 1992). As in tooth replantation, the original attachment apparatus is broken down following surgery. Views in the literature regarding the subsequent regeneration of the attachment apparatus in the peri-implant epithelium remain conflicting. The aim of the final part of this section is to describe the ultrastructure of the dentogingival border of the dental implant in detail.

3.5.1 Interface between dental implant and epithelium

A number of authors observed eventual restoration of the junctional epithelium at the surface of implants using light microscopy (Abrahamsson et al., 1996, 1999, 2002; Berglundh et al., 1991, 2007; Fujii et al., 1998; Moon et al., 1999; Schüpbach et al., 1994). A few reports dealt with the *in vivo* reconstruction of the attachment apparatus at the electron microscopic level (Gould et al., 1984; Hashimoto et al., 1989; McKinney et al., 1985). Hashimoto et al. (1989) demonstrated that the innermost cells of the peri-implant epithelium in monkey gingiva attached to a single-crystal sapphire dental implant surface by means of basal lamina-like structures and hemidesmosomes at 3 months after implant insertion. In addition, they showed a lack of attachment apparatus at the apical portion of the peri-implant epithelium.

On the other hand, no attachment apparatus was formed between plasma-sprayed ITI implants and the peri-implant epithelium of dogs, and the nature of the epithelium was closer to that of oral mucosal epithelium than to that of junctional epithelium, based on immunohistochemical results (Fujiseki et al., 2003). In their electron micrograph, many microvilli were evident at the periphery of the cells at the implant sites in place of hemidesmosomes and basal lamina after 6 months implantation. In another recent group research, formation of both internal basement membrane and hemidesmosomes was observed only in the lower region of the boundary (Ikeda et al., 2000). The presence of laminin 5, known to be important in epithelial cell adhesion and reported to be localized in the basement membrane of the junctional epithelium in normal tooth (Hormina et al., 1998; Oksanen et al., 2001), was observed by immunoelectron microscopy in the cells of the innermost layer and basal layer of peri-impant mucosa (Atsuta et al., 2005). Internal basement membrane, which also contained laminin 5 and hemidesmosomes, formed an adhesive structure at the apical portion of the interface between implant and peri-implant epithelium (Atsuta et al., 2005). These observations indicate the importance of laminin 5 in the attachment of an implant to the peri-implant epithelium. This notion may be supported by a recent study showing that a laminin-5-derived peptide coating strongly favored *in vitro* formation of adhesion structures (Werner et al., 2009).

We have demonstrated that peri-implant (pure-titanium) epithelium was formed at 1 week after implantation in rat. At 8 weeks after implantation, the leading edge of the peri-implant epithelium receded in the direction of the gingival crest, and this epithelium showed the characteristics of oral sulcular epithelium at the light microscopic level (Fig. 11a). In detailed examination, we showed that binding of the pure-titanium implant and the peri-implant epithelium was imperfect at the ultrastructural level. That is, neither hemidesmosomes nor basal lamina were present at the interface between the epithelium and the implant (Fig. 11b). No cells with the morphology of junctional epithelium were observed in the peri-implant epithelium, unlike with tooth replantation.

The discrepancies between these results were probably caused by a number of factors, including implant diameter, contact surface topology, surgical protocol, experimental period, and animal model used. A preliminary animal experiment was performed to determine whether regeneration of the attachment apparatus was influenced when $CaTiO_3$ implants were replaced with pure-titanium implants.

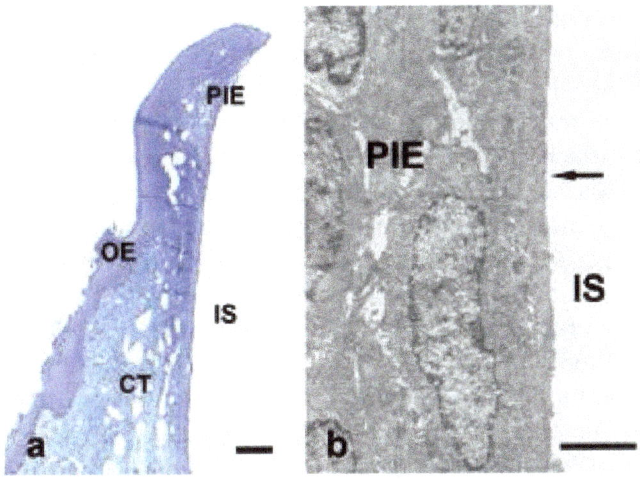

(a) Coronal side of pure titanium implant was covered by peri-implant epithelium (PIE). (b) Peri-implant epithelial-cells (PIE) resembled oral sulcular epithelial cells of control rat. Note no attachment apparatus at implant surface (arrow). CT, connective tissue; IS, implant space; OE, oral epithelium. Scale bars = 100 µm (a), 2 µm (b). Modified from Shioya et al., 2009 © Clinical Oral Implants Research.

Fig. 11. Light micrograph (a) and electron micrograph (b) of peri-implant epithelium

The results showed that no attachment apparatus was organized between the peri-implant epithelium and the $CaTiO_3$ implant (Fig. 12: unpublished data). This suggests that the surface topography of an implant does not, at least, influence the regeneration of the basal lamina or hemidesmosomes at the interface between the dental implant and the epithelium. Attachment of soft tissue to titanium implants was found not to be influenced by the roughness of the surface of the implant (Abrahamsson et al, 2002). These findings are consistent with a recent report by de Sanctis et al. (2009) showing that different implant designs and implant surfaces did not significantly influence bone healing at fresh extraction sockets.

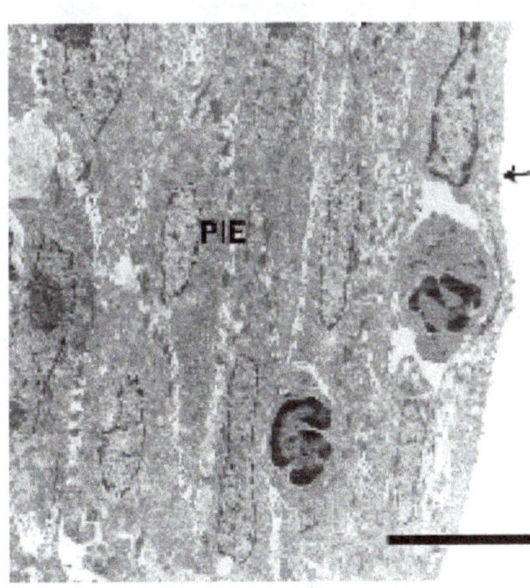

Peri-implant epithelium (PIE) lacked attachment apparatus at interface with implant surface (arrow). Scale bar = 5 µm.

Fig. 12. Electron micrograph of peri-implant epithelium at 8 weeks after implantation ($CaTiO_3$ implant)

3.5.2 Interface between dental implant and connective tissue

Alternative structures of peri-implant tissues were reported (Abrahamsson et al., 2002; Berglundh et al., 2007; Moon et al., 1999; Shioya et al., 2009). A layer of aligned, epithelial-like cells emerged within peri-implant tissue, and this cell layer was unaccompanied by any structures related to attachment apparatus, including hemidesmosomes or basement membrane (Fig. 13). This cell layer was surrounded by bundles of collagen fibrils and elongated fibroblasts oriented parallel to the long axis of the implant. This structure was thought to seal the peri-implant tissue from the oral environment. The biological significance of the epithelium-like layer of cells is not clear, but it may, as Abrahamsson et al. (2002) suggested, cooperate with fibroblasts to help stabilize peri-implant tissues.

In a very recent study, Rinaldi & Arana-Chavez (2010) investigated the ultrastructure of the interface between periodontal tissues and orthodontic titanium mini-implants in rat mandibles. The results demonstrated that a thin cementum-like layer was formed at longer times after implantation at the interface between the surface of the implant and the periodontal ligament. The cementum-like layer contained some collagen fibrils, although it did not contain collagen fiber bundles such as Sharpey's fibers from the periodontal ligament.

Therefore, the next step of our study is to elucidate the origin of epithelial-like cells and their possible functional role in the formation of the cementum-like structure forming at the interface with the implant surface.

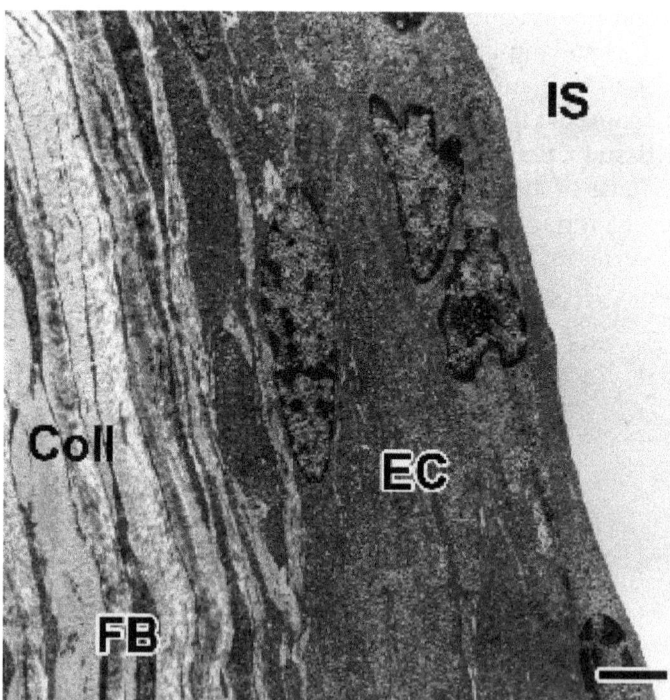

Cells (EC) showing epithelial-like alignment with narrow intercellular spaces were observed in peri-implant connective tissue, which was closely attached to implant. Cells had numerous ribosomes and a large amount of rough endoplasmic reticulum. Fibroblasts (FB) among bundles of collagen fibers (Coll) were oriented parallel to long axis of implant. IS, implant space. Scale bar = 2 μm. Modified from Shioya et al., 2009 © Clinical Oral Implants Research.

Fig. 13. Interface of peri-implant connective tissue 8 weeks after implantation

4. Conclusion

The internal basement membrane of the junctional epithelium at the dentogingival border in normal tooth is specialized for mechanical strength by means of its much wider lamina densa with unusually thick cords. In addition, strong gingival-tooth adhesion is established by partial mineralization of the internal basement membrane.

Newly formed internal basement membrane and numerous hemidesmosomes were observed between regenerated junctional epithelium and replanted teeth. On the other hand, peri-implant epithelium was preserved in the form of oral sulcular epithelium, and neither junctional epithelium nor attachment apparatus was restored after implantation. An alternative structure in peri-implant tissues was observed, comprising a layer of aligned, epithelial-like cells surrounded by collagen fiber bundles. The role of this epithelium-like layer may be stabilization of peri-implant tissues together with fibroblasts.

5. Acknowledgment

The authors would like thank Associate Professor Jeremy Williams, Tokyo Dental College, for his assistance with the English of this manuscript.

6. References

Abrahamsson, I., Berglundh, T., Wennström, J., & Lindhe, J. (1996). The peri-implant hard and soft tissues at different implant systems. A comparative study in the dog. *Clin Oral Implants Res*, 7(3):212-219.

Abrahamsson, I., Berglundh, T., Moon, I.S., & Lindhe, J. (1999). Peri-implant tissues at submerged and non-submerged titanium implants. *J Clin Periodontol*, 26(9):600-607.

Abrahamsson, I., Zitzmann, N.U., Berglundh, T., Linder, E., Wennerberg, A., & Lindhe, J. (2002). The mucosal attachment to titanium implants with different surface characteristics: an experimental study in dogs. *J Clin Periodontol*, 29(5):448-455.

Andreasen, J.O. (1981). Relationship between cell damage in the periodontal ligament after replantation and subsequent development of root resorption. A time-related study in monkeys. *Acta Odontol Scand*, 39(1):15-25.

Atsuta, I., Yamaza, T., Yoshinari, M., Goto, T., Kido, M.A., Kagiya, T., Mino, S., Shimono, M., & Tanaka, T. (2005). Ultrastructural localization of laminin-5 (γ2 chain) in the rat peri-implant oral mucosa around a titanium-dental implant by immuno-electron microscopy. *Biomaterials*, 26(32):6280-6287.

Berglundh, T., Lindhe, J., Ericsson, I., Marinello, C.P., Liljenberg, B., & Thomsen, P. (1991). The soft tissue barrier at implants and teeth. *Clin Oral Implants Res*, 2(2):81-90.

Berglundh, T., Abrahamsson, I., Welander, M., Lang, N.P., & Lindhe, J. (2007). Morphogenesis of the peri-implant mucosa: an experimental studt in dogs. *Clin Oral Implants Res*, 18(3):1-8.

Bosshardt, D.D. & Lang, N.P. (2005). The junctional epithelium: from health to disease. *J Dent Res*, 84(1): 9-20.

de Sanctis, M., Vignoletti, F., Discepoli, N., Zucchelli, G., & Sanz, M. (2009). Immediate implants at fresh extraction sokets: bone healing in four different implant systems. *J Clin Periodontol*, 36(8)705-711.

Eady, R.A. (1994). The hemidesmosome: a target in auto-immune bullous disease, *Dermatology*, 189(Suppl 1):38-41.

Eide, B., Lie, T., & Selvig, K.A. (1983). Surface coatings on dental cementum incident to periodontal disease. I. A scanning electron microscopic study. *J Clin Periodontol*, 10(2):157-171.

Frank, R.M. & Cimasoni, G. (1970). Ultrastructure de l epithelium cliniquement normal du sillon et la junction gingivo-dentaires. *Z Zellforsch Mikrosk Anat*, 109(3):356-379.

Friedman, M.T., Barber, P., & Newman, H.N. (1993). Ultrastructure and histochemistry of the dental cuticle in adult periodontitis. *J Periodontol*, 64(6):520-528.

Fujii, N., Kusakari, H., & Maeda, T. (1998). A histological study on tissue responses to titanium implantation in rat maxilla: the process of epithelial regeneration and bone reaction. *J Periodontol*, 69(4): 485-495.

Fujiseki, M., Matsuzaka, K., Yoshinari, M., Shimono, M., & Inoue, T. (2003). An experimental study on the features of peri-implant epithelium: immunohistochemical and electron-microscopic observations. *Bull Tokyo Dent Coll*, 44(4):185-199.

Garrod, D.R. (1993). Desmosomes and hemidesmosomes. *Curr Opin Cell Biol*, 5(1):30-40.

Gould, T.R.L., Westbury, L., & Brunette, D.M. (1984). Ultrastructural study of the attachment of human gingiva to titanium in vivo. *J Prosthet Dent*, 52(3):418-420.

Hashimoto, M., Akagawa, Y., Nikai, H., & Tsuru, H. (1989). Ultrastructure of the peri-implant junctional epithelium on single-crystal sapphire endosseous dental implant loaded with functional stress. *J Oral Rehabil*, 16(3):261-270.

Hodson, J.J. (1966). A critical review of the dental cuticle with special reference to recent investigations. *Int Dent J*, 16(3):350-384.

Hormina, M., Sahlberg, C., Thesleff, I., & Airenne, T. (1998). The epithelium-tooth interface - a basal lamina rich in laminin-5 and lacking other known laminin isoforms. *J Dent Res*, 77(7):1479-1485.

Ihara, I., Miake, Y., Morinaga, K., Yatsuhashi, T., Nakagawa, K., & Yanagisawa, T. (2007). Calcification of pulp canal space after replantation of immature rat molars. *J Hard Tissue Biol*, 16(2):54-60.

Ikeda, H., Yamaza, T., Yoshinari, M., Ohsaki, Y., Ayukawa, Y., Kido, M.A., Inoue, T., Shimono, M., Koyano, K., & Tanaka, T. (2000). Ultrastructural and immunoelectron microscopic studies of the peri-implant epithelium-implant (Ti-6Al-4V) interface of rat maxilla. *J Periodontol*, 71(6): 961-973.

Inoue, S. (1989). Ultrastructure of basement membranes. *Int Rev Cytol*, 117:57-98.

Inoue, S. (1994). Basic structure of basement membranes is a fine network of "cords," irregular anastomosing strands. *Microsc Res Tech*, 28(1):29-47.

Inoue, S. & Leblond, C.P. (1988). Three-dimensional network of cords: The main component of basement membranes. *Am J Anat*, 181(4):341-358.

Inoué, S., Leblond, C.P., & Laurie, G.W. (1983). Ultrastructure of Reichert's membrane, a multilayered basement membrane in the parietal wall of the rat yolk sac. *J Cell Biol*, 97(5 Pt 1), 1524-1537.

Ito, H., Enomoto, S., & Kobayashi, K. (1967). Electron microscopic study of the human epithelial attachment. *Bull Tokyo Med Dent Univ*, 14(2): 267-277.

Jollie, W.P. (1968). Changes in the fine structure of the parietal yolk sac of the rat placenta with increasing gestational age. *Am J Anat*, 122(3):513-531.

Kobayashi, K. & Rose, G.G. (1978). Ultrastructural histochemistry of the dento-epithelial junction. II. Colloidal thorium and ruthenium red. *J Periodontal Res*, 13(2):164-172.

Kobayashi, K. & Rose, G.G. (1979). Ultrastructural histochemistry of the dento-epithelial junction. 3. Chloramine T-silver methenamine. *J Periodontal Res*, 14(2):123-131.

Kobayashi, K., Rose, G.G., & Mahan, C.J. (1976). Ultrastructure of the dento-epithelial junction. *J Periodontal Res*, 11(6):313-330.

Lie, T. & Selvig, K.A. (1975). Formation of an experimental dental cuticle. *Scand J Dent Res*, 83(3):145-152.

Line, S.E., Polson, A.M., & Zander, H.A. (1974). Relationship between periodontal injury, selective cell repopulation and ankylosis. *J Periodontol*, 45(10):725-730.

Listgarten, M.A. (1966). Electron microscopic study of the gingivo-dental junction of man. *Am J Anat*, 119(1):147-177.

Listgarten, M.A. (1967). Electron microscopic features of the newly formed epithelial attachment after gingival surgery. A preliminary report. *J Periodontal Res*, 2(1):46-52.

Listgarten, M.A. (1970). Changing concepts about the dento-epithelial junction. *J Can Dent Assoc*, 36(2): 70-75.

Listgarten, M.A. (1972). Electron microscopic study of the junction between surgically denuded root surfaces and regenerated periodontal tissues. *J Periodontal Res*, 7(1):68-90.

López, N.J., Gigoux, C., & Canales, M.L. (1990). Morphologic and histochemical characteristics of the dental cuticle in teeth affected by prepubertal periodontitis. *J Periodontol*, 61(2): 95-102.

Maríková, Z. (1983). Ultrastructure of normal and newly formed dento-epithelial junction in rats. *J Periodontal Res*, 18(5):459-468.

Marks, S.C.Jr., McKee, M.D., Zalzal, S., & Nanci, A. (1994). The epithelial attachment and the dental junctional epithelium: ultrastructural features in porcine molars. *Anat Rec*, 238(1):1-14.

Masaoka, T., Hashimoto, S., Kinumatsu, T., Jung, H.S., Yamada, S., & Shimono, M. (2009). Immunolocalization of laminin and integrin in regenerating junctional epithelium of mice after gingivectomy. *J Periodontal Res*, 44(4):489-495.

Matsson, L., Theilade, J., & Attström, R. (1979). Electron microscopic study of junctional and oral gingival epithelia in the juvenile and adult beagle dog. *J Clin Periodontol*, 6(6):425-436.

McKinney, R.V. Jr., Steflik, D.E., & Koth, D.L. (1985). Evidence for a junctional epithelial attachment to ceramic dental implants. A transmission electron microscopic study. *J Periodontol*, 56(10): 579-591.

Moon, I.S., Berglundh, T., Abrahamsson, I., Linder, E., & Lindhe, J. (1999). The barrier between the keratinized mucosa and the dental implant. An experimental study in the dog. *J Clin Periodontol*, 26(10): 658-663.

Nagatsuka, M. (1983). Ultrastructure of the odonto-gingival junction of Japanese monkey (*Macaca fuscata*). *Shikwa Gakuho* 83(11):1387-1435.

Oksanen, J., Sorokin, L.M., Virtanen, I., & Hormina, M. (2001). The junctional epithelium around murine teeth differs from gingival epithelium in its basement membrane composition. *J Dent Res*, 80(12): 2093-2097.

Rinaldi, J.C. & Arana-Chavez, V.E. (2010). Ultrastructure of the interface between periodontal tissues and titanium mini-implants. *Angle Orthod*, 80(3):459-465.

Sato, T. (1973). An electron microscopic observation on epithelial attachment. Epithelial attachment of early stage of inflammed gingiva. *J Jpn Soc Periodontol*, 15(1):3-28.

Sawada, T. & Inoue, S. (1996). Ultrastructural characterization of internal basement membrane of junctional epithelium at dentogingival border. *Anat Rec*, 246(3), 317-324.

Sawada, T. & Inoue, S. (2000). Specialized basement membrane of monkey maturation stage ameloblasts mediates firm ameloblast-enamel association by its partial calcification. *Calcif Tissue Int*, 66(4), 277-281.

Sawada, T. & Inoue, S. (2001a). Ultrastructure and composition of basement membranes in the tooth. *Int Rev Cytol*, 207,151-194.

Sawada, T. & Inoue, S. (2001b). High resolution ultrastructural reevaluation of dental cuticle in monkey tooth. *J Periodontal Res*, 36(2):101-107.

Sawada, T. & Inoue, S. (2003). Mineralization of basement membrane mediates dentogingival adhesion in mammalian and nonmammalian vertebrates. *Calcif Tissue Int*, 73(2):186-195.

Schroeder, H.E. (1969). Ultrastructure of the junctional epithelium of the human gingiva. *Helv Odontol Acta*, 13(2), 65-83.

Schroeder, H.E. (1986). The periodontium, *in* A.Oksche & L. Vollrath (eds.), *Handbook of Microscopic Anatomy*,Vol. v/5., Springer-Verlag, Berlin, pp. 233-313.

Schroeder, H.E. & Listgarten, M.A. (1971). Fine structure of the developing epithelial attachment of human teeth, *in* A. Wolsky (ed.), *Monographs in developmental biology*, Vol. 2, Karger, Basel, pp. 1-134.

Schroeder, H.E. & Listgarten, M.A. (1977). Fine structure of the developing epithelial attachment of human teeth, *in* A. Wolsky (ed.), *Monographs in Developmental Biology*, Vol. 2, 2nd ed., Karger, Basel, pp. 1-136.

Schüpbach, P., Hürzeler, M., & Grunder, U. (1994). Implant-tissue interfaces following treatment of peri-implantitis using guided tissue regeneration: a light and electron microscopic study. *Clin Oral Implants Res*, 5(2):55-65.

Shioya, K., Sawada, T., Miake, Y., Inoue, S., & Yanagisawa, T. (2009). Ultrastructural study of tissues surrounding replanted teeth and dental implants. *Clin Oral Implants Res*, 20(3):299-305.

Stern, I.B. (1981). Current concepts of the dentogingival junction: the epithelial and connective tissue attachments to the tooth. *J Periodontol*, 52(9):465-476.

Taylor, A.C. & Campbell, M.M. (1972). Reattachment of gingival epithelium to the tooth. *J Periodontol*, 43(5):281-293.

Weber, H.P. & Fiorellini, J.P. (1992). The biology and morphology of the implant-tissue interface, *Alpha Omegan*, 85(4):61-64.

Werner, S., Huck, O., Frisch, B., Vautier, D., Elkaim, R., Voegel, J.C., Brunel, G., & Tenenbaum, H. (2009). The effect of microstructured surfaces and laminin-derived peptide coatings on soft tissue interactions with titanium dental implants. *Biomaterials*, 30(12):2291-2301.

6

Current Concept of Densitometry in Dental Implantology

Dragana Gabrić Pandurić, Marko Granić, Mato Sušić and Davor Katanec
Department of Oral Surgery, School of Dental Medicine, University of Zagreb
Department of Oral Surgery, Clinical Hospital Center Zagreb
Croatia

1. Introduction

Bone density measurement have an important clincal role in the evaulation of bone quality and volume pre-operative and bone loss during dental implant treatment. It can be based on intra-oral and panoramic radiographs, cone beam and micro-computed tomography (CBCT and CT), dual-energy X-ray absorptiometry (DEXA), magnetic resonance imaging (MR), quantitative ultrasound and laser Doppler flowmetry. DEXA is recognized by some clinicians as the gold standard for bone density analysis. Bone densitometry performed by DEXA have provided the foundation for treatment of patients with osteoporosis. However, the equipment needed is usually not available in dental clinics and its units are quite expensive. A major challenge is to develop a widespread, low cost, user- and patient-friendly tool for bone density evaulation. The most widely used densitometric method in implantology is Computer Assisted Densitometric Image Analysis (CADIA). CADIA is computer program based on densitometric interpretion of digitalised radiografic images. CADIA is most commonly used for periapical and panoramic images. Due to inexpensive, non-invasive diagnostic method, CADIA is capable to detect minimal variations of the mineralized tissue density, such as bone remodeling after flap surgery, peri-implant tissue variations after flap surgery, the healing process in the furcation area after regenerative procedures. Before digital era was introduced in clinical diagnostic practise (where images are automatically digitalized), conventional radiographic images were digitalized mostly using scanner or video camera, which resulted in 10% reduced quality of images. CADIA analysis has been reported to be highly sensitive and specific, showing a diagnostic accurecy of 87%. Digitalized 2D images are presented in pixels and 3D images in voxels. A image quality (i.e. resolution) changes according to increasing or decreasing pixel/voxel size. The three parameters of image quality are contrast, sharpness and noise. The contrast describes differences in dose, brightness or intensity in an image, the sharpness refers to the transitions between the different densities. Since densitomeric evaluation is used for comparing images, in attempt to achieve more objective and precise interpretation, it is of utmost importance to standardize criteria in radiografic imaging. For the standardisation of the intraoral radiogfraphs following criteria should be considered:

- The procjection used should minimize distortion of the anatomic structures of interest
- The method should provide information about the degree of standardization achieved

- The ionizing radiation exposure should be the minimum necessary to provide diagnostic information
- The method should be flexible enought to allow monitoring of all sites in the mouth
- The method should not be uncomfortable to the patient
- The method should not require extensive training for use
- The method should use readly avaible meterials

The most common method in standardizing densitometric technique is by using a copper calibrating stepwedge which consists of 5 layers, with the first layer presented by 0,1 in width and visible on a particular and predetermined site of the image (Figure 1). Copper is chosen due to its effective atomic number which is similar to bone. In the past aluminium

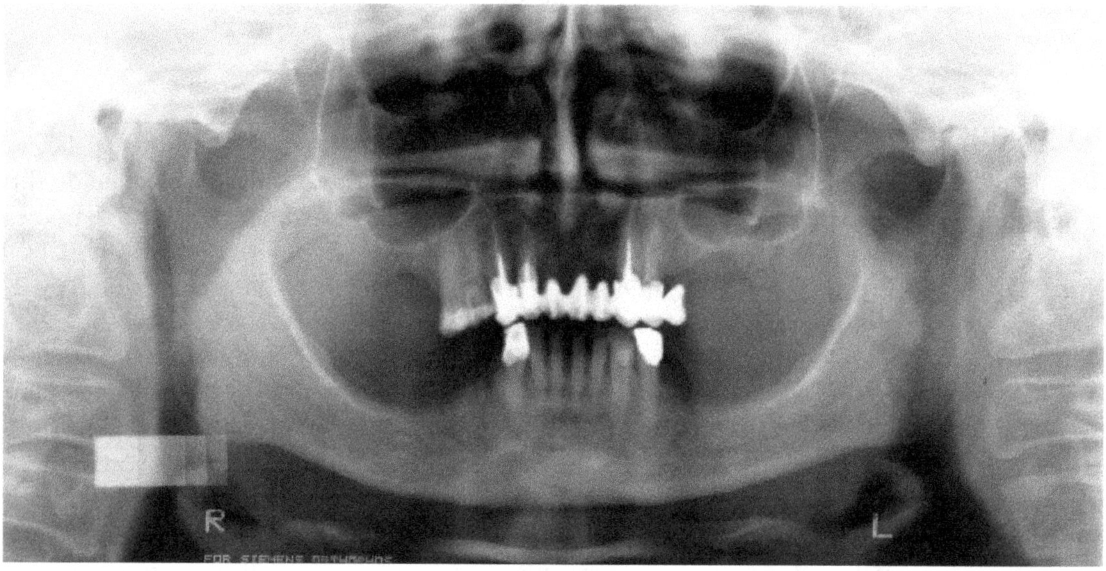

Fig. 1. Position of copper calibrating stepwedge on digital panoramic image.

was used instead, but was found to be too massive for positioning when used in retroalveolar images. In the manner of the easiest X-ray-film manipulation, many other materials such as a nickel in various thicknesses, hydroxyapatite, barium sulfate or some solutions such as CsCl or CaCl2 to simulate bone density, ethanol for fat and water for soft-tissue equivalent are in use. Stepwedge is used for linearisation, contrast-brightness adaptation and contrast optimisation for every measured image. Densitometric evaluation is based on intensity of gray shadows, which is predetermined on a scale varying from 0 (zero=black) to 255 (white) for intra-oral and panoramic radiographs. Recent CT scan devices can distinguish up to 4000 different gray shadows and therefore are far more precise, objective and reliable in comparison with periapical and panoramic images. Gray shadows determined by CT machines and its software programs are called Houndsfield Units (HU) representing a radiation attenuation for every pixel of the computer slice image. An HU value of 0 is equivalent to the radiation attenuation value of water, while an HU scale starts at value of -1000 corresponds to the value of air and generaly ends at around 3000 HU corresponding to the enamel. The density of structures within the images using CT scan is absolute and quantitative and can be used to differentiate tissuas in a region (i.e. muscle, 35-70 HU; fibrous tissue, 60-90 HU; cartilage, 80-130 and bone 150-1800 HU depending of the gradation of the bone quality). CT enables the evaulation of proposed implant sites and provides diagnostic information that other imaging methods could not. Recent CBCT scans have few advantages in a comparasion to CT witch are lower effective dose of the radiation, better device avaibility for dentist (size and price), 3D view of images insted of 2D, simple computer software device and better tool for implant placement. A lack of CBCT ,due to lower effective dose, is resolution of images compared to CT device. MR is used in implant imaging as a secondary imaging technique when primary imaging techniques such as CT or CBCT fails. MR is a technique to image the protons of the body using magnetic fields. MR depicts trabecular bone as a negative image by virtue of the strong signal generated by the abundant fat and water protons in the sorrounding tissue, whereas bone mineral lacks free protons and generates no MR signal and its not useful in charecterizing bone density. It is reasonable to say that the preoperative densitometric evaulation of bone undergoing implant placement using CT scans are far more precise than any avaible devices. When it comes to postprosthetic imaging whose purpose is to evaulate the status and prognosis of dental implant, method of choice is CADIA. Periapical or panoramic radiography produces high resoultion images of the dental implant and sorounding alveolar bone (Figure 3). CADIA have limitations in determining buccal and linqual changes in alveolar bone and depiction of the 3D relationship between dental implant and soruonding bone. CT is able to determine that changes but it cannot match the resolution of periapical image due to artifacts which produse titanium implant (Figure2).

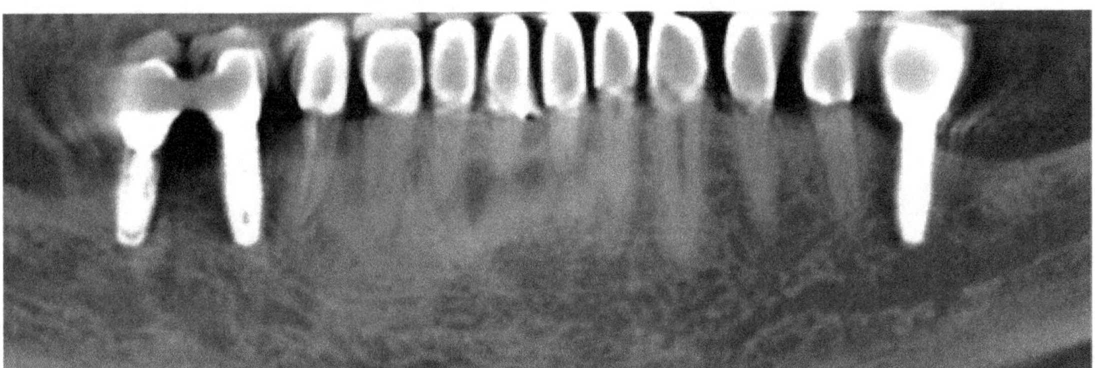

Fig. 2. CBCT scan used after implant placement shows lower resoultion of bone around dental implant due to interaction with titanium implant

2. CADIA modification

In this chapter densitometric measurement will be shown throught the modification of conventionally used CADIA and DIGORA software. Digital periapical and panoramic images were used, due to their minimal radioactive emission and high image quality that are not lost upon digitalization. Main task was to measure bone density around inserted dental implants using titanium implant itself as a stepwedge. This modification contains 12 measurement points for periapical and 10 points for panoramic images. They are precisely located in positions in and around dental implants. The measurement of bone density is obtained automatically due to performed software package after entering the RVG image. Positions of the 12 points are specified in advance and inserted in the software database,

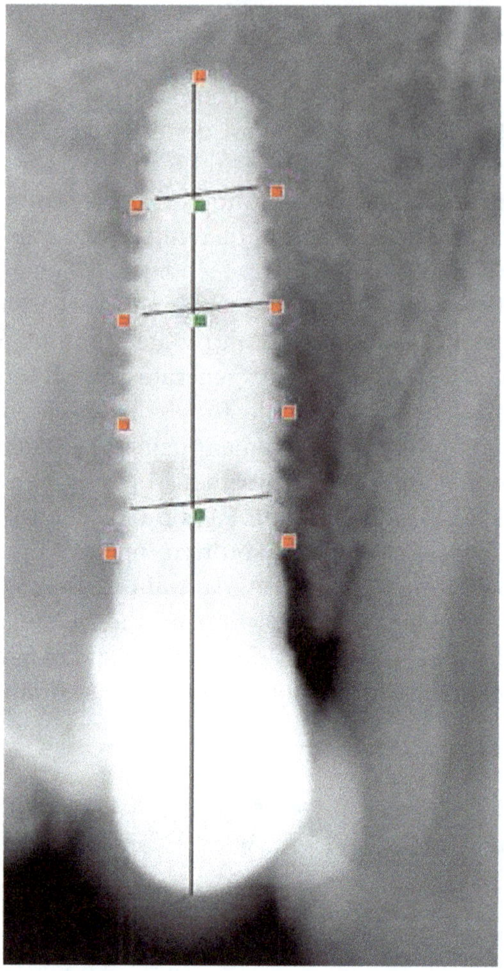

Fig. 3. Position of the correction (green) and measurement (red) points.

so the points remain in the same location for all evaluated images (Figure 3). The first 3 points are regarded as correction factors (modified stepwedge) which are situated on different parts of the implant. The first correction point is located in the apical part of the implant, where density of the gray shadows was the highest; the second correction point is located in the middle part of the implant where density of gray shadows have minimal intensity due to the perforated structure of the implant and the third correction point is located in the cervical part of the implant where density of gray shadows have midium intensity in the position where the crown screw is attached to the implant. Correction points served for revision of density change in measurements which occured due to discontinuity of the x-rays (i.e. distortion of x-rays present in each image in the series of follow-ups, as well as difference in exposition in the same series of images that were taken during a follow-up period). Measuring points are positioned as follows: the first point was placed in the middle line 1mm apically to the implant, and the remaining 8 points were placed in the bone surrounding the implant in precisely determined positions. This CADIA modification is designed to monitor changes in bone density around implants and to compare it with other images. If there is a need to precisely determine a densitometric value, original stepwedge is inevitable.

3. Usage of modificated CADIA in clinical purpose

Current modification of CADIA is in use since 2008. and there are few publications describing its use in clinical purpose about various tehniques of implant placement. In the first study complete densitometric measurement with images, grapfhs and tables will be shown while in the other cases only final images will be presented.

3.1 Comparison between flapless and two-stage techique of dental implant placement

Minimally invasive surgical techniques are a current trend, not only in dental implantology but in all surgical fields. It gives an atraumatic approach for the patients which results in better and easier accomplishment of treatment, not only for the patient but for the surgeon as well. Both of surgical techniques, two-stage and flapless, are safe methods with a long

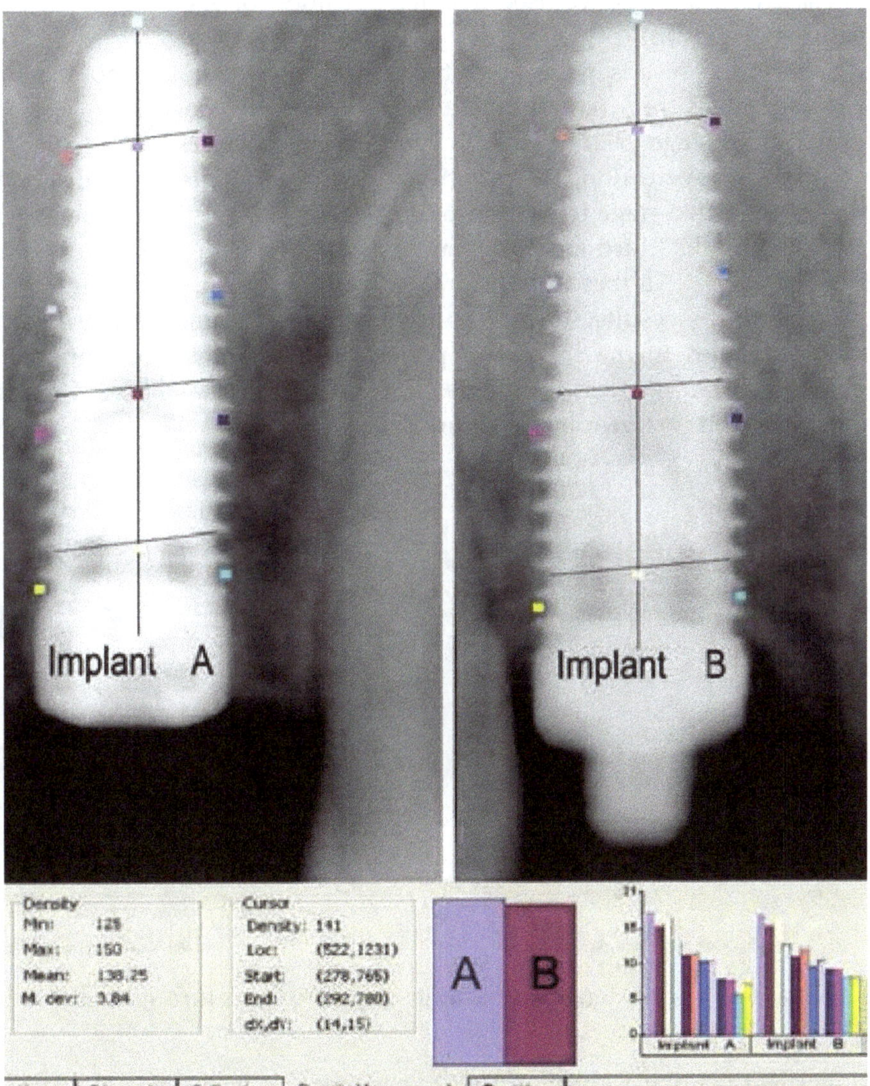

Fig. 4. CADIA comparison between two stage(left) and flapless (right) technique.

term success and satisfaction for the patients. Further cases describes radiographic assessment of flapless technique and determination of its clinical values in comparison with two-stage dental implant technique through computerized densitometric analysis. Values of densities were measured in all 10 patients through 3 months in certain time interval in 12 determined points. The first point was placed in the middle line 1mm apically to the implant, and the rest of 8 points were placed on the precise positions between 4. and 5., 9. and 10., 13. and 14., and between 18. and 19. of the screw thread, on each side of the dental implant (Figure 4).

The validaity of results in measured densities for all 5 patients, in which the implants were inserted using two-stage technique, throught all 3 measurements are shown in Table 1. The validaity of results in measured densities throught 3 measurements in all 5 patients, in which the implants were inserted using flapless technique are shown in Table 2. For easier analogy of measured densities, we used average densities for each technique according to stage of measurement.

Due to pilot study, the results were notstatistically analyzed, but compared through the values of average densities. Average value of density in period of 3 months (first measurement) in two-stage technique was 174.1, and in flapless technique were 158.8. Second measurements were done 12 months after the implants were inserted, and the results were: 172.18 in two-stage technique, and 158.47 in flapless technique. Average value of density after 18 months (third measurement) was for two-stage technique 170.86, and for flapless technique 157.57. All these results are shown in Figure 5. After mutual comparison of average densities, the results showed approximately the same decrease of density for both surgical techniques in the follow-up period of 18 months, conventional two-stage technique shown 3.24 and flapless technique 1.23. It shows minimal loss of density in both surgical techniques, as it is shown in the Figure 6.

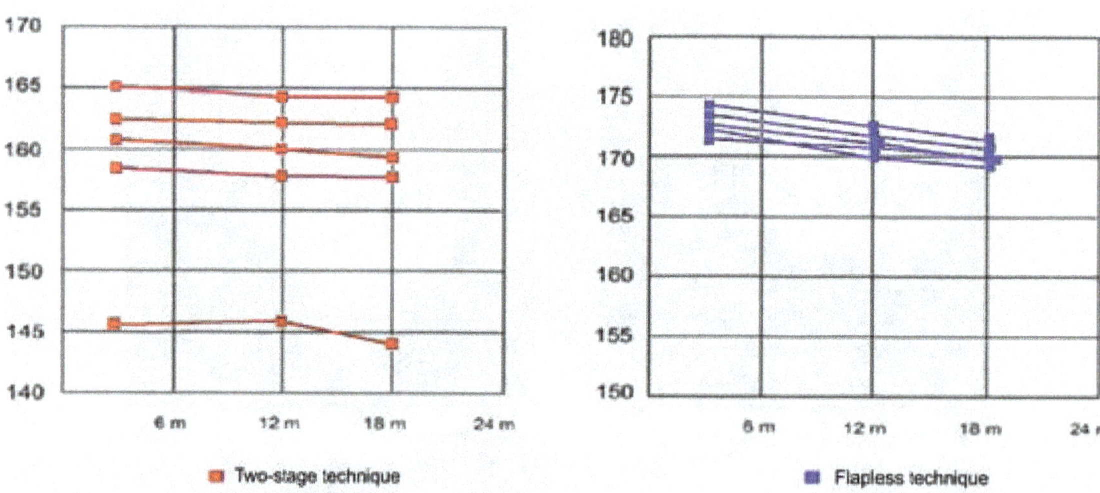

Fig. 5. Average values of bone density around inserted implants throught all 3 measurements.

After dental implant loading, values of density changes due to masticatory forces. Effect of masticatory forces can be enrolled in the changes of the bone around inserted implant with the help of densitometric analysis.

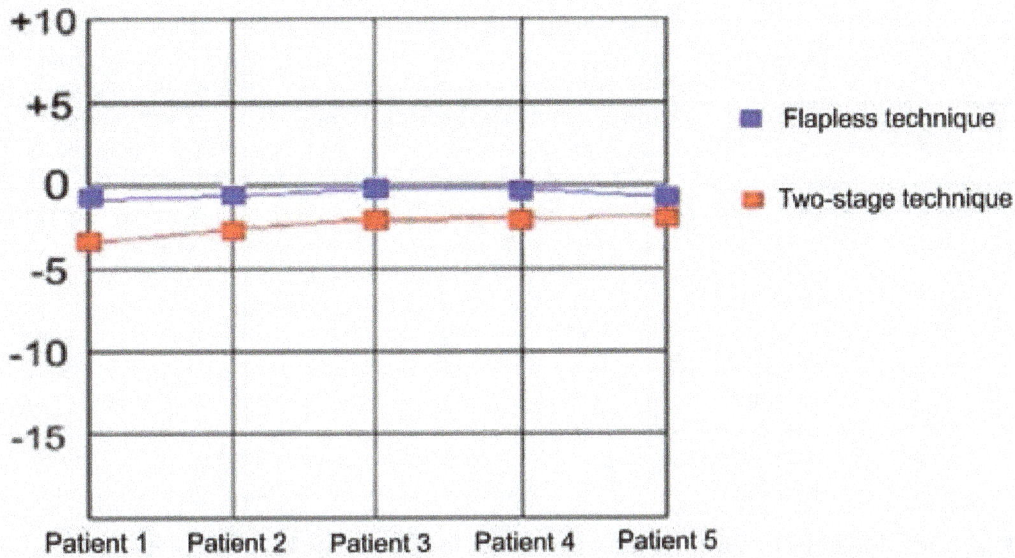

Fig. 6. Comparation of average bone densities showed approximately the same decrease of density for both surgical techiques in the follow-up period.

	Patient 1			Patient 2			Patient 3			Patient 4			Patient 5		
Point	3. month	12. month	18. month	3. month	12. month	18. month	3. month	12. month	18. month	3. month	12. month	18. month	3. month	12. month	18. month
1	254.96	255.14	254.19	254.52	255.41	254.99	254.42	254.85	254.12	253.99	254.12	254.01	253.84	254.04	253.94
2	248.23	244.21	245.74	247.91	244.82	245.83	248.35	247.68	246.07	244.25	244.58	244.56	242.38	243.15	242.67
3	247.43	251.25	250.69	249.95	251.36	251.44	250.81	251.04	251.83	248.08	247.84	247.92	247.09	246.44	246.89
4	204.16	200.31	198.22	204.16	203.54	202.38	194.69	192.42	192.1	200.74	199.86	197.94	198.53	197.69	196.99
5	190.12	187.21	183.72	191.29	189.36	188.45	193.53	191.34	189.79	185.65	186.41	184.27	184.33	183.04	182.85
6	192.82	216.23	205.14	190.21	191.24	190.41	193.74	190.95	190.41	193.54	192.85	192.41	186.37	184.65	184.22
7	177.2	179.43	179.12	172.28	174.67	173.56	177.6	177.52	177.08	174.91	175	173.57	180.7	178.31	177.68
8	180.74	176.78	172.1	181.84	180.05	179.68	184.9	182.37	181.69	184.67	180.49	179.62	182.57	179.91	179.56
9	171.4	155.62	151.12	170.69	167.66	166.95	168.67	167.44	166.55	168.55	167.21	165.74	174.39	171.24	170.77
10	166.53	162.23	169.72	169.88	163.59	160.06	174.18	175.73	174.28	178.79	177.12	174.83	174.95	172.58	171.72
11	144.71	132.87	134.21	141.41	138.48	134.59	144.69	140.25	134.52	134.07	133.43	132.07	140.55	138.69	137.41
12	143.42	137.44	140.59	140.97	137.26	133.08	141.64	138.92	136.95	144.61	140.81	138.4	139.84	138.29	137.59
Average	174.57	172.01	170.44	173.64	171.76	169.91	174.85	172.99	171.49	173.95	172.58	170.98	173.58	171.6	170.98

Table 1. Bone densities throught 3 measurements for 5 patients in the two-stage technique group.

Changes of the bone around inserted implant were mostly expressed on the points 7, 8, 9 and 10 which are located on the 9., 10., 13. and 14. thread of the implant. In the two-stage and flapless surgical technique, average values of bone density change (with the same indications) were approximately the same. Decrease of 3.24, and in flapless technique was 1.23. Due to our knowledge, there are no published results in the recent literature regarding densitometric comparison between these two surgical techniques. Most of the authors use the minimally invasive surgical techniques in everyday practice, including the flapless

	Patient 1			Patient 2			Patient 3			Patient 4			Patient 5		
Point	3. month	12. month	18. month	3. month	12. month	18. month	3. month	12. month	18. month	3. month	12. month	18. month	3. month	12. month	18. month
1	231.76	228.05	232.8	255	251.56	253.21	254.17	254.56	254.8	254.8	253.73	254.01	253.88	254.2	253.65
2	208.79	219.69	217.45	226.07	227.22	226.69	229.3	229.44	230.04	231.59	230.67	231.58	235.67	236.47	232.91
3	222.6	215.41	212.92	240.13	242.42	240.9	240.08	241.42	242.17	244.12	243.77	243.99	247.53	248.33	247.93
4	189.65	185.35	185.01	196.96	185.56	184.54	197.58	196.96	196.35	190.37	188.38	188.17	190.77	188.2	187.69
5	188.84	187.3	186.92	169.11	169.65	163.01	180.42	178.6	178.22	185.9	184.93	184.56	185.39	184.62	183.74
6	186.97	185.63	184.9	171.36	180.13	178.63	181.64	181.04	180.74	184.55	183.41	183.2	184.06	183.93	183.53
7	164.52	164.08	163.96	157.68	155.75	155.44	163.27	164.28	164.16	174.71	175.36	175.06	173.61	173.07	171.49
8	157.15	160.43	158.24	159.76	159.13	158.41	164.88	164.58	164.4	173.43	174.11	173.58	171.94	172.38	171.15
9	151.28	150.27	149.53	120.07	120.46	118.3	141.09	140.9	140.84	163.27	163.24	162.89	155.07	154.75	153.57
10	149.71	150.42	148.71	122.76	125.58	123.17	142.37	141.89	141.79	160.76	161.39	160.85	153.26	153.57	152.94
11	133.1	132.07	130.56	105.01	108.06	107.63	125.99	125.74	125.47	127.69	126.5	126.23	130.43	129.76	128.4
12	131.58	130.01	128.72	108.5	109.5	107.21	126.07	125.94	125.86	124.95	125.49	124.73	128.82	128.7	128.07
Average	161.42	160.62	159.62	145.69	145.98	144.04	158.15	157.77	157.54	165.07	164.76	164.36	163.71	163.22	162.29

Table 2. Bone densities throught 3 measurements for 5 patients in the flapless technique group.

approach in dental implantology. Becker et al. have found that implants placed without flap reflection remained stable and exhibited clinically relevant osseointegration similar to when implants were placed using conventional flap procedures. Campelo and Camara have published the most extensive study about using one-stage flapless surgical technique in dental implantology. In their 10-year retrospective study the cumulative success rate, for 770 implants using a flapless surgical technique, have varied from 74.1% to 100%, relative to the year of placement, which can be explained with a learning curve combining technology and material development in dental implantology. Survival rates in other reported studies, for flapless surgical approach, are between 91% and 98.7%5 which indicate successful results of this technique application. Based on our results, we can say that both of examined groups, and two different techniques in dental implantology show the same clinical values after 18 months of follow-up.

3.2 Comparation between two different techniques of sinus floor elevation

Prior to planning implant surgery and prosthetic reconstruction in the posterior maxillar region, it is not uncommon not to consider sinus floor elevation surgery first, which can be achieved using either open or closed technique approach, or minimal invasive baloon sinus lifting thechnique which has recently been in use. Two clinical cases presented in the literature, in which densitometric measurements were compared by both techniques of sinus elevation, the baloon sinus lifting with open and closed access. In the first case elavation of the right maxillary sinus was done by the balloon controled technique (transcrestal approach). The augmentation was done with alloplastic bone filler (tricalcium phosphate). Lifting of the left maxillary sinus was performed by forming lateral fenestration on the buccal cortical plate followed by augmentation with the mixture of xenogenic bone filler and autologous bone graft. After 6 months of augmentation 3 implants on each side were placed and prosthetic suprastructure was completed within next 4 mounths. Values of bone density were measured in 10 points around each inserted implant compared with RFA measurements of implant stability before loading and 3 and 12 mounths after prosthetic loading. After mutual comparison of average densities, the results showed approximately the same decrease of density for both surgical techniques in the follow-up period of 12 mounths. It shows minimal loss of density around inserted implants in grafted maxillary sinus areas elevated by both surgical techniques. Gained data results are showing that sinus lifting method with enclosed balloon approach techique can result in gaining enough area for implant placement as well as with opened approach technique. Furthermore balloon technique is more over less traumatic experience for patient with a much fewer side effects and postoperational problems. In addition if there is a sufficient bone width for the purpose of sinus lifting in favour of placing of two up to 3 implants in that area it can equaly sufficient use enclosed balloon technique instead of open lateral approach which is causing much more traumatised experience for patient and much more postoperative problems (Figures 7, 8 and 9).

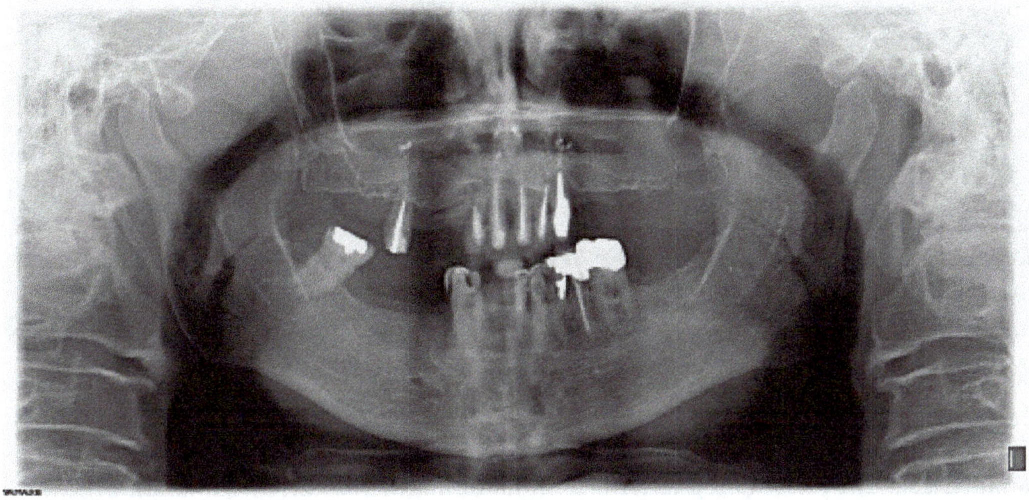

Fig. 7. Initial radiograph before surgical treatment

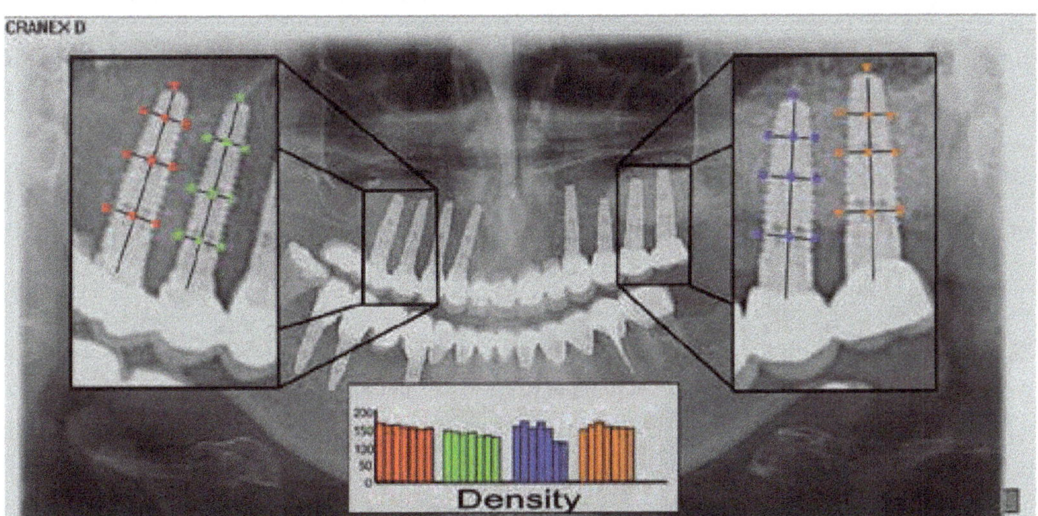

Fig. 8. Densitometric measurement of two different approaches, open sinus lift technique (red and green points) and ballon technique (blue and orange points).

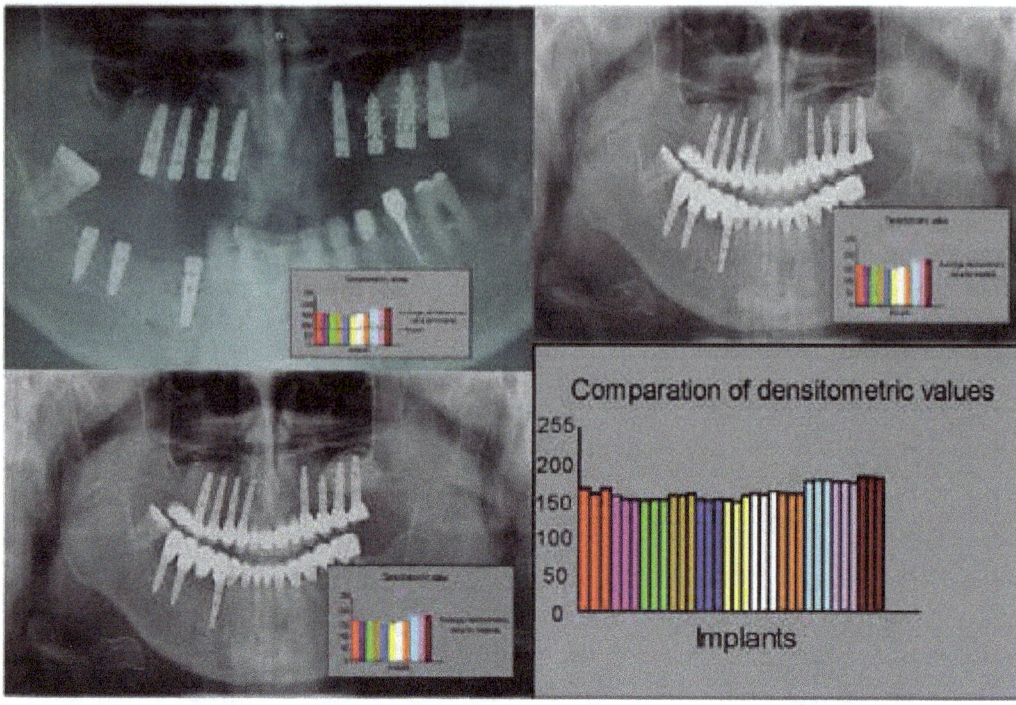

Fig. 9. Densitometric comparison between two different approaches, open sinus lift technique (left upper molar region) and ballon technique (right upper molar region). Lower right molar region was augmented using splitting technique (2 implants)

In the second case elevation of the right maxillary sinus was done by close sinus lift technique and on the left side by the ballon controled technique filled with alloplastic material (tricalcium phosphate). After 6 months of augmentation one implant on each side were placed and prosthetic suprastructure was completed within next 4 mounths. Values of bone density were measured in 10 points around each inserted implant compared with RFA measurements of implant stability before loading and 3 and 12 mounths after prosthetic loading, same as int he first case. First densitometric measurement showed, that the bone

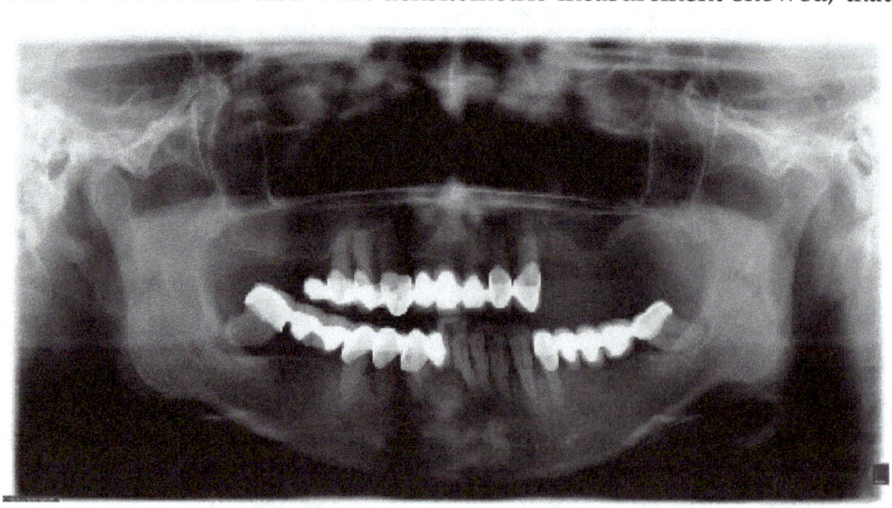

Fig. 10. Initial radiograph before surgical treatment

around dental implants augmented by ballon sinus lift technique, had twice more value in comparation with close sinus lift techinque due to bone filler. After follow-up period of 12 mounths, like in the first case, the same decrease of density for both surgical techniques were observed (Figures 10 and 11).

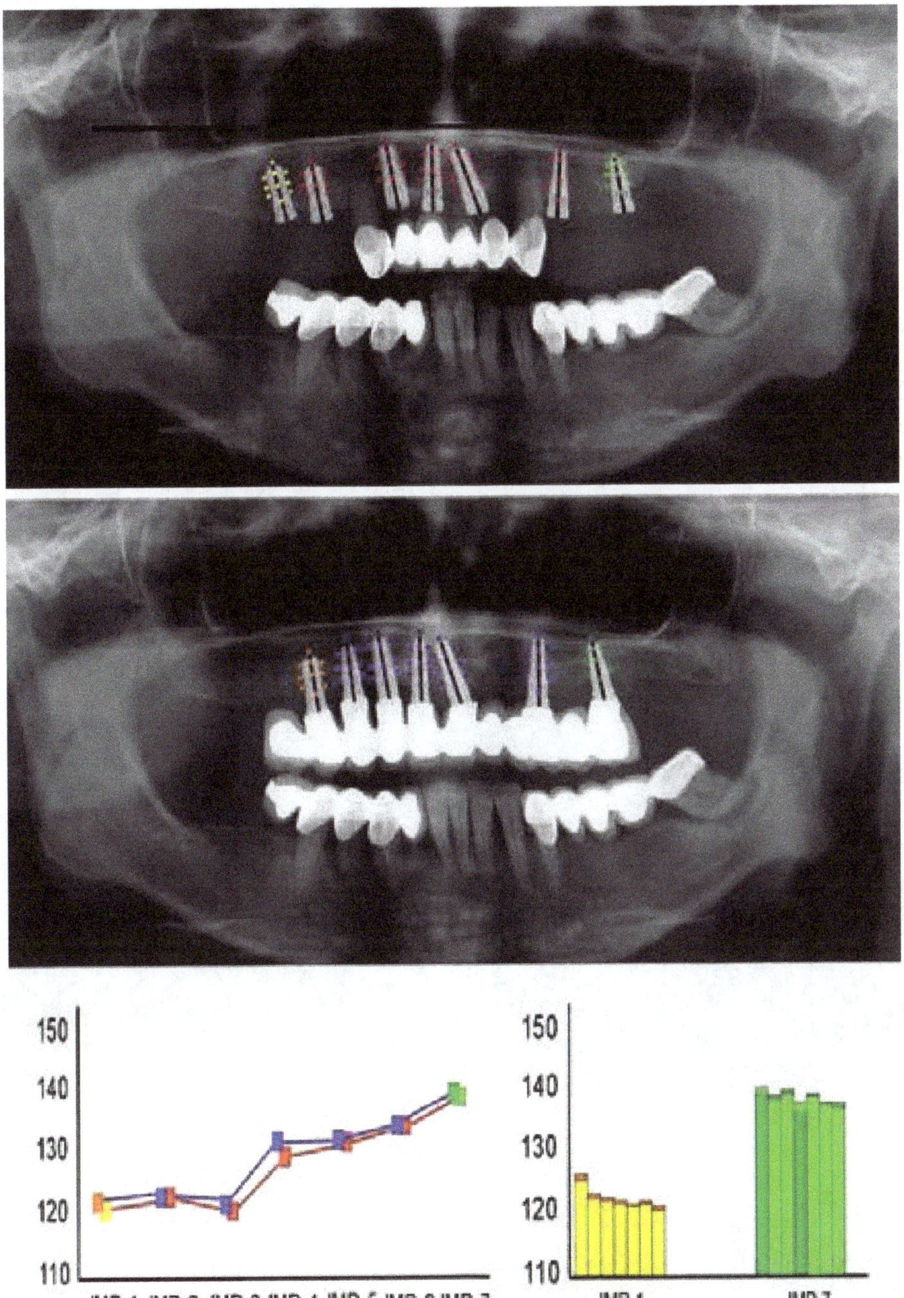

Fig. 11. Densitometric comparison between two different transcrestal approaches, close sinus lift technique (left implant and yellow graph) and ballon technique (right implant and green graph).

3.3 Alveolar ridge augmentation using splitting technique

In oral implant surgery, in order to widen the alveolar ridge and avoid horizonatal ridge augmentation by using autologous bone transplants, splitting and spreading techniques are indicated instead. These two methods are regarded as minimally invasive surgical techniques which reduce the number of surgical interventions, and result in minimally present postoperative complications, such as the patient's discomfort during the procedure. They also minimize the healing period in which it is expected to accomplish final prostetic reconstruction. Two clinical cases are shown in which densitometric measurements were compared by splitting technique and cllasic two-stage technique of dental implants placement. In the first case two implants in lower molar region using splitting technique and one implant in premolar lower region using two-stage technique were placed (Figure 8). Prosthetic suprastructure was completed within next 4 mounths. Values of bone density were measured in 10 points around each inserted implant after placement, after 4 and 12 mounths. After mutual comparison of average densities, the results showed almost nearly the same decrease of density for both surgical techniques in the followup period of 12 mounths. In the second case splitting technique is used in lower premolar and molar region, placing 3 dental implants (Figure 12). Values of bone density were measured in 10 points around each inserted implant after placement, after 4 and 12 mounths. The results showed again the same decrese of density compared with two-stage technique.

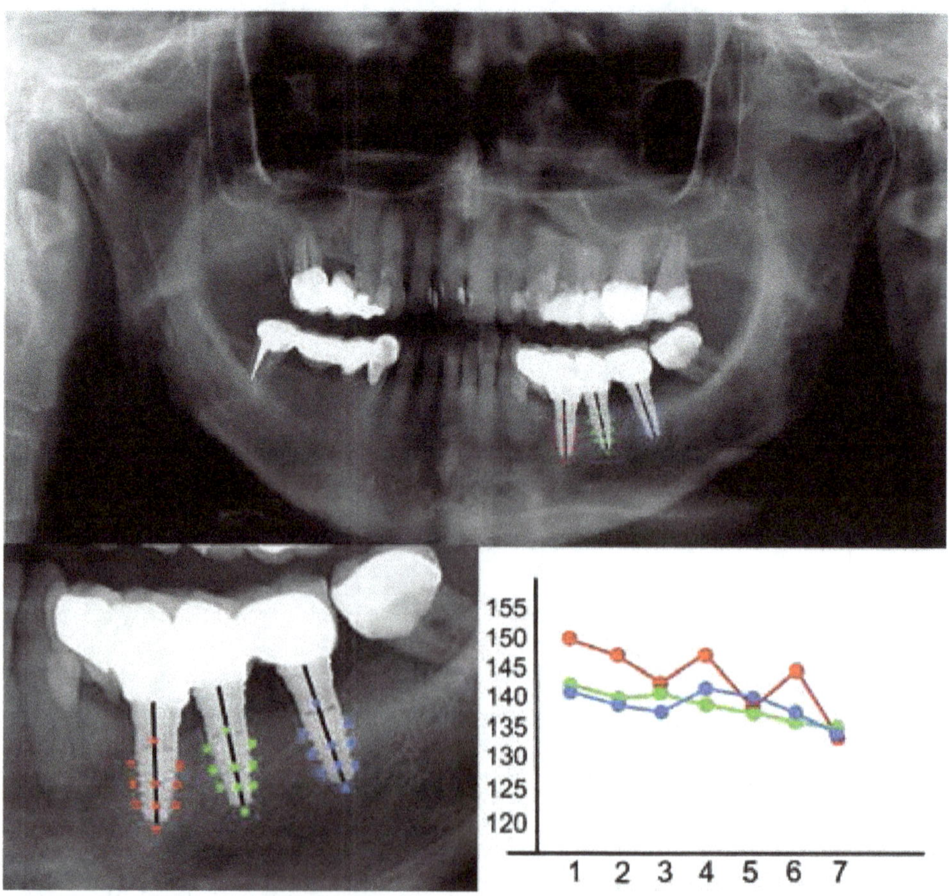

Fig. 12. Densitometric measurement of bone around 3 implants using splitting technique

3.4 Augmentation with autologous bone graft with simultaneous dental implant placement

Defect of the alveolar ridge of the left maxilla remained after extractions of the central and lateral incisors due to vertical root fractures (Figure 13) were augmented with the autologous bone block harvested from the retromolar area after two dental implants placement. Primary stability of the inserted implants was satisfactory. The gap between autologous graft and bone defect walls were filled with autologous bone chips harvested with bone scraper from the same harvesting site in the retromolar area. Augmented area was covered with the xenogenic bone substitude and resorbable collagen membrane. Densitometric measuremnt was performed six months after surgical procedure (Figure 14).

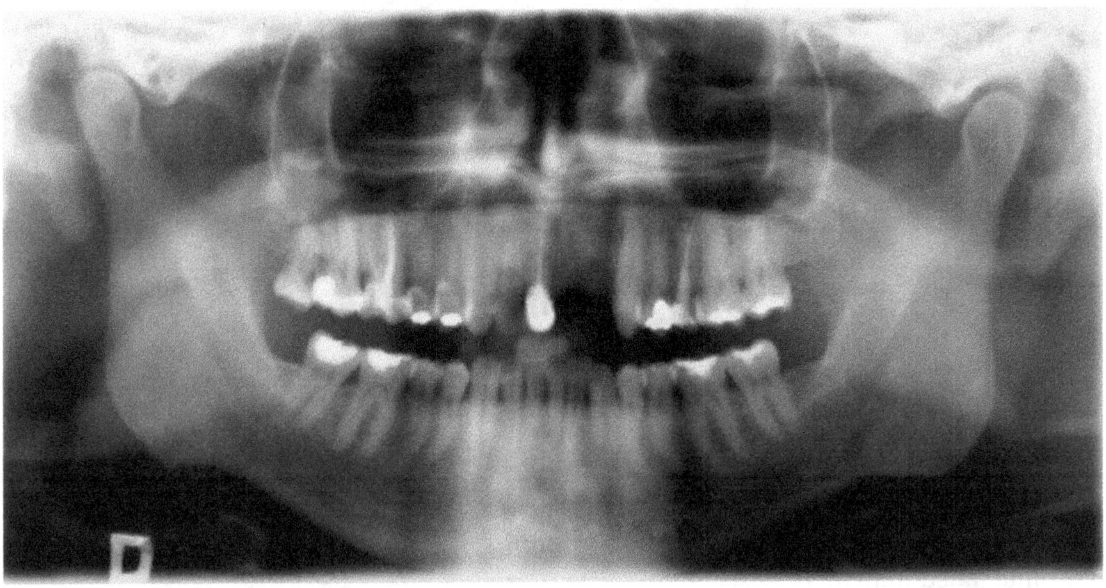

Fig. 13. Initial radiograph before surgical treatment

The results showed the higher decrese of density on bone grafts in comparation with bone alone.

3.5 Spreading technique in combination with autologous bone graft

Dental implant was placed after spreading the alveolar ridge bone due to long edentulous period (Figure 15). After implant placement infraction of the buccal cortical plate has remained. Defect was augmented with the autologous bone chips harvested with the bone scraper from the retromolar area, covered with β-tricalcium phosphate bone substitude and resorbable collagen membrane. Densitometric measurement was performed six months after surgical procedure, directly before final prosthetic restoration, and 12 months after surgery and 6 months after loading (Figures 16 and 17).

3.6 Alveolar ridge augmataion using rhBMP-2

In recent years, the delivery of osteoinductive factors such as bone morphogenic proteins (BMPs) have become an alternative approach to traditional bone grafting due to their capacity to enhance the natural ability of the surrounding tissues to produce bone healing and new bone and cartilage formation. In following case densitometric measurements were compared between bone induced by rhBMP-2 and normal bone (Figure 19). Substantial loss of vertical ridge height was noted bilaterally in both the mandibular molar regions and were deemed insufficient without augmentation to enable placement of dental implants. Bone was augmented using human recombinant BMP-2 and 3 dental implant were placed 6 mounths after. Values of bone density were measured in 10 points around each inserted

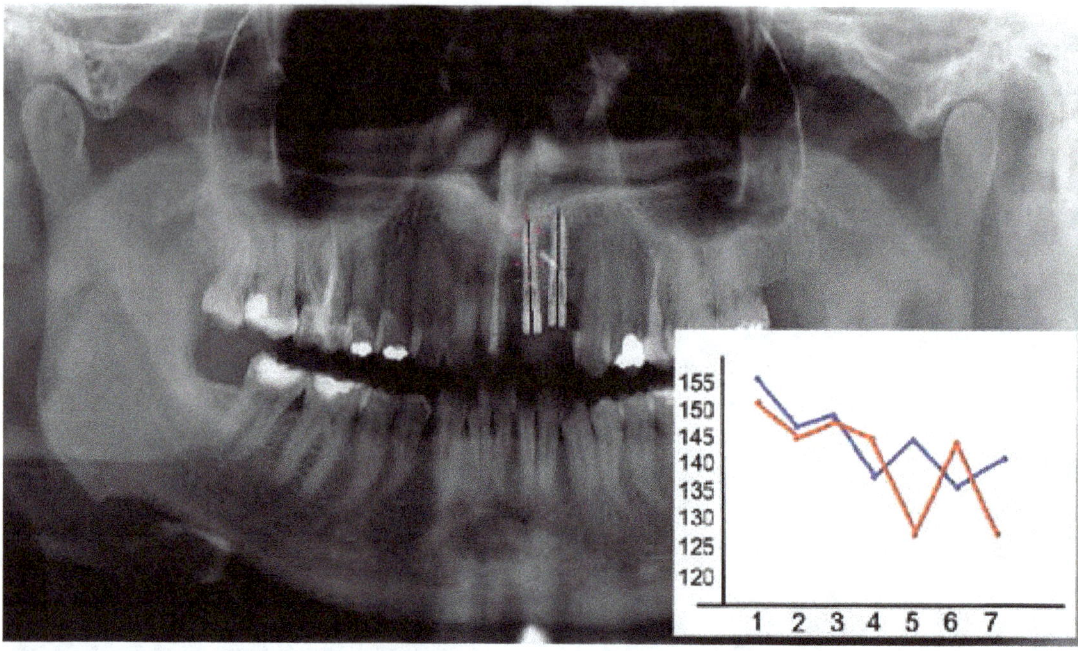

Fig. 14. Densitometric measurement of augmented bone around 2 implants placed simultaneouslly with the autologous bone graft (the fixation screw is positioned between the osseointegrated implants)

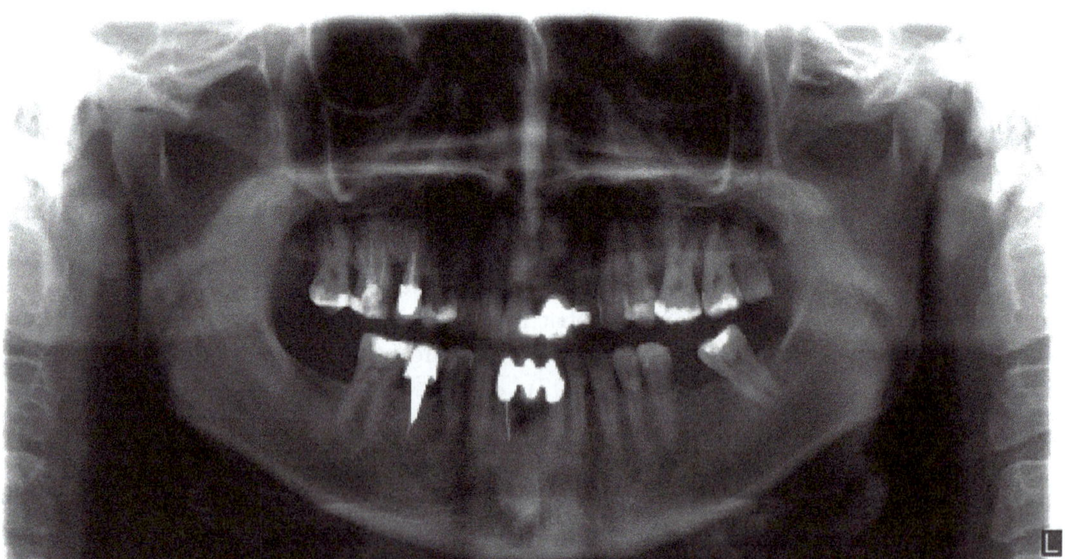

Fig. 15. Initial radiograph before surgical treatment

implant after placement, after 4 and 12 mounths. In this case, the results shows slighty decrease of density in bone induced with rhBMP-2 in comparison with classic two-stage technique of dental impalnts placement in the follow-up period of 12 mounths.

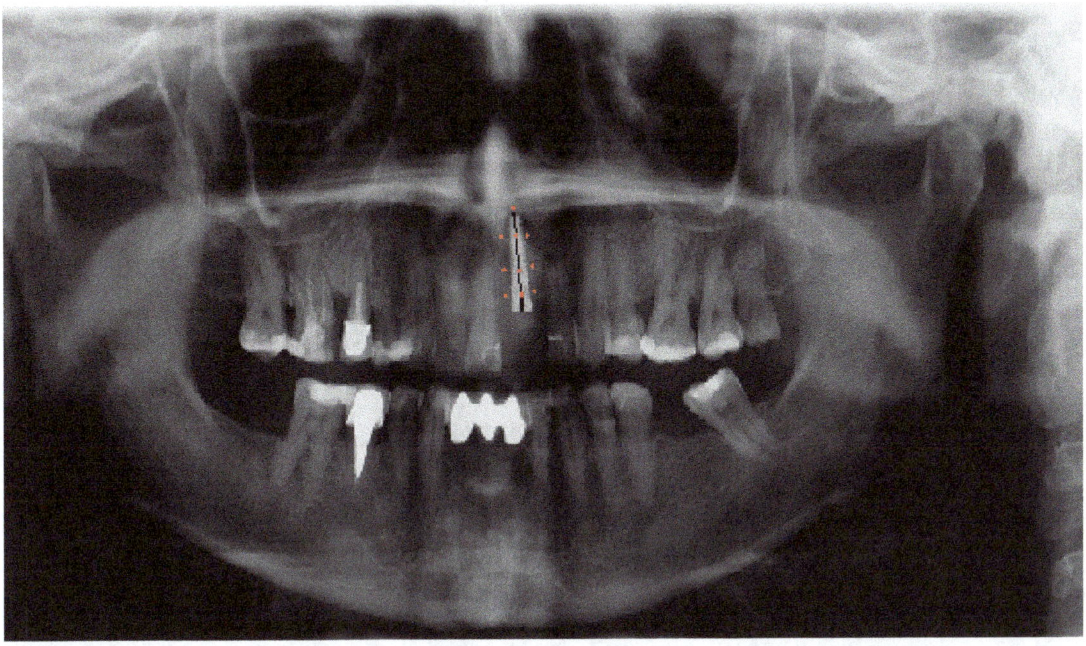

Fig. 16. Densitometric measurement of augmented bone around dental implant after spreading technique, 6 months after surgical procedure

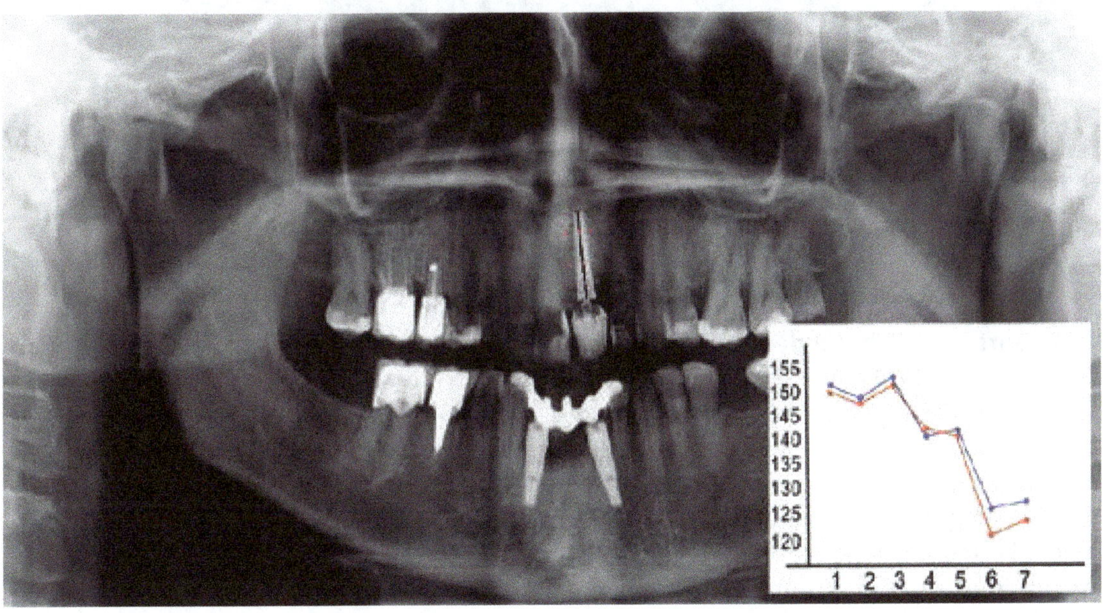

Fig. 17. Densitometric measurement of augmented bone around dental implant after spreading technique, 12 months after surgical procedure

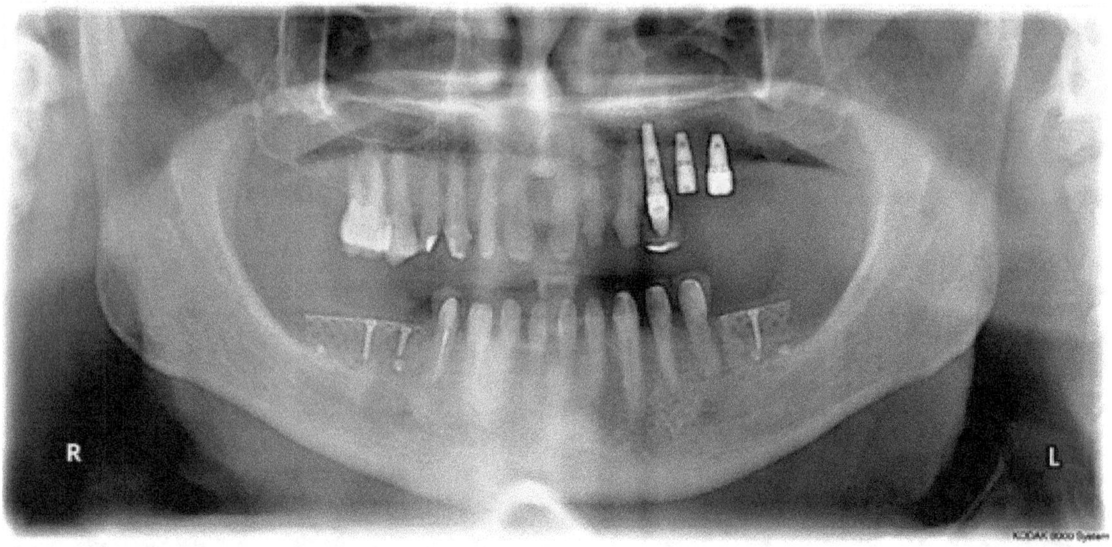

Fig. 18. Radiograph taken after placement od rhBMP-2

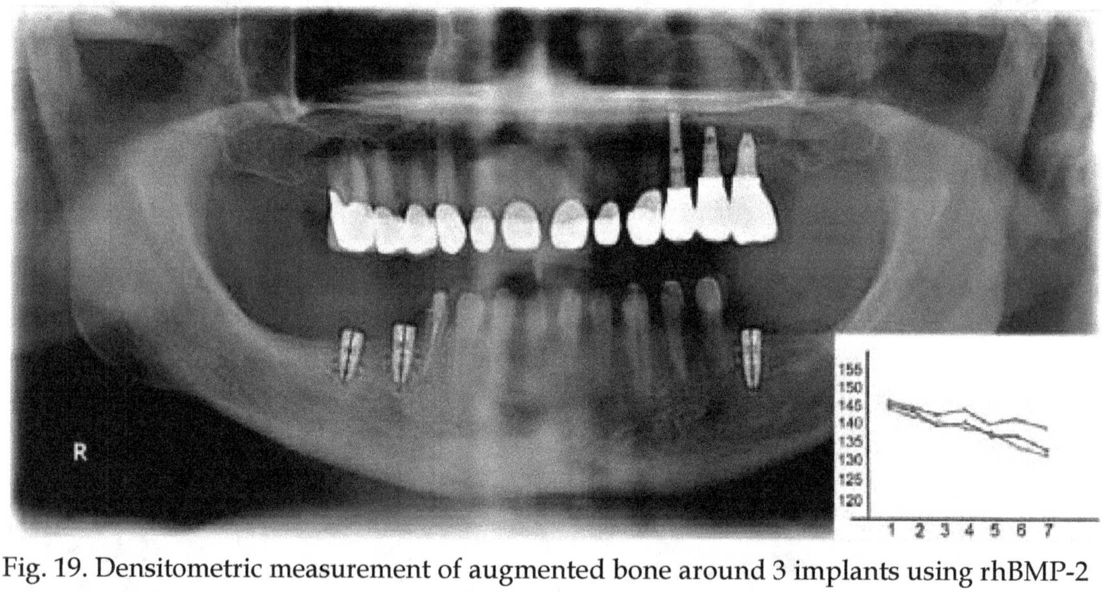

Fig. 19. Densitometric measurement of augmented bone around 3 implants using rhBMP-2

3.7 Importance of bone density in implant dentistry

Currently the use of osseointegrated implants to treat partially or completely the endentulous arch is considered realible and predictable, with a success rate of 98% or higher. The success of dental implant treatment is associated with good primary implant stability. Primary stability corresponds with bone density and it has been determining factor in treatment planing, implant design, surgical approach, healing time and initial progressive bone loading during prostetic reconstruction. Secondary implant stability results after formation of secondary bone contact of woven and lamellar bone. Bone density is related directly to the strenght of the bone and it seems to be a vital factor in the achievement of osseointegration. For assessing bone quality several classification systems and method were introduced. The most popular method was introduced by Lekholm and Zarb

Quality 1	Homogenous compact bone
Quality 2	Thick layer of cortical bone surrounding dense trabecular bone
Quality 3	Thin layer of cortical bone surrounded by dense trabecular bone of favorable strenght
Quality 4	Thin layer of cortical bone surrounding a core of low-density trabecular bone

Table 3. Classification of bone density by Lekholm and Zarb

who listed four bone qualities found in the anterior regions of the jawbone (Table 3). Their scale of bone quality ranges from 1 where is composed of homogeneuous compact bone to 4 where is a thin layer of cortical bone surrounding a core of low density trabecular bone. Their classification has recently been questioned due to poor objectivity and reproductibility because it provides only a rought mean value of the entire jaw. Misch proposed five bone density groups independet of the regions of the jaws based on macroscopic cortical and trabecular bone characteristic, their tactile sence during implant placement, location and CT values. (Table 4). The percentage of bone contact is significantly greater in cortical bone than in trabecular bone. An antherior mandible (D1, D2) provides the highest percentage of bone in contact with implant compared with posterior maxilla (D4) which offer less areas of bone contact with implant. Its reasonable to say that the period of osseointegration is longer in maxilla (4-6 months) than in mandible (3-4 months) and it coresponds with implant success. The male patients had higher average bone density value than that in female patients. That constatation could be explained with the hormonal peculliarities in females and generally higher bone mass in males.

Bone density	Description	Tactile analog	Typical Anatomical Location	CT values
D1	Dens cortical	Oak or maple wood	Anterior mandible	>1250 HU
D2	Porous cortical and coarse trabecular	White pine or spruce wood	Anterior mandible posterior mandible Anterior maxilla	850-1250 HU
D3	Porous cortical and fine trabecular	Balsa wood	Anterior maxilla Posterior maxilla Posterior mandible	350-850 HU
D4	Fine trabecular	Styrofoam	Posterior maxilla	150-350 HU
D5	Soft bone with incomplete mineralisation	Styrofoam		<150 HU

Table 4. Classification of bone density by Misch

Another bone classification by Tomaso and Vercellotti has universal application and can be used in all fields of bone surgery expecially in implantology. The classification outlines the quantitative characteristics of the cortical crest and separately the density of spongy bone mineralization (Table 5).

Quantitative cortical thickness classification	
0 mm	Thickness of cortical crest at the site of recent tooth extraction after few months
1 mm	Thickness of cortical crest at the site of tooth extraction after several months
2 mm	Thickness of cortical crest at the site of tooth extraction after a few years
3 mm or more	Thickness of cortical crest at the site of tooth extraction after several years and characterized by a reduction in spongy bone resulting in partial merging oft he buccal cortical and lingual cortical bone
Qualitative spongy bone density classification	
High density	The tomographic image is prevalently radiopaque and grayish-whitish in color
Medium density	The tomographic image is rather radiopaque and grayish in color
Low density	The tomographic image is radiolucent and grayish-blackish in color

Table 5. Classification of bone density by Tomaso and Vercellotti

Implant stability can be measured by non-invasive clinical test methods (i.e. insertion torque, the periotest, resonance frequency anaysis). Insertion torque is a method that records the torque required to place the implant. The Periotest M (Figure 20) is a measuring device for use in dental practises and is designed for the following range of applications:

1. Assessment oft he osseointegration of dental implants
2. Diagnosis and assessment of periodontopathies (the Periotest Mmeasuers the damping characteristics oft he periodontium and, indirectly, tooth mobility, which it outputs In the form of a Periotest value)
3. Assessment oft he occlusal load
4. Control of the treatment's progress

The unit scale ranges from -08 to +50. The measuring procedure is electromechanical. An electrically driven and electrically monitored tapping head percusses the test object (tooth or implant) 16 times. The entire measuring procedure requires approximatelly 4 seconds. The tapping head is pressure sensitive and records the duration of contact with the test object. Loose teeth or implants display a longer contact time and the Periotest values are correspondingly higher, while sturdy teeth and implants have a short contact time and result in low Periotest values. The Periotest M should not be applied in the following cases:

all types of acute apical periodontitis and acute trauma (dislocation, root fracture, alveolar process fracture).
Another method, resonance frequency anaysis (RFA) and their instrument called Osstell mentor are commonly used in clinical studies (Figure 20). The technique is contactless, non-invasive, patients experience no pain sensation from the measurement and the measurement takes 1-2 seconds.The unit of Osstell measurement is the implant stability quotient (ISQ) that is calculated from the resonance frequency and ranges from 0 to 100 units.

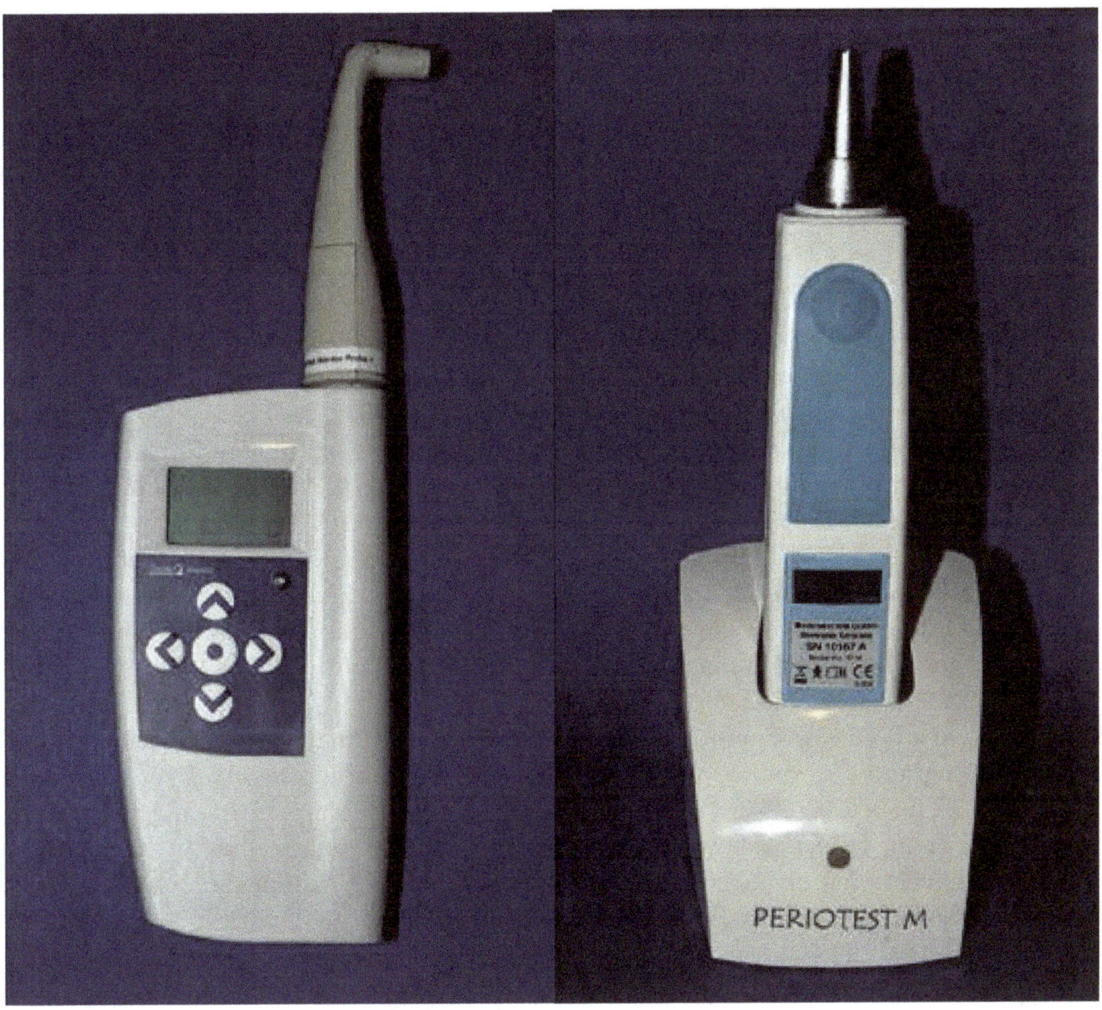

Fig. 20. Osstell mentor (left) and Periotest M (right)

Turkyilmaz et al found strong correlations between mean bone density scaned by CT, insertion torque and resonance frequency analsysis for the early loading protocols of dental implants. Autors suggested that primary stability is achived for early loading of dental implants when CT value is over 528 HU, insertion torque value is 32 Ncm or 45 Ncm and RF values higher than 65 ISQ.

In the end of this chapter there is a need for discusion of implant success criteria which were proposed by Albrektsson et al. Implant treatment, to be regarded as successful, need to meet the following criteria:

1. No radiolucent zone around the implant
2. The implant is acting as an anchor for the functional prosthesis
3. Confirmed individual implant stability
4. No suppuration, pain or ongoing pathologic processes

4. Conclusion

In this chapter CADIA measurement were described and its values were in strong correlation with CT values. Described CADIA modification is designed to monitor changes in bone density around implants and to compare it with other images. If there is a need to precisely determine a densitometric value, original stepwedge is inevitable, CADIA measurement were follow-up with Osstell device witch was helpful tool for determination of primary stability. Primary implant stability is in strong correlation with implant success.

5. References

Albrektsson, T. et al. (1986). The long-term efficacy of currently used dental implants: a review and proposed criteria of success. . *The International Journal of Oral & Maxillofacial Implants*, Vol. 1, pp. 11-25, ISSN 0882-2786.

Aranyarachkul, P. et al. (2005). Bone density assessments of dental implant sites: 2. quantitative cone-beam computerized tomography. *The International Journal of Oral & Maxillofacial Implants*, Vol. 20 pp. 416–424, ISSN 0882-2786.

Becker, W. et al. (2005). Minimally invasive flapless implant surgery. *Clinical implant dentistry and related research*, Vol. 7, No. 1, pp. 21-27, ISSN 1523-0899.

Becker, W. et al. (2006). Histologic evaluation of implants following flapless and flapped surgery: a study in canines. *Journal of periodontology*, Vol. 77, No. 10, pp. 1717-1722, ISSN 0022-3492.

Bragger, U. et al. (1988). Computer-assisted densitometric image anaysis in periodontal radiography. A methodological study. *Journal of clinical periodontology*, Vol. 15, pp. 27-37, ISSN 0303-6979.

Bragger, U. et al. (1989). Computer-assisted densitometric image anaysis (CADIA) for assessment of alveolar bone density change sin furcations. *Journal of clinical periodontology*, Vol. 16, pp. 46-52, ISSN 0303-6979.

Bragger, U. et al. (1992). Image processing for the evaulation of dental implants. *Dentomaxillofacial radiology*, Vol. 21, pp. 208-212, ISSN 0007- 1285

Bolotin, H.H. (2001). Inaccuracies inherent in dual-energy X-ray absorptiometry in vivo bone mineral densitometry may flaw osteopenic/osteoporotic interpretations and mislead assessment of antiresorptive therapy effectiveness. *Bone*, Vol. 28, pp. 548-555, ISSN 8756-3282.

Bouxsein, M.L. et al. (1997) Precision and accuracy of computed digital absorptiometry for assessment of bone density of the hand. *Osteoporosis International*, Vol. 7, pp. 444-449, ISSN 1433-2965.

Campelo, L.D. & Camara, J.R. (2002). Flapless implant surgery: a 10-year clinical retrospective analysis. *International Journal of Oral & Maxillofacial Implants*, Vol. 17, pp.271-276, ISSN 0882-2786.

Casap, N. et al. (2006). Flapless approach for removal of bone graft fixing screws and placement of dental implants using computerized navigation. *The International journal of oral & maxillofacial implants*, Vol. 21, pp. 314-319, ISSN 0882-2786.

Choel, L. et al. (2004). Trabecular alveolar bone microarchitecture in the human mandible using high resolution magnetic resonance imaging. *Dentomaxillofacial Radiology*, Vol. 33, pp. 177–182, ISSN 0007-1285.

Christgau, M. et al. (1998). Accuracy of quantitative digital subtraction radiography for determining changes in calcium mass in mandibular bone: an in vitro study. *Journal of periodontal research.*, Vol. 33, pp. 138-149, ISSN 0022-3484

Cochran, D.L. et al. (1998). Bone response to unloaded and loaded titanium implants with sandblasted and acid-etched surface: A histometric study in the canine mandible. *Journal of Biomedical Materials research*, Vol. 40, pp. 1-11. ISSN 1549-3296.

Corten, F.G. et al. (1993). Measurement of mandibular bone density ex vivo and in vivo by dual-energy X-ray absorptiometry. *Archives of Oral Biology*, Vol. 38, pp. 215–219, ISSN 0003-9969.

Devlin, H. & Horner K. (1991). Measurement of mandibular bone mineral content using the dental panoramic tomogram. *Journal of Dentistry*, Vol. 19, pp. 116-120, ISSN 0300-5712.

Dove, S.B. et al. (2000). Analysis of sensitivity and specificity oft he new digital subtraction system: an in vitro study. *Oral surgery, oral medicine, oral pathology, oral radiology, and endodontics*, Vol. 89, pp. 771-776, ISSN 1079-2104.

Duckworth, J.E. et al. (1983). A method for the geometric and densitometric standardization of intraoral radiographs. *Journal of periodontology*, Vol. 54, pp. 435-440, ISSN 0022-3492.

Dural, S. et al. (2005). Evaluation of mandibular bone density to predict osteoporosis in adolescents with constitutional delayed growth. *Saudi Medical Journal*, Vol. 26, pp. 1235–1239, ISSN 0379-5284.

Friberg, B. et al. (1991). Early failures in 4641 consecutively placed Branemark dental implants: a study from stage I surgery to the connection of completed prostheses. *The International journal of oral & maxillofacial implants*, Vol. 6, pp. 142-146, ISSN 0882-2786.

Fujita, H. et al. (1986). Investigation of basic imaging properties in digital radiography. 5. Characteristic cures of II-TV digital systems. *Medical Physics*, Vol. 13, pp. 13-18, ISSN 0094-2405.

Gabric Panduric, D. et al. (2008) Densitometric analysis of dental implant placement between flapless technique and the two-stage techique – a pilot study. *Collegium Antropologicum*, Vol. 32, No. 2, pp. 315-319, ISSN 0350-6134.

Hahn, J. (2000). Single-stage, immediate loading, and flapless surgery. *Journal of Oral Implantology*, Vol. 26, pp. 193-198, ISSN 0160-6972.

Horner, K. & Devlin, H. (1992). Clinical bone densitometric study of mandibular atrophy using dental panoramic tomography. *Journal of Dentistry*, Vol. 20, pp. 33-37, ISSN 0300-5712.

Inaba, D. et al. (1997). A computer-assisted videodensitometric method to visualize mineral distributions in vitro and in vivo formed rooth caries lesions. *European journal of oral sciences*, Vol. 105, pp. 74-80, ISSN 0909-8836.

Jean, A. et al. (1996). Digital image ratio: a new radiographic method for quantifying changes in alveolar bone. Part 1: theory and methodology. *Journal of periodontal research.*, Vol. 31, pp. 161-167, ISSN 0022-3484.

Jemt, T. et al. (1989). Osseointegrated implants in the treatment of partially edentulous patients: a preliminary study on 876 consecutively placed fixtures. *The International Journal of Oral & Maxillofacial Implants*, Vol. 4, pp. 211-217, ISSN 0882-2786.

Johansson, P. & Strid, K.G. (1994). Assessment of bone quality from placement resistance during implant surgery. *The International Journal of Oral & Maxillofacial Implants*, Vol. 9, pp. 279-288, ISSN 0882-2786.

Kan, J.Y. et al. (2003). Immediate placement and provisionalization of maxillary anterior single implants: 1-year prospective study. *The International journal of oral & maxillofacial implants*, Vol. 18, No. 1, pp. 31-39, ISSN 0882-2786.

Katanec, D. (1997). Evaulation of HA bone implants using Computer Assisted Densitometric Image Analysis. *Dissertation*, University of Zagreb

Katanec, D. et al. (1998). Computer Assisted Densitometric Image Analysis (CADIA) of Bone Density in Periradicular Bone Defects Healing. *Collegium Antropologicum*, Vol. 22, pp. 7-13, ISSN 0350-6134.

Klemetti, E. et al. (1993). Trabecular bone mineral density of mandible and alveolar height in postmenopausal women. *Scandinavian journal of dental research*. Vol. 101, pp. 166-170, ISSN 0029-845X.

Knezovic-Zlataric, D. & Celebic, A. (2003). Mandibular bone mineral density changes in complete and removable partial denture wearers: a 6-month follow-up study. *The International Journal of Prosthodontics*, Vol. 16, pp. 661–665, ISSN 0893-2174.

Kribbs, P.J. et al. (1983). Oral findings in osteoporosis. Part I: Measurement of mandibular bone density. *The Journal of prosthetic dentistry*, Vol. 50, pp. 576-579, ISSN 0022-3913.

Kribbs, P.J. et al. (1989). Relationships between mandibular and skeletal bone in an osteoporotic population. *The Journal of prosthetic dentistry*, Vol. 62, pp. 703-707, ISSN 0022-3913.

Kribbs, P.J. (1990). Comparison of mandibular bone in normal and osteoporotic women. *The Journal of prosthetic dentistry*, Vol. 63, pp. 218-222, ISSN 0022-3913.

Kribbs, P.J. et al. (1990). Relationships between mandibular and skeletal bone in a populatio of normal women. *The Journal of prosthetic dentistry*, Vol. 63, pp. 86-89, ISSN 0022-3913.

Kribbs, P.J. (1992). Two-year changes in mandibular bone massin an osteoporotic population. *The Journal of prosthetic dentistry*, Vol. 67, pp. 653-655, ISSN 0022-3913.

Kupeyan, H.K. et al. (2006). Definitive CAD/CAM-guided prosthesis for immediate loading of bone-grafted maxilla: a case report. *Clinical implant dentistry and related research*, Vol. 8, pp. 161-167, ISSN 1523-0899.

Landini, G. (1991). Videodensitometrical study of the alveolar bone crest in periodontal disease. *Journal of periodontology*, Vol. 62, pp. 528-534, ISSN 0022-3492.

Lekholm, U. & Zarb, G.A. (1985). Patient selection and preparation, In: Tissue integrated prostheses: osseintegration in clinical dentistry, P.I. Branemark, (Ed.), pp. 199-209, Quintessence Publishing Company, ISBN 0-86715-129-3, Chicago, USA.

Meredith, N. et al. (1996). Quantitative determination oft he stability oft he implant-tissue interface using resonance frequency analysis. . *Clinical Oral Implants Research*, Vol. 7, pp. 261-267, ISSN 0905-7161.

Meredith, N. (1998). Assessment of implant stability as a prognostic determinant. *The International Journal of Prosthodontics*, Vol. 11, pp. 491-501, ISSN 0893-2174.

Misch, C.E. (2005). Bone density: Diagnostic Imaging and Techniques, In: *Dental implant prosthetics*, C.E. Misch (Ed.), pp. 53-70, Elsevier Mosby, ISBN 978-0-323-01955-2. St. Louis, USA.

Misch, C.E. (2005). Bone density: A key determinant for clinical success, In: *Dental implant prosthetics*, C.E. Misch (Ed.), pp. 130-141, Elsevier Mosby, ISBN 978-0-323-01955-2. St. Louis, USA.

Nicholson, P.H.F. et al. (1996). A comparison of time-domain and frequency domain approaches to ultrasonic velocity measurements in trabecular bone physics in medicine biology. *Physics in Medicine and Biology*, Vol. 41, pp. 2421–2435, ISSN 0031-9155.

Oh, T.J. et al. (2006). Effect of flapless implant surgery on soft tissue profile: a randomized controlled clinical trial. *Journal of periodontology*, Vol. 77, pp. 874-882, ISSN 0022-3492.

Petrungaro, P.S. (2005). Immediate restoration of implants utilizing a flapless approach to preserve interdental tissue contours. *Practical procedures & aesthetic dentistry*, Vol. 17, No. 2, pp. 151-158, ISSN 1534-6846.

Rocci, A. et al. (2003). Immediate loading in the maxilla using flapless surgery, implants placed in predetermined positions, and prefabricated provisional restorations: a retrospective 3-year clinical study. *Clinical implant dentistry and related research*, Vol. 5, No. 1, pp. 29-36, ISSN1523-0899.

Shapurian, T. et al. (2006). Quantitative evaluation of bone density using the Hounsfield index. *The International Journal of Oral & Maxillofacial Implants*, Vol. 21, pp. 290–297, ISSN 0882-2786.

Steigmann, M. & Wang, H.L. (2006). Esthetic buccal flap for correction of buccal fenestration defects during flapless immediate implant surgery. *Journal of periodontology*, Vol. 77, pp. 517-522, ISSN 0022-3492.

Stoppie, N. et al. (2006). Structural and radiological parameters for the characterization of jawbone. *Clinical Oral Implants Research*, Vol. 17, pp. 124–133, ISSN 0905-7161.

Todisco, M. & Trisi, P. (2005). Bone mineral density and bone histomorphometry are statistically related. *The International Journal of Oral & Maxillofacial Implants*, Vol. 20, pp. 898-904, ISSN 0882-2786.

Trouerbach, W.T. et al. (1984). A study of the radiographic aluminium equivalent values of the mandible. *Oral surgery, oral medicine, and oral pathology*, Vol. 58, pp 610-616, ISSN 0030-4220.

Turkyilmaz, I. et al. (2008). Is there a lower threshold value of bone density for early loading protocols of dental implants? *Journal of Oral Rehabilitation*, Vol. 35, pp. 775-781, ISSN 0305-182X.

Turkyilmaz, I. & McGlumphy, E. (2008). Influence of bone density on implant stability parameters and implant success: a retrospective clinical study. *BMC Oral Health*, Vol. 8, pp. 32, ISSN 1472-6831.

Vercellotti, T. (2009). New bone classification for analysis of the single sargical site, In: *Essentials in piezosurgery*, T. Vercellotti, (Ed.), pp. 91-93, Quintessenza Edizioni, ISBN 978-1-85097-190-0, Milano, Italy.

Verdonck, H.W.D. et al. (2008). Implant stability during osseointegration in irradiated and nonirradiated minipig alveolar bone: an experimental study. *Clinical Oral Implants Research*, Vol. 19, pp. 201-206, ISSN 0905-7161.

White, S.C. et al. (2005). Change in mandibular trabecular pattern and hip fracture rate in elderly women. *Dentomaxillofacial Radiology*, Vol. 34, pp. 168–174, ISSN 0007- 1285.

7

Biomaterials Applicable for Alveolar Sockets Preservation: In Vivo and In Vitro Studies

Christiane Kunert-Keil[1], Tomasz Gredes[2] and Tomasz Gedrange[1]
[1]*University of Greifswald, Department of Orthodontics*
[2]*University of Wroclaw, Department of Orthodontics*
Germany
Poland

1. Introduction

Bone density and quantity are primary conditions for the insertion and stability of dental implants. In cases of a lack of adequate maxillary or mandibulary bone, e.g. in terms of front to back depth or thickness, bone augmentation will be necessary. Lack of bone or bone defects can be caused by inflammation, congenital malformation, trauma or oncological surgery. Several procedures and materials for augmenting bone height have been developed to overcome the problem of a reduced amount of bone. In dentistry, bone substitution materials were used for the following applications: (1) socket preservation; (2) periodontal defects; (3) third molar extraction sites to support 2nd molars; (4) ridge augmentation; (5) defects following cyst removal / apicoectomies; (6) sinus lifts; (7) distraction osteogenesis; and (8) implant dentistry. The treatment of bone-defects and socket preservation include autografting (from one location to another within the same individual), xenografting (from a donor of another species) and allografting (from a genetically dissimilar member of the same species) cancellous bone. After blood, bone is the most commonly transplanted tissue. Worldwide, an estimated 2.2 million grafting procedures are performed annually to repair bone defects in orthopaedics, neurosurgery, and dentistry (Giannoudis et al. 2005). The increasing number of grafting procedures and the disadvantages of current autograft and allograft treatments (e.g. limited graft quantity, risk of disease transmission) drive the quest for alternative methods to treat bone defects.

The use of synthetic bioactive bone substitute materials is of increasing importance in modern dentistry as alternatives to autogenous bone grafts. Various alloplastic bone substitution materials of different origin, chemical composition, and structural properties have been investigated in the last years. The materials commonly used in all approaches are ceramics, polymers or composites (Burg et al. 2000). These alloplastic materials are either absorbable or non-absorbable, as well as naturally derived or synthetically manufactured (Figure 1).

Various types of biomaterials (minerals and non-mineral based materials as well as natural and artificial polymers) with different characteristics have been used for studying ossification and bone formation. For example, calcium phosphate ceramics include a variety of ceramics such as hydroxyapatite, tricalcium phosphate, calcium phosphate cement, etc. These mentioned ceramics have excellent biocompatibility and bone bonding or bone regeneration properties. Recently non-biodegradable and degradable membranes have been tested for their appliance in bone defects (Zhao et al. 2000). Cell-biomaterial interactions depend on surface characteristics, e.g. chemistry or topography. Surface characteristics determine the ionic exchange dynamics and the protein attachment as well as cell attachment, cell proliferation and cell differentiation.

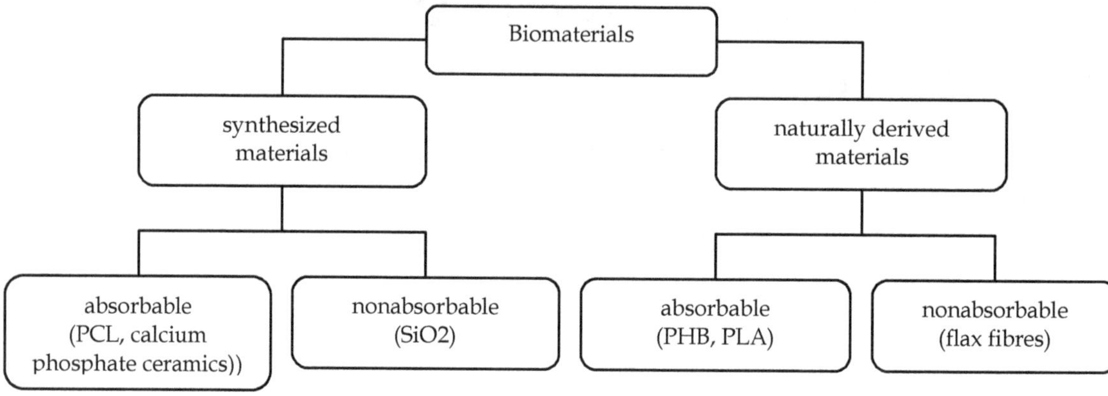

Fig. 1. The classification of used biomaterials for bone tissue engineering modified according to Burg (Burg et al. 2000)

Xenogenic grafting has been shown to be one of the most effective methods of creating bone in areas where there is none, whereas alloplastic graft material constitutes the second of the most popular forms of bone grafting material in dentistry.

2. Bone regeneration

Bone is a dynamic tissue that constantly undergoes remodelling. The signal that initiates bone remodelling has not been identified, but there is evidence that mechanical stress can alter local bone architecture. This can be sensed by osteocytes followed by secretion of paracrine factors such as insulin-like growth factor (IGF-1) in response to mechanical forces (Lean et al. 1996). Bone formations result from a complex cascade of events that involves proliferation of primitive mesenchymal cells (osteoinduction), differentiation into osteoblast precursor cells, maturation of osteoblasts, formation of matrix, and finally mineralization. Osteoblasts converge at the bottom of the resorption cavity and form osteoid which begins to mineralize after 13 days. The osteoblasts continue to form and mineralize osteoid until the cavity is filled (Hill 1998). Some of the osteoblasts differentiate into osteocytes and become embedded in the matrix.

Even if pre-existing osteoblasts may help to form new bone, it is generally agreed that such osteoblasts only contribute a minor portion of the new bone needed in a fracture-healing situation. The initial event must be the chemotactic attraction of osteoblasts or their precursors to sites of the resorption defect. This is likely to be mediated by the release of local, biochemical and biophysical messengers. The second event involved in the formation phase of the coupling phenomenon is proliferation of osteoblast precursors. This is likely to be mediated by osteoblast-derived growth factors and those growth factors released from bone during the resorption process. The third event of the formation phase is the differentiation of the osteoblast precursor into the mature cell. The differentiating osteoprogenitor cells express several bone matrix macromolecules, namely alkaline phosphatase, type I collagen, bone sialoprotein, osteopontin, Cbfa1 and osteocalcin (Hill 1998).

It is a balance between the amount of bone resorbed by osteoclasts and the amount of bone formed by osteoblast (Frost 1964). Bone remodelling occurs in small packets of cells called basic multicellular units (BMU), which turn bone over in multiple bone surfaces (Frost 1991). BMU consist of osteoblasts, other bone-forming cells such as osteocytes and bone-lining cells, bone-resorbing cells - osteoclasts, the precursor cells of both, and their associated cells like endothelial cells and nerve cells (Papachroni et al. 2009). Osteoblasts are key components of the bone multicellular unit and have a seminal role in bone remodelling, which is an essential function for the maintenance of the structural integrity and metabolic capacity of the skeleton. Osteoblasts originate from the non-hematopoietic part of bone marrow, which contains a group of fibroblast-like stem cells with osteogenic differentiation potential, known as the mesenchymal stem cells (MSCs) and also referred as skeletal stem cells (SSCs), bone marrow stromal cells (BMSCs) and multipotent mesenchymal stromal cells (MMSCs) (Abdallah and Kassem 2008; Heino and Hentunen 2008). MSCs are capable of multi-lineage differentiation into mesoderm-type cells such as osteoblasts, adipocytes and chondrocytes (Dezawa et al. 2004; Luk et al. 2005). Osteoblast growth and differentiation is determined by a complex array of growth factors and signalling pathways. The following three families of growth factors influence the main aspects of osteoblast activity and induce, mediate or modulate the effects of other bone growth regulators:

- the transforming growth factor-β (TGF-β) family
- the insulin-like growth factors (IGFs)
- bone morphogenetic proteins (BMPs) (Zhou et al. 1993; Mundy 1994; Bikle 2008).

Furthermore, other growth factors, such as the vascular endothelial growth factor (VEGF), fibroblast growth factor (FGF) as well as platelet derived growth factor (PDGF) are involved in bone formation.

Many growth factors involved in the natural process of bone healing have been identified and tested as potential therapeutic candidates to enhance the regeneration process. *In vitro*, BMPs can differentiate mesenchymal stem cells into the osteoblastic phenotype (Cheng et al. 2003; Luu et al. 2007). Furthermore, the osteoinductive BMPs (e.g. BMP-2/-4/ and BMP-5 to -8) can initiate the complete cascade of bone formation when implanted ectopically (Wozney 2002). In general, TGF-β stimulates migration of skeletal stem cells and regulates cell proliferation, cell differentiation, and extra cellular matrix synthesis (Bostrom and Asnis 1998; Janssens et al. 2005). Stimulatory effects on bone healing and bone formation have been evaluated in various experimental settings (Janssens et al. 2005). FGFs are considered potent regulators of cell growth and wound healing and have mitogenic effects. The best studied member of FGFs is FGF-2. Although FGF-2 alone is not capable of inducing ectopic bone formation, it plays an important role in the regulation of normal bone healing (Marie 2003). In various animal studies exogenous recombinant FGF-2 enhances callus formation and stimulates bone healing (Kato et al. 1998; Nakamura et al. 1998; Radomsky et al. 1998). IGFs are the most abundant growth factors produced by bone cells and are stored at the highest concentration of all growth factors in the bone matrix. It was shown that IGF has an anti-apoptotic effect on pre-osteoblast cells and enhances bone matrix synthesis (Niu and Rosen 2005). In animal models and clinical trials of osteoporosis, systemic IGF infusion showed an increase in bone formation, bone volume, and / or bone turnover (Rosen 2004). VEGF is considered one of the key regulators of angiogenesis during bone formation

(Gerstenfeld et al. 2003). In various experimental models the stimulation of the bone regeneration process has been shown in response to VEGF administration (Street et al. 2002; Eckardt et al. 2005). In addition, PDGF regulates general tissue repair as well as enhances proliferation of various bone cell types and angiogenesis (Hollinger et al. 2008).

Mechanisms that promote skeletal tissue specificity are necessary, because none of these growth factors are specific for cells in the osteoblastic lineage and these involve interactions with other circulating hormones in addition to the action of specific intracellular mediators on bone-specific transcription factors. It is certain that bone remodelling is regulated by systemic hormones and by local factors (Canalis 1983), which affect cells of both the osteoclast and osteoblast lineages and exert their effects on the replication of undifferentiated cells, the recruitment of cells, and the differentiated function of cells (Hill 1998). The following hormones are involved in bone formation:

- Calcitonin (CT) – decreases the reabsorption of calcium from bones thereby lowering blood calcium levels. It can inhibit osteoclastic bone resorption and probably osteocytic osteolysis (Weiss et al. 1981; Wallach et al. 1993).
- Estrogens and androgens - slow the rate of bone remodelling and protect against bone loss. They help retain calcium in bones, thereby maintaining a strong bone matrix. Sex steroids not only influence the accrual of bone mass and bone mineral density but also bone growth (Manolagas et al. 2002; Bertelloni et al. 2010).
- Growth hormone (GH) - is one of the most important regulator substances for both bone growth and bone remodelling. It directly increases longitudinal bone growth by stimulating prechondrocites. GH is a polypeptide complex that regulates the processes of bone physiology, increases the rate of mitosis of chondrocytes and osteoblasts, and increases the rate of protein synthesis (collagen, cartilage matrix, and enzymes for cartilage and bone formation) (Ohlsson et al. 1998; Calvo-Guirado et al. 2011).
- Insulin – increases energy production from glucose. It has been established as an osteoblast regulator. In bone organ culture, insulin stimulates collagen synthesis at periphysiological hormone concentrations (Wettenhall et al. 1969; Cornish et al. 1996).
- Parathyroid hormone (PTH) - a major systemic regulator of bone metabolism, increases the reabsorption of calcium from bones to the blood, thereby raising blood calcium levels and increases the absorption of calcium by the small intestine and kidneys. The anabolic effect of intermittent PTH on bone has made it an effective treatment for osteoporosis in humans, where it was shown to increase bone mass and reduce fracture rate (Neer et al. 2001).
- Thyroxine – increases the rate of protein synthesis and increases energy production from all food types. It directly stimulates the metabolic activity of bone cells and profoundly affects bone turnover. Thyroxine influences the responsiveness of bone cells to 1,25-dihydroxycholecalciferol, parathyroid hormone, and calcitonin (High et al. 1981).

Besides growth factors and regulating hormones, expression of transcription factors is necessary and sufficient for mesenchymal cell differentiation. Runx2 is an essential bone-specific transcription factor. It was recently shown, that the complete Runx2 gene inactivation in transgenic mice leads to complete lack of intramembraneous and endochondral ossification owing to lack of mature osteoblasts (Komori et al. 1997). In addition, heterozygous Runx2 mice demonstrate specific skeletal abnormalities that are characteristic of the human heritable skeletal disorder cleidocranial dysplasia (Otto et al. 1997).

3. Pre-conditions of bone surrogates

Selection of graft materials is based on operator preference, type and size of the bone defect, resorbability of graft material as well as cost and patient acceptance. Furthermore, bone graft materials are generally evaluated based on their osteogenic, osteoinductive, or osteoconductive potential. Osteoinduction is a basic biological mechanism that occurs regularly, e.g. in fracture healing but also in implant incorporation (Albrektsson and Johansson 2001). Osteoconduction means that bone grows on a surface and is defined as the ability to stimulate the attachment, migration, and distribution of vascular and osteogenic cells within the graft material (Albrektsson and Johansson 2001). Several physical characteristics can affect the graft osteoconductivity, including porosity, pore size, and three-dimensional architecture. In addition, direct interactions between matrix proteins and their appropriate cell surface receptors play a major role in the host response to the graft material. An osteoconductive material guides repair in a location where normal healing will occur if left untreated (Kulkarni et al. 1971; Helm and Gazit 2005).

The ability of a graft material to independently produce bone is termed its direct osteogenic potential. The main critical considerations in bone tissue-engineering scaffold design are:

- Promotion of bone in-growth
- Average pore sizes approximately 200-400 μm
- Sterilization without loss of properties
- Absorbation with biocompatible components
- Good bony apposition
- Correct mechanical and physical properties for application
- Maximal bone growth through osteoinduction and/or osteoconduction
- Adaptation to irregular wound site (malleableness)
- Absorbation in predictable manner in concert with bone growth
- Availability to surgeon on short notice (Peter et al. 1998; Burg et al. 2000)

To have direct osteogenic activity, the graft must contain cellular components that directly induce bone formation. Polymers have been shown to be an excellent substrate for cellular or bioactive molecule delivery. They can differ in their molecular weight, polydispersity, crystallinity, and thermal transitions, allowing different absorption rates. Their relative hydrophobicity and percent crystallinity can affect cellular phenotype (Hollinger and Schmitz 1997). Various types of biomaterials (minerals and non-mineral based materials as well as natural and artificial polymers) with different characteristics have been used for studying ossification and bone formation. For example, calcium phosphate ceramics include a variety of ceramics such as hydroxyapatite, tricalcium phosphate, calcium phosphate cement, etc. Local tissue responses to polymers *in vivo* depend on the biocompatibility of the polymer as well as its degradative by-products (Hollinger and Battistone 1986). The mentioned ceramics have excellent biocompatibility and bone bonding or bone regeneration properties. They have been widely used in no or low load-bearing applications (Milosevski et al. 1999). Furthermore, natural polymers like collagen have been used for bone tissue engineering purposes (Hutmacher et al. 2001a; Lauer et al. 2001). Recently non-biodegradable and degradable membranes have been tested for their appliance in bone defects (Zhao et al. 2003). Scores of artificial polymers of diverse character are already in use for bone supply. One of them, poly(3)hydroxybutyrate (PHB) due to its form stability combined with little inflammatory response after implantation, may serve as a scaffold for tissue engineering (Gogolewski et al. 1993; Schmack et al. 2000).

4. Alloplastic materials in dentistry

Today, the above-mentioned clinical problems are solved by bone grafting. Autogeneic bone graft from the iliac crest is the main source of trabecular bone. It has a good osteoinductive capacity, but the sources are limited and the harvest procedure causes postoperative discomfort to the patient. Allogeneic bone is also widely used but provides mainly osteoconductive properties. Moreover, despite of extensive testing, there are still potential risks for transmitting diseases. Synthetic or alloplastic materials are alternative materials to avoid the drawbacks of autografts or allografts, because alloplastic materials show very little risk of morbidity and mortality. Alloplastic materials are divided into two main groups: (1) non-resorbable materials that acts as replacement bone and (2) resorbable frameworks or scaffolds for bone to grow into at its normal rate. A large percentage of alloplastic biomaterials are based on one raw material, such as hydroxyapatite (HA) and tri-calcium phosphate (TCP) or bioactive silicates (SiO2). Recent developments have focused on composites with different chemical phases, such as HA+TCP (Straumann® BoneCeramic, Straumann, Freiburg, Germany), SiO2+HA (Nanobone®,Artoss, Rostock, Germany) or SiO2+Ha+TCP (BonitMatrix®, DOT, Rostock, Germany).

4.1 Homogenous chemical composition

Until now HA-based biomaterials are the most abundant materials used in modern bone substitution. At the moment calcium phosphate cements play a secondary role in dentistry, although they often have an excellent biocompatibility (Noetzel and Kielbassa 2005). For HA scaffolds both pore size and porosity have effects on mineralisation and bone formation (Harris and Cooper 2004; Kruyt et al. 2004).

In vitro testing is used primarily as a first stage test for acute toxicity and cytocompatibility. A precondition for osteoconductivity and osteoinductivity are proliferating cells. Reichert and coworkers could show that neither Cerasorb® (TCP; Curason AG, Sonneberg, Germany), Geistlich Bio-Oss® (HA; Geistlich Pharma, Wolhusen, Germany) nor Perioglas® (SiO2; Novabone, Jacksonville, U.S.A.) has a negative influence on cellular proliferation, as compared to the control (Reichert et al. 2009). In fact, the tested bone substitution materials led to an increased AlamarBlue reduction over the observation period of 7d. Only PerioGlas® showed slight, but not significant decrease in AlamarBlue reduction, compared to controls (Reichert et al. 2009). The effect on the proliferation of osteoblast *in vitro* was investigated using phytogene HA (Algipore®), TCP (Bio-Base®) and bovine HA (Bio-Oss®). Kübler et al. have found that human osteoblast cells seeded with Bio-Oss® showed the lowest proliferation and differentiation rate after comparison with the other tested bone graft materials (Kubler et al. 2004). Furthermore, there were no obvious differences in cell migration and growth behaviour between BioOss® and Vitoss® scaffolds, but significantly higher osteocalcin expression in cells seeded on BioOss® scaffolds (Payer et al. 2010). In contrast, DNA content, LDH (lactate dehydrogenase) and alkaline phosphatase activity as well as expression of bone-related genes, such as alkaline phosphatase, osteonectin, osteopontin and bone sialoprotein II revealed proliferation and osteogenic differentiation of osteoblasts on Cerasorb®, but not on BioOss® during cultivation over 28 days (Bernhardt et al. 2010).

Bioactive glass ceramic was seeded with human primary osteoblasts and evaluated after 2, 6 and 12 days. Incubation with Bioglass 45S5 increased human osteoblast proliferation to 155% as shown by flow cytometric analysis (Xynos et al. 2000b). Analysis of osteoblast specific markers, such as alkaline phosphatase and osteocalcin indicate that Bioglass

advanced osteoblast augmentation. Furthermore, expression of IGF2 was 2,9fold increased compared to control cells (Xynos et al. 2000a).
However, *in vitro* characterization is not able to demonstrate the tissue response to materials. Animal models are essential for evaluating biocompatibility. Bone substitution materials, such as hydroxyapatite and β-tricalcium phosphate were shown to be osteoinductive (Okumura et al. 1997; Habibovic et al. 2008; Sun et al. 2008). The *in vivo* bone-regenerative capacity of calcium silicate was investigated in rabbits and results were compared with TCP. Micro-CT and histomorphometric analysis showed resorption and newly formed bone with both materials, but resorption as well as bone formation of calcium silicate was higher than that of TCP (Xu et al. 2008). Wistar rats were used to histologically evaluate the healing of surgically created defects on the tibia after implantation of bioactive glass. Bioactive glass promoted comparable bone formation independently of the size of glass granules (Macedo et al. 2005). Also new bone formation was found after implantation of NovaBone 45S5 bioglass particulate (NovaBone, Jacksonville, USA) in sheep. In addition, acute as well as chronic inflammatory reactions were associated with the use of these glass granules (Kobayashi et al. 2010). Furthermore, cylindrical porous hydroxyapatite implants were implanted in rabbit femurs. Histological analyses of bone sections with toluidine blue showed new bone formation (Damien et al. 2003). Various publications discussed the use of porous hydroxyapatite in maxillary sinuses. Histologically, the grafted sinuses exhibited a significant amount of new bone formation. The porous hydroxyapatite granules appeared integrated with the new formed bone (Browaeys et al. 2007).
To date, predominantly histological staining and immunohistochemical analyses were used to study the behaviour of bone substitute materials on bone graft healing. Only a few numbers of studies present the molecular mechanisms of bone formations associated with bone substitutes. Recently it was shown, that bovine hydroxyapatite (HA) and β-tricalcium phosphate (β-TCP) up-regulate the expression of Runx2, Alpl and osteocalcin in biopsies from human jaws (Gotz et al. 2008).
Calcium phosphate cements and sintered ceramics as well as calcium sulphate cements and bioglass have been used as BMP carriers (del Real et al. 2002; den Boer et al. 2003; Kroese-Deutman et al. 2005). Synthetic porous hydroxyapatite might be providing a delivery system for bioactive agents. It was recently shown that the supplementation of a synthetic porous hydroxyapatite with IGF-1 significantly increased new bone formation and bone mineral apposition rate compared with hydroxyapatite alone (Damien et al. 2003). In contrast, the resorption of IGF1, TGFbeta1 or bFGF onto a carrier of TCP does not enhance new bone formation (Clarke et al. 2004). A multi-centre, randomized clinical trial using recombinant human platelet-derived growth factor with β-TCP for the treatment of intra-osseous periodontal defects showed significantly higher extent of linear bone growth and per cent bone fill compared to β-TCP alone after six months (Jayakumar et al. 2011).
An example for commercially available products containing growth factors is Gem 21S™ (Osteohealth, Shirley, USA), β-tricalciumphosphate and recombinant human PDGF.

4.2 Composites with different chemical phases

Advances in biomaterial fabrication have introduced numerous innovations in designing scaffolds for tissue engineering. The combination of different bone substitution materials is an important research topic. Biomaterials on the basis of calcium phosphates are most widely used in craniofacial bone surgery and considered to be biocompatible, nonimmunogenic and osteoconductive (Ruhé et al. ; Abukawa et al. 2006; Weinand et al. 2006). It is well know that the surface topography has an influence on cell attachment. Figure 2 showed surface topographies of three different commercially available bone substitution materials, especially Cerasorb®, Straumann® BoneCeramic and NanoBone®.

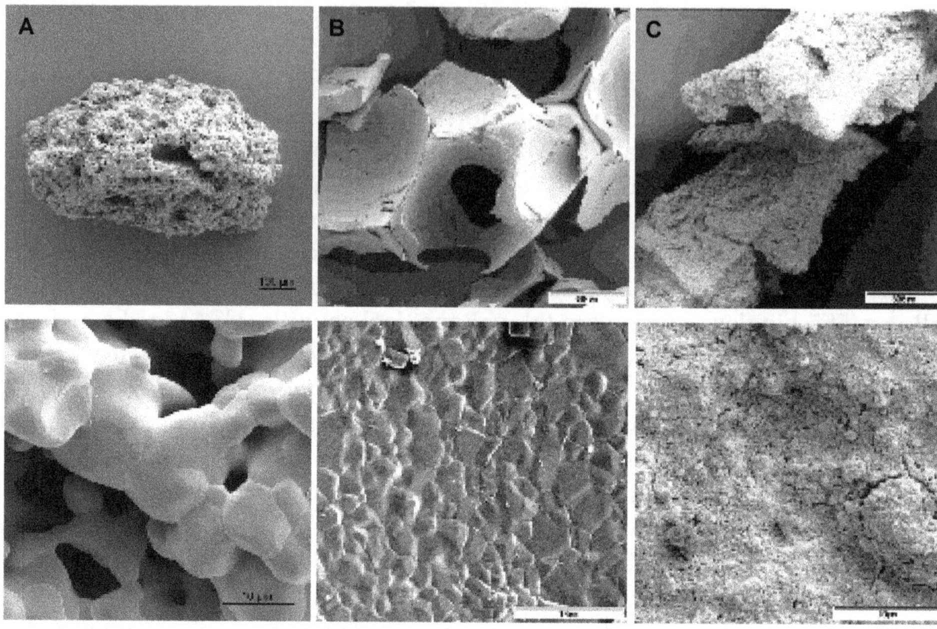

Fig. 2. Scanning electron micrographs of different biomaterials on the basis of calcium phosphates at different magnifications. (A) Cerasorb® (Curason AG, Germany), (B) Straumann® BoneCeramic (Straumann, Freiburg, Germany), (C) NanoBone® (Artoss, Rostock, Germany)

The composition of bioceramics influences the cell attachment and proliferation. It was shown that incorporation of zinc or silicate in calcium phosphate ceramics is followed by an increase of osteoblast attachment and proliferation (Ishikawa et al. 2002; Thian et al. 2005), whereas carbonate had contradictory effects on these cells (Redey et al. 2000).

Viability, proliferation and growth characteristics of fibroblasts cultured together with NanoBone® and Straumann® BoneCeramic were analysed over a period of 28 days. Fibroblast viability does not show any differences between cells incubated with the different bone graft materials and the control cells. Electron microscopy showed that fibroblast cells grew and proliferated at the surface of both bone graft materials (Kauschke et al. 2006). The same results could be observed by Reichert and coworkers (Reichert et al. 2009). They show no differences in the cellular proliferation between control cells and cells incubated with Straumann® BoneCeramic, NanoBone® and BonitMatrix® (Reichert et al. 2009). Furthermore, endothelial cells predominantly spread on BonitMatrix® and cells expressed endothelium-specific surface marker proteins (Thimm et al. 2008).

The biocompatibility of Straumann® BoneCeramic, NanoBone® and BonitMatrix® were tested using different animal models. A rapid vascularization and good integration within the peri-implant tissue was shown for BonitMatrix® after subcutaneously implantation in Wistar rats (Ghanaati et al. 2010).

In vivo studies using the mouse dorsal skinfold chamber model revealed a high biocompatibility comparable to that of cancellous bone for NanoBone®. Both NanoBone granules and plates do not show any venular leucocyte activation after implantation. Furthermore, signs of angiogenesis could be observed (Abshagen et al. 2009). Vascularization as well as osteoneogenesis after implantation of NanoBone® was observed using guinea pigs (Punke et al. 2008). Our own group could establish a FE model of remodelling processes occurring in a bone area provided with bone graft substitutes (Gedrange et al. 2008). MicroCT images revealed specimen changes in the spongious and compact areas provided with the bone substitution material (Figure 3). The use of NanoBone® as bone substitution material seems to decrease the bone atrophy after teeth extraction in pigs as compared to untreated alveolars, but the reduction is not significant (Figure 4).

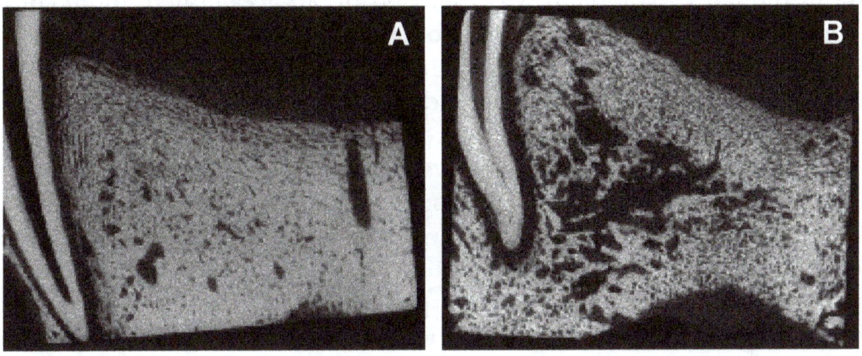

Fig. 3. MicroCT images of embedded bone specimens showing the remodelling of the area provided with NanoBone®. (A) NanoBone treated animal; (B) control animal (Gedrange et al., 2008).

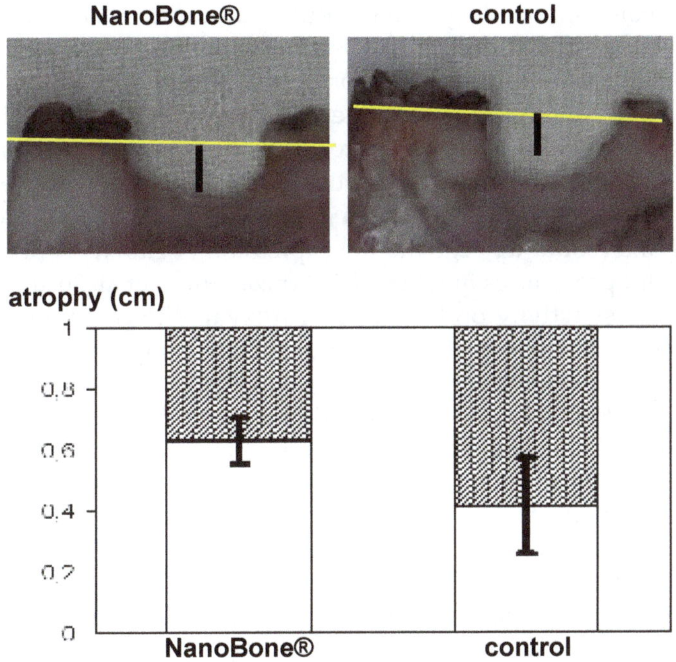

Fig. 4. Measurement of alveolar bone atrophy 70 days after teeth extraction and animal treatment with or without NanoBone®

The ideal substrate for the synthesis of bone should be able to promote the expression of the osteoblastic phenotype as well as provide a template for bone deposition (Kaufmann et al. 2000). An osteoblastic phenotype expression on the surface of hydroxyapatite ceramics, with subsequent gene expression of osteocalcin was found (Okumura et al. 1997). Recently it has been shown that OSSA NOVA and BONITmatrix® could stimulate bone regeneration of surgically created cranial defects in rats, but OSSA NOVA leads, in comparison with granular BONITmatrix®, to an accelerated more comprehensive bone regeneration (Kunert-Keil et al. 2009). Studies from our lab demonstrated an increased expression of the IGF1 mRNA in cranial defects treated with BONITmatrix® and OSSA NOVA (Gredes et al. 2010a). The increase in the IGF1 expression was followed by an accelerated, more comprehensive bone regeneration using both synthetic biomaterials consisting of calcium phosphates embedded in a silica matrix (Gredes et al. 2010a). Furthermore, Real-time RT-PCR analyses showed that the amount of the osteocalcin and Alpl mRNA was significantly increased after treatment with BONITmatrix®. It was recently shown that mesenchymal stem cells differentiated to osteoblasts within 14 days on hydroxyapatite and BONITmatrix® in expansion medium with and without osteogenic differentiation additives (Muller et al. 2008). Cells revealed a higher Alpl activity and increased mRNA expression of osteocalcin and collagen 1 (Muller et al. 2008). Another bone graft material consisting of nanocrystalline hydroxyapatite embedded in a porous silica gel matrix, Nanobone® was implanted in the mandible of minipigs. It was shown that Nanobone® is able to stimulate the differentiation of bone cells into osteoblasts and osteoclasts, because osteocalcin, alkaline phosphatase, osteopontin and BMP-2 were located in newly formed bone and focally in particles (Gerber et al. 2006). Furthermore, the matrix of all Nanobone® granules showed very strong immunoreactivity of osteocalcin and alkaline phosphatase in human jaw bone augmented with Nanobone® (Gotz et al. 2008). In addition, two other common markers for osteogenesis, mineralization and bone remodelling, namely Runx2 and Phex were analysed. Similar to the outcomes of other bone substitution materials like NanoBone® and their influence on bone healing process (Gotz et al. 2008), the expression of Runx2 gene was unaltered after application of BONITmatrix® and OSSA NOVA. Otherwise BONITmatrix® slightly increased the expression of the osteogenic transcription factor Runx2 in mesenchymal stem cells (Muller et al. 2008). In addition, it was suggested that diverse forms of hydroxyapatite nanoparticles may differentially affect the osteoblast cell function as shown on gene and protein levels (Xu et al. 2009). That NanoBone® could up-regulate the expression of Runx2, Alpl and osteocalcin was also shown in sinus lift procedures in rabbits (De Souza Nunes et al. 2010).

The degree of osteoclast activity on the most hydroxyapatite containing scaffolds depends on material qualities such as crystal size and surface roughness (Rumpel et al. 2006). Therefore the silica gel matrix granules of NanoBone® were replaced by an organic matrix by accompanying osteoblastic and osteoclastic relationships. Bio-Oss®, another type of hydroxyapatite material derived from bovine bone, is also degraded by osteoclasts with ruffled borders and acid phosphatase activity (Rumpel et al. 2006). The osteoclast-like cells are not only localized along the surface of the newly formed bone but also directly on the biomaterial. In the case of Bio-Oss® signs of osteoclastic resorption were evident in the formerly vascular osteon channels not surrounded by bone lamellae. Contrastingly, osteoclast attached to NanoBone® granules also occurred in defect regions without visible bone formation (Rumpel et al. 2006). Similar findings showed osteoclast-like cells on the surface of the NanoBone® bodies as well as on newly formed bone in human jaw bone augmented with Nanobone®. An osteoclastic as well as osteoblastic compartment could be observed after TRAP staining (Gotz et al. 2008).

Results of clinical studies using bone graft materials have recently shown that the implant success rate was 100% after three years when NanoBone® was used as grafting material. Furthermore the periotest values indicated a solid osseointegration (Heinemann et al. 2009).

4.3 Polymers

Tissue repair and regeneration by tissue engineering is dependent on the use of biodegradable polymer scaffolds which serve as a carrier matrix for bioactive substances or for incorporated cells. The adhesion of cells to bioresorbable scaffolds and the proliferation of cells on these scaffolds are important components for tissue engineering projects and play a fundamental role in regulating cell differentiation, growth and survival. Biodegradable polymers have displayed several properties of a suitable implant scaffold for the growth of osteoblast precursor cells. The ideal polymer would satisfy the following criteria: i) fill defects of various sizes and shapes, ii) mechanical and physical properties for a particular application, iii) a long shelf life, and iv) biocompatible degradation products.

Polymers are large organic macromolecules composed by many monomers in a regular pattern (structural units). Cellulose, collagen, agarose, chitin or hyaluronan are members of natural polymeric materials or so-called biological polymers. Natural polymers like collagen have been used for bone tissue engineering purposes (Hutmacher et al. 2001a). The most widely used bioresorbable materials are polymers of monocarboxylic acid derivates. A number of natural and synthetic polymers, such as poly-lactid acid (PLA), poly-glycolic acid (PGA), polyurethane (PU), and polycaprolactone (PCL), are in use as tissue scaffolds (Kiremitci and Piskin 1990; Vunjak-Novakovic et al. 1998; Hayashi et al. 2008). Recently these materials have been joined by linear polyesters of microbiological origin - polyhydroxykanoates (PHA). Local tissue responses to polymers *in vivo* depend on the biocompatibility of the polymer as well as its degradative by-products (Hollinger and Battistone 1986).

At the moment, two polymers are commercially available as a bone substitution material, first a PLA granulate (TruGraft™, Osteobiologics, San Antonio, U.S.A.) and second NovoSorb™ (PolyNovo Biomaterials, Port Melbourne, Australia).

The poly(α-hydroxy acid) polymers such as PLA, polygylcolide (PLG) and their copolymers PLGA are the most commonly used synthetic polymers to deliver BMPs (Isobe et al. 1999). Additional polymers used as BMP delivery systems include polyanhydrides, polypropylene fumurate, polyethylene glycol-PLA as well as polyphosphate (Lucas et al. 1990; Miyamoto et al. 1992; Renier and Kohn 1997; Behravesh et al. 1999). Incorpoartion of BMP-2 and BMP-7 in polycaprolactone suppressed bone marrow mesenchymal stem cell proliferation and increased the alkaline phosphatase activity (osteogenic differentiation) (Yilgor et al. 2010). An *in vivo* study determined the effects on osseointegration when polycaprolactone with BMP-2 coating was applied to bone screws. BMP-2 within the polycaprolactone coating did not stimulate osteogenesis (Niehaus et al. 2009). In contrast, using PCL scaffold, platelet-rich plasma and recombinant human BMP-2, a critical-size defect in the anterior mandible of a 71-years-old female patient was regenerated using de novo-grown bone (Schuckert et al. 2009).

4.3.1 Poly-3-hydroxybutyrate (PHB)

The most widespread and best studied polyhydroxyalkanoat (PHA) is the lipidic polymer, poly-3-hydroxybutyrate (PHB), which is found in the plasma membranes of Escherichia coli complexted to calcium polyphosphorate (Reusch and Sadoff 1983). Different bacterial types of microorganisms produce PHB from renewable sources, e.g. sugar and molasses, as intracellular storage materials. PHB is an ideal biomaterial, because it is a biodegradable polyester and completely degrades in D,L-b-hydroxybutyrate (HB), a normal component of blood and tissue (Miller and Williams 1987; Suwantong et al. 2007). PHB is perfectly isotactic viz. the monomers have all branch groups on the same side of the polymeric chain and are oriented in the same way (Figure 5).

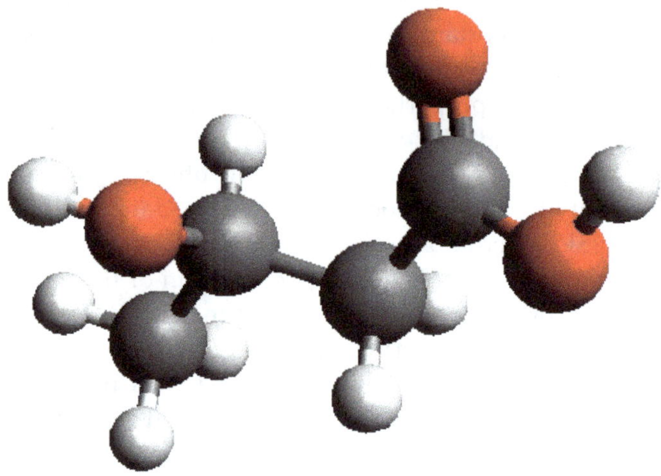

Fig. 5. Schematically illustration of a PHB monomer. The PHB monomer consists of hydroxybutyric acid ($C_4H_6O_2$ units) and a methyl group as side chain. Grey = carbon molecule; white = hydrogen molecule, red = oxygen molecule.

The biocompatibility of PHB has been confirmed *in vitro*, in cell cultures of various origins. It was found that mouse fibroblast cells and chondrocytes do not grow very well on microbial PHB films (Deng et al. 2002; Yang et al. 2002). PHB showed a high degree of crystallization and this rapid crystallization generates pores and protrusions on the PHB surface film. It was speculated that this surface could prohibit the attachment and growth of mammalian cells (Zhao et al. 2003). It is well known that biocompatibility of bio materials depends not only on the chemical structure but, to a large extent, on the size. Suwantong and coworker could show using indirect cytotoxicity assessment that PHB fibre mats were acceptable to both mouse L929 fibroblast cells and mouse Schwann cells (RT4-D6P2T) (Suwantong et al. 2007). Mouse fibroblast cells cultured with polymeric PHB microspheres revealed no cytotoxic effects which were indicated by the absence of changes in the cell morphology, cell viability and proliferative activity (Shishatskaya and Volova 2004). In addition, human osteoblast cells grow very well on PHB embroidery (Mai et al. 2006).

Several *in vivo* studies have shown that PHB may serve as a scaffold for tissue engineering due to its excellent biocompatibility as evidenced by lack of toxicity and compatibility with tissue and blood (Saito et al. 1991; Clarotti et al. 1992; Gogolewski et al. 1993; Schmack et al. 2000; Mai et al. 2006; Mack et al. 2008; Gredes et al. 2009). PHB sheets did not caused any inflammation in the chorioallantoic membrane of the developing egg (Saito et al. 1991). In mouse tissues no acute inflammation, abscess formation, or tissue necrosis was observed after subcutaneously implantation. In contrast, mononuclear macrophages, proliferating fibroblasts, and mature vascularized fibrous capsules were typically found (Gogolewski et al. 1993). Furthermore, PHB sutures implanted intramuscularly did not cause any acute vascular reaction or inflammation, necrosis calcification of the fibrous capsule or malignant tumour formation in rats (Shishatskaya et al. 2004). On the other hand, implantation of PHB implants significantly increased the mRNA expression of VEGF (vascular endothelial growth factor), IGF1 and IGF2 (insulin-like growth factor) and decreased the GDF8 (growth differentiation factor 8; myostatin) mRNA amount in Musculus latissimus dorsi of rats (Table 1) (Gredes et al. 2009).

Tested gene	mRNA expression (gene/β-actin)		
	controls	6 weeks of treatment	12 weeks of treatment
VEGF	3.9 ± 1.0	6.2 ± 1.6 *	
IGF1	14.2 ± 3.0	29.0 ± 7.0 *	19.2 ± 3.0 *
IGF2	5.5 ± 1.8	8.2 ± 1.8 *	
GDF8	4.8 ± 1.6	2.9 ± 1.0 *	3.3 ± 0.8 *

Table 1. Relative expression of the VEGF, IGF1, IGF2 and GDF8 mRNA in M. latissimus dorsi of control rats and in M. latissimus dorsi of rats 6 and 12 weeks after PHB scaffold implantation. Mean ± S.E.M. are given. Students t-test * = $p < 0.05$.

In addition, PHB scaffolds showed synergistic effects with the surrounding muscle, because of an increase in the slow myosin isoform after implantation (Mack et al. 2008). Another study showed ectopic bone formation in nude rats after intramuscular implantation of PHB embroidery seeded with human osteoblast cells (Mai et al. 2006). The osteogenic potential of different PHB scaffolds was also shown in nude rats (Rentsch et al. 2009). In mini pigs PHB was used for covering defined bone defects in the anterior skull base including a Dura mater lesion. The anterior skull base bone defect was completely closed after 9 months. Furthermore no reaction or adhesions between brain and PHB or Dura mater and PHB was observed (Bernd et al. 2009).

PHB patches were used to close experimentally induced atrial septal defects in calves. Twelve months postoperatively no shunt or sign of infection was found. This experimental model thus prompted formation of regenerated endothelial tissue and complete degradation of the PHB patches (Malm et al. 1992). Recently it was shown that PHB can be used as an alternative to epineural suturing in the treatment of peripheral nerve injuries at the wrist/forearm level of the arm (Aberg et al. 2009).

4.3.2 Polylactid (PLA)

Among the family of biodegradable polyesters, polylactides have come to the fore because, they are produced from renewable resources, they are biodegradable, have high mechanical performance and very low or no toxicity. The degradable material PLA is applied in dentistry as Guided Tissue/Bone Regeneration membranes even though these membranes do not have any significant biological function such as the facilitation of cell adhesion. Polylactic acid or polylactide (PLA) is the most commonly used biodegradable, thermoplastic, aliphatic polyester derived from renewable resources in surgery especially in osteosynthesis (Ashammakhi et al. 2003). PLA can be used for biomedical purposes because of its biodegradability in contact with biological tissues (Rimondini et al. 2005). Polylactide acid is degraded by hydrolysis or specific cleavage of oligopeptides (Drury and Mooney 2003). It is known that the degradation product of PLA, lactic acid, is normally present in the body, can enter the tricarbonxylic acid cycle and is excreted as H_2O and CO_2 (Gunatillake and Adhikari 2003). On the other hand degradation products of PLA are partially cytotoxic (Nesic et al. 2006).

In our own experiments we could show that cultivation of L929 mouse fibroblast cells with PLA membranes significantly decreased cell proliferation and increased the amount of death cells compared to control cells. Our results are in agreement with findings from Yang et al (Yang et al. 2002). They show that growth of L929 cells was poor on PLA films. The numbers of adhered cells cultured on PLA were significantly lower than those on control disks in early periods of incubation but became comparable after 21 days (Iwamatsu-Kobayashi et al. 2005). Human keratinocytes delayed growth has been shown on a PLA film with respect to culture on standard tissue culture polystyrene, even though the same plateau level was observed after 2 weeks (Garric et al. 2005). Former *in vitro* studies have shown that osteoblast cells are able to attach well to PLA or poly-glycolic acid (PGA) (Ishaug et al. 1994). We could demonstrate that primary osteoblast cells growth on PLA membranes (Figure 6).

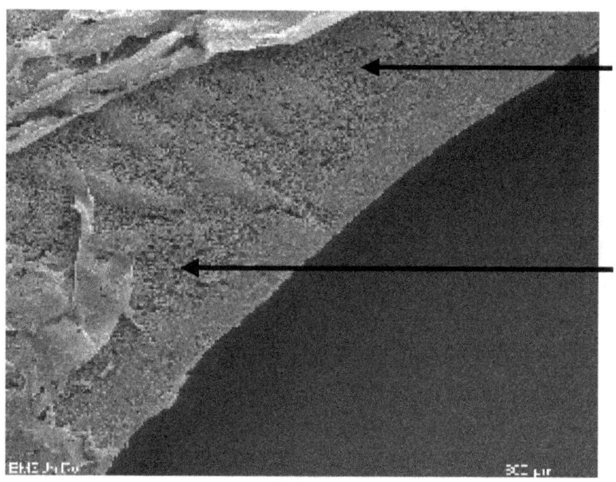

Fig. 6. Scanning electron micrograph of osteoblast cells (PO62) growing on a PLA membranes. Heterogenous morphology of these cells was observed after 10 days of cell culture. Bars = 300 μm

Collagen coating and NaOH treatments of the PLA film improved skin cell adhesion and proliferation but their extent depends usually on the culture time (Garric et al. 2005). Furthermore, an enhanced 3-dimensional porous structure of PLA coated with collagen showed a significantly higher amount of initial cell attachment than PLA porous scaffold without collagen immobilization (Fuse et al. 2009). Other PLA surface modifications with chloric acid mixture solution increased the surface wettability and with it the cell adhesion on the surface (Lee et al. 2002). In contrast, human RT-112 cells did not show any differences in the proliferation rate after incubation with PLA alone or PLA-copolymers (Holzl et al. 2000).

In vivo biocompatibility of poly(L-lactide) resorbable mesh was shown in rats. It was found that PLA induces important immunological reaction. Amongst others PLA caused mild

inflammatory response by infiltrating mononuclear and polynuclear inflammatory cells in animals (de Tayrac et al. 2008). Furthermore, stereocomplexed PLA nanofibers induced milder inflammatory reaction than poly(L-lactide) nanofibers after subcutaneous implantation in rats (Ishii et al. 2009).
To date, predominantly histological staining and immunohistochemical analyses were used to study the behaviour of bone substitute materials on bone graft healing. Only a few numbers of studies present the molecular mechanisms of bone formations associated with bone substitutes. Recently it was shown that the expression of type I and type II collagen was increased in human mesenchymal progenitor cells as well as adipose stem cells seeded on PLA (Heckmann et al. 2007; Maenpaa et al. 2010). PLA nanofibres possessed a growth inhibitory effect on human tendon derived fibroblasts and no meaningful influence on the gene expression of collagen I was observed (Theisen et al. 2010). Furthermore, PLA nanofibres tend to result in a down-regulation in bone morphogenetic protein 2 (BMP-2) and VEGF expression during the period of human mesenchymal stem cell differentiation towards osteoblasts (Schofer et al. 2009). On the other hand PLA membranes do not have any influence on the gene expression of different growth factors, collagen I and II as well as myostatin after subcutaneously implantation in rats (Gredes et al. 2010b).

4.3.3 Polycaprolactone (PCL)

Polycaprolactone (PCL), a thermoplastic polymer derived from the chemical synthesis of crude oil, has a very low melting point of about 60°C and degrades by hydrolysis of its ester linkage under physiological conditions. Polycaprolactone has also been regarded as a tissue-compatible biodegradable polymer with good mechanical properties (Khor et al. 2003). PCL has been proven to be a tissue-compatible biodegradable polymer with satisfying mechanical properties although it is not very favourable for cell growth because of its intrinsic hydrophobicity and lack of bioactive functional groups (Zhu et al. 2002). *In vitro* studies showed that human calvarial periosteal cells attached and proliferated on PCL membranes with the formation of extracellular matrix (Schantz et al. 2002). Further studies were conducted with primary human fibroblast cells. Light, environmental scanning electron, and confocal laser microscopy as well as immunohistochemistry showed cell proliferation and extracellular matrix production on the polycaprolactone surface in the first culturing week. Over a period of 3-4 weeks in a culture, the fully interconnected scaffold architecture was completely 3D-filled by cellular tissue (Hutmacher et al. 2001b). Human primary craniofacial cells proliferated on PCL as shown by DNA-assay and collagen-I staining. Short- and long-term attachment studies demonstrated the expression of osteoblast cell markers on the PCL (Gough et al. 2003). Figure 7 illustrates a natural cover of a PCL membrane with primary osteoblast cells after 10 d of cell culture.
On the other hand, decreased fibroblast cell density was present by Vance et al. after 5 days of treatment with NaOH-modified PCL (Vance et al. 2004). These findings are in agreement with our own observations that mouse fibroblast cells incubated with PCL membranes showed a significantly decreased proliferation rate and a higher amount of death cells as compared to control cells.
The ability of PCL to repair bone defects were tested in white rabbits. Bone defects of 4.5 x 12 mm in the bilateral femoral condyle were prepared and PCL cylinders implanted into the defects. After 3 to 12 months of implantation, it was shown that bone defects were filled with new bone on the PCL-surface, and no inflammatory reaction appeared. Furthermore, the bone mineral density was greater in the PCL treated animals compared to untreated control group (Aahmat et al. 2005). PCL has a good biocompatibility and high osteoinductivity.

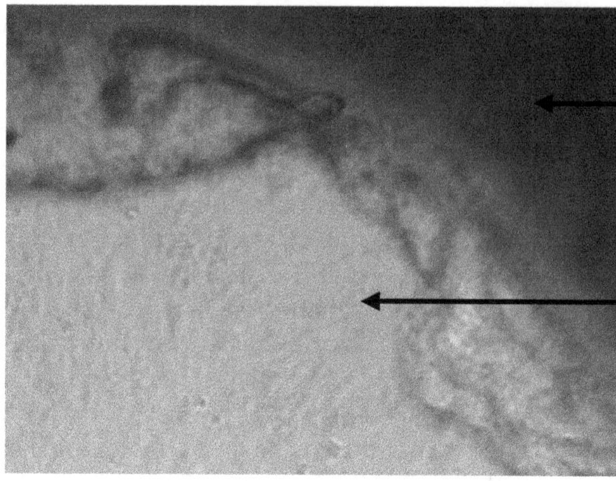

Fig. 7. Transmission microscopy of osteoblast cells (PO62) growing on a PCL membrane. Normal morphology of these cells was observed after 10 days of cell culture. Magnification: x 200.

To increase the osteoinductivity and osteoconductivity of PCL scaffolds, the PCL surface was modified. Previously, PCL-tricalcium phosphate scaffolds were developed and implanted into rat femoral defects. Histological evaluation illustrated infiltration of vascularized connective tissue and bone in treated rats, whereas the bone in-growth of untreated defects is minimal (Rai et al. 2007a). Polycaprolactone-20% tricalcium phosphate (PCL-TCP) scaffolds were assessed for the treatment of critical-sized defects of the mandible. Micro-CT measurements showed an increase in the bone volume fraction in defects grafted with scaffolds. The increase in the bone volume fraction was more pronounced after combination of the PCL-TCP scaffolds with platelet-rich plasma (Rai et al. 2007b). Another modification is the incorporation of hydroxyapatite (HA) particles in PCL scaffolds. These PCL/HA scaffolds increase the expression of osteogenic differentiation markers, such as type I collagen and osteocalcin in an in vitro model. Furthermore, the use of the PCL/HA scaffolds in a mouse calvarial model showed significantly greater amounts of new bone compared to pure PCL scaffolds (Chuenjitkuntaworn et al. 2010).

4.3.4 Collagen

Natural polymers used in bone tissue engineering include collagen, fibrin, alginate, silk, hyaluronic acid, and chitosan (Hutmacher et al. 2001a). Many of the naturally occuring animal-derived polymers are components of the extracellular matrix. They are biocompatible, bioresorbable and can be formulated into many configurations with variable residence time using enzymatic treatment and chemical crosslinking. Collagen is the most abundant extracellular matrix protein and component of connective tissue. Collagen, in the form of elongated fibers, is mostly found in tendon, ligament and skin, as well as in cartilage and bone. The collagen used in dental procedures is readily isolated and purified from various animal species by enzyme treatment. Collagen type I is the main organic component that is originally secreted by osteoblasts, which then becomes mineralized at a later stage of bone development. Collagen has been actively investigated as a favourable artificial environment for bone ingrowth. It was shown that endothelial cells adherent, spread and proliferated on a collagen membrane (Lycoll®, Resorba, Nuernberg, Germany) (Breithaupt-

Faloppa et al. 2006). Twardowski and co-workers found that type I collagen potently stimulates angiogenesis *in vitro* and *in vivo* (Twardowski et al. 2007). Furthermore, mesenchymal stem cell osteogenic differentiation was demonstrated on collagen scaffolds (Donzelli et al. 2007; Schneider et al. 2010; Jurgens et al. 2011). Alveolar ridge augmentation was found utilizing collagen wound dressing, so called COLLACOTE® (Zimmer Dental, Carlsbad, USA) (Ceravolo et al. 1987).

Type I collagen gel matrix was used for nasal reconstruction in rats. Histological sections of the collagen implant revealed restoration of the nasal anatomy with a thin plate of immature bone (Lindsey et al. 1996; Toung et al. 1999). Recently it was shown that resorbable collagen membranes can be used for guided bone regeneration after apicectomy or around dental implants. Both studies demonstrate that quantity and quality of new bone formation were much better in bone defects covered with collagen compared to untreated bone defects (Fei et al. 2008; Dominiak et al. 2009). At the moment two collagen-based bone augmentation materials are commercially available: Foundation™ (J. Morita USA, Inc.) and COLLAPLUG® (Zimmer Dental, Carlsbad, USA). Foundation™, an absorbable atelo-collagen sponge consists of 85 to 95% bovine collagen type I and 5 to 15% bovine collagen type III and has been used with great success since 1998 in Japan. Using rats it was shown that TERUPLUG® (different brand name for Foundation™) is able to stimulate endochondral ossification within two weeks after implantation into the calf muscle. Alkaline phosphatase activity and the calcium content had increased markedly in treated rats (Shinji et al. 2003). In addition, four weeks after implantation of TERUPLUG® in rabbit cranial defects a lot of newly formed collagen fibers around the inserted material were observed. Newly formed and matured bone was found eight weeks after implantation of TERUPLUG® compared to untreated animals (Kim et al. 2008). TERUPLUG® was used for maxillary sinus augmentation in rabbits. Gradually increased new bone formation was observed after 4, 12 and 24 weeks (Marukawa et al. 2011). In contrast, little or no new bone formation was observed on the maxillary sinus floor at six months following sinus membrane elevation and support with COLLAPLUG® in humans (Ahn et al. 2011).

Despite the good *in vitro* and *in vivo* biocompatibility, collagen undergoes rapid degradation upon implantation within 4-5 weeks (Donzelli et al. 2007). Furthermore, commercial collagen sponge (COLLAPLUG®) and membrane (BioGuide®, Geistlich Pharma, Wolhusen, Germany) induced considerable cell death, impaired initial function, and generated extraordinary intracellular reactive oxygen species in attached osteoblast cells. These effects substantially ameliorated after N-acetyl cysteine pre-treatment of the collagen sponge and membrane (Yamada et al. 2010).

Collagen is very often used as matrix for application of growth factors, e.g. TGF-β or BMP-2. Intramuscular application of TGF-β-loaded collagenous matrix is resulted in bone induction in primates (Ripamonti et al. 1997; Duneas et al. 1998). TERUPLUG®, as a carrier for Escherichia coli-derived recombinant human bone morphogenetic protein-2 (ErhBMP-2), was implanted into the calf muscle of Wistar rats. After 21 days, mature bone was formed and on days 14 to 21 after implantation, alkaline phosphatase activity and calcium content increased (Shinji et al. 2003).

Examples for a commercially available product containing growth factors is INFUSE® Bone Graft (Medtronic GmbH, Meerbusch, Germany), recombinant human bone morphogenetic protein 2 in an absorbable collagen sponge.

4.4 Biocomposites containing flax fibers in a polyester matrix

The usage of barrier membranes for osteogenesis has increased in the last years. Small bony defects seem not to depend on the application of membranes to regenerate bone, but large bone defects benefit from membranes, because they reduce the indispensable resorption of bone grafts when used alone. The application of barrier membranes to promote bone regeneration was described in orthopedic research. However, the clinical potential of these membranes was recognized some years ago for periodontal regeneration (Hermann and Buser 1996; Sculean et al. 2008).

Fibre-reinforced plastics have successfully proven their value in various applications because of their excellent specific properties, such as high strength and stiffness. The use of natural fibres for fabrication of composites in combination with biodegradable polymers is an excellent approach for biomedical application. Natural fibres are of basic interest since they have the capability to replace glass, ceramics or carbon fibres (Bax and Müssig 2008). Natural fibres combined with biodegradable polymers like polyhydroxyalkanoate (PHA), polylactic acid (PLA), polycaprolactone (PCL) and starch polymers frequently used as a matrix resulted in composites called "green" because of their complete biodegradability (Mohanty et al. 2005). The influence of plant fibres like flax, jute, ramie, oil palm fibres or cellulose fibres on the mechanical properties of biodegradable polymers was tested several years ago. Wollendorfer and Bader found in increased tensile strength as well as a four times better wheat starch of the reinforced polymer compared to the polymers without fibres (Wollendorfer and Bader 1998) Composites reinforced with natural fibres have been used in several branches of industry (i.e. automobile) and medicine with special focus on tissue artificial scaffold, drug-release systems, cardiovascular patches and nerve cuffs (Williams and Martin 2002; Misra et al. 2006). Flax fibres are amongst the oldest fibre crops in the world. The use of flax for the production of linen goes back at least to ancient Egyptian times. It is known that flax fibres are stronger than cotton fibres but less elastic. Flax fibres provide natural raw materials for composites and pulp / paper (van Dam et al. 1996). Former studies have shown an increased biological reaction around linen threads compared to synthetic threads (Jarosz-Cichulska 1988). Recently, the cytotoxicity of flax fibres, oil emulsion, and seedcake extract from transgenic flax overproducing various antioxidative compounds was determined in a culture of mouse fibroblasts. No changes in the total number of fibroblasts and comparable numbers of dead cells were shown in the presence of each type of flax material (Skorkowska-Telichowska et al. 2010).

In order to improve the biochemical and mechanical properties of flax fibres, transgenic flax over-expressing the bacterial polyhydroxybutyrate (PHB) gene was produced (Wrobel et al. 2004; Wrobel-Kwiatkowska et al. 2007). Composites containing fibres from transgenic plants did not differ from the control plants in the level of major fibre constituents (i.e. cellulose, lignin and pectin content) but was significantly stronger and more elastic than those containing fibres from control flax plants (Szopa et al. 2009). Furthermore, genetically modified flax plants producing PHB showed significantly increased parameters such as strength, Young´s modulus, energy for failure of flax fibres and phenolic acid level, a reason for improved plant resistance to pathogen infection (Wrobel-Kwiatkowska et al. 2007; Wrobel-Kwiatkowska et al. 2009).

We found that composites containing flax fibres from transgenic flax plants producing polyhydroxybutyrate (M50) and control (wt-Nike) plants in a polylactid (PLA) or polycaprolactone (PCL) matrix showed a good *in vitro* biocompatibility despite the cell viability of mouse fibroblast cells treated with these composites being slightly reduced and the amount of dead cells significantly increased compared to untreated cells after incubation for 12h to 48h. The biocompatibility of composites from transgenic flax plant fibres producing PHB did not differ from composites of non-transgenic flax plant fibres. Both linen membranes coated with PLA showed a significant increase in the proliferation rate of fibroblast cells compared to cells treated with membranes composed of PLA alone, whereas both flax membranes in the PCL matrix significantly decreased the proliferation rate of mouse fibroblast cells compared to cells treated with membranes composed of PCL alone. No differences were found between genetically modified and non-modified flax (Figure 8).

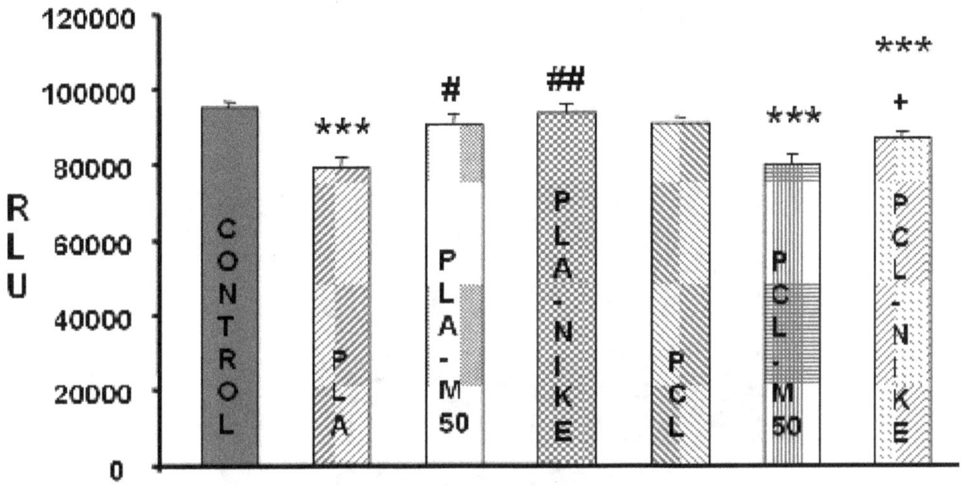

Fig. 8. Determination of cell viability by measurement of ATP. Viability of mice fibroblast cells (L929) cultured without and with membranes produced of polylactide (PLA), linen from PHB producing flax fibres coated with PLA (PLA-M50), linen from normal flax fibres coated with PLA (PLA-NIKE), polycaprolactone (PCL), linen from PHB producing flax fibres coated with PCL (PCL-M50) and linen from normal flax fibres coated with PCL (PCL-NIKE) for 24h was analysed using the CellTiter-Glo® assay. Means ± S.E.M. are given in all cases for n = 14-48 samples. Stars indicate significant differences: ***) $p < 0.005$, membrane-treated cells versus control; $^{\#\#}$) $p < 0.01$, $^{\#\#\#}$) $p < 0.005$, PLA versus linen membrane, $^{+}$) $p < 0.05$, PCL versus linen membrane, unpaired t-test. RLU = relative luminescence units.

Beside macroscopically and histological examination the biocompatibility can be assessed by analyses of the biomaterial influence on the gene expression. Because of this we analysed the gene expression of growth factors such as vascular endothelial growth factor (VEGF) and insulin-like growth factor (IGF) as well as myostatin also known as growth differentiation factor 8 (GDF8) after subcutaneous implantation. We found that subcutaneously insertion of the different biocomposites had no influence on the gene expression of the most tested genes. The constantly happening muscle contraction of the Musculus latissimus dorsi is not followed by stress-induced changes in muscle growth factor expression (Gredes et al. 2010b). The influence of the new biocomposites on bone regeneration must be checked using *in vitro* models. Cell culture experiments with primary osteoblast cells and these biocomposites showed that osteoblast cells are able to attach and proliferate on these membranes. The proliferation is much better on PLA-biocomposites compared to PCL-flax membranes (Figure 9).

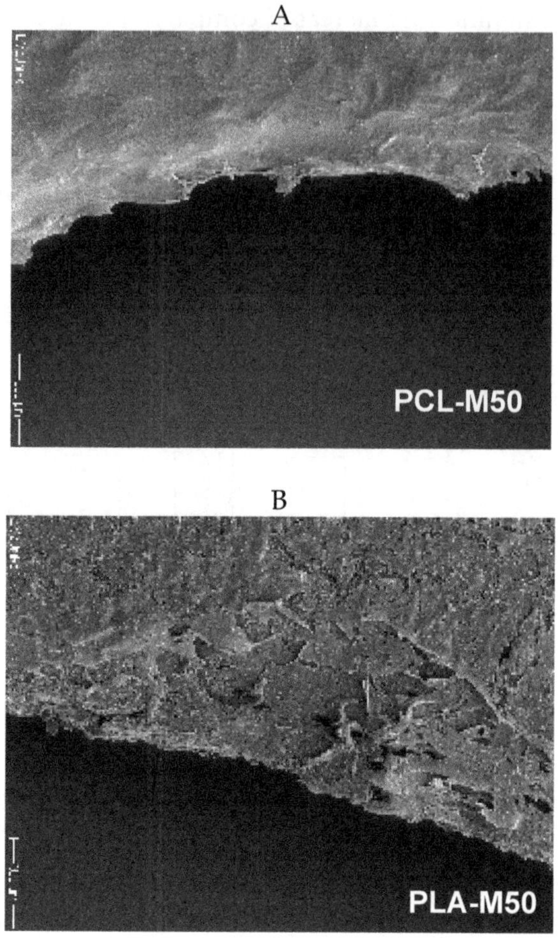

Fig. 9. Scanning electron micrographs of osteoblast cells (PO62) growing on a PCL-M50 (A) or a PLA-M50 membrane (B). After 10 days of cell culture on PCL-M50 membranes moderate natural cover with osteoblast cells could be observed, whereas culturing on PLA-M50 increased the amount of growing cells. Bars = 300 μm

4.5 Carrier for growth factors

As described earlier in this chapter bone formation is mediated by the release of local, biochemical and biophysical messengers, e.g. growth factors. In therapeutic use the bone growth factors need a carrier. Carrier requirements for most bone repairs are also simplified by the concurrent use of either internal or external fixation or coaptation, eleminating the need for mechanical strenght or resistance to motion. Furthermore, the carrier should assure local, sustained release of the growth factors which may otherwise be rapidly absorbed before instituting their effect. Bone is also highly vascular and carriers used for bone repair have to be capable of supporting vascular in-growth. Several biodegradable materials have been investigated as carriers for bone growth factors, including (1) organic materials such as inactive demineralized bone proteins, collagen, fibrin, squalene, and coral; (2) ceramics, including tricalcium phosphate, hydroxyapatite, calcium-sulphate composites, and bioactive glasses; and (3) synthetic polymers such as polylactide, polylactide-polyglycolide co-polymer, polyanhydride, and polyorthoester (Table 2).

Biodegradable materials as carriers for bone growth factors		Quality characteristics	References
organic materials	collagen	Collagen molecules assemble into heterotypic aggregates that define the biological and mechanical properties of most tissues and organs. Type I collagen, the major component of the organic bone matrix can bind osteoblasts via specific cell surface receptors, the integrins.	(Burgeson and Nimni 1992; Tzaphlidou 2005)
	fibrin	High adhesion to many biological surfaces, excellent seeding effects and good tissue development. It is not toxic, allergenic or inflammatory.	(Ye et al. 2000)
	coral	Natural coral is radiodense, it resorbs more rapidly than ceramic materials and the natural pore size of native coral facilitates osteoconduction and bone growth.	(Sciadini et al. 1997)
ceramics	tricalcium phosphate	Porous beta-tricalcium phosphate scaffolds are employed for local drug delivery in bone. It is used alone or in combination with resorbable polymer or autologous materials.	(Bansal et al. 2009; Kundu et al. 2010)
	hydroxyapatite	An identical composition to the bone tissue of living organisms and has similar physical, mechanical, and other properties. It shows high biocompatibility, does not give rise to inflammatory phenomena, and is non-toxic.	(Yarosh et al. 2001)
	calcium-sulphate composites	Calcium sulfate (plaster of Paris) is an absorbable, moldable material that has easy handling properties. It promotes osseous formation.	(Pecora et al. 1997)
	bioactive glass	This material has osteoconductive and osteo-promotive abilities in the biocompatible interface for osseous migration, and a bioactive surface colonized by osteogenic cells free in the surgical wound. It bonds to soft and osseous tissues.	(Wilson and Low 1992; Macedo et al. 2004)

synthetic polymers	polylactide (PLA)	Prosperities of PLA depend on the component isomers, processing temperature and molecular weight. In nature, polymer degradation is induced thermal activation, hydrolysis, biological activity, oxidation, photolysis, or radiolysis. In biomedical fields it is also used as bone fixation material and drug delivery microsphere.	(Zhao et al. 2004; Madhavan Nampoothiri et al. 2010)
	polylactide-polyglycolide copolymer	It promotes specific cell adhesion, differentiation and bone formation. Its degradation depends on the formulation, amorphous/crystalline structure, isomeric characteristics, molecular weight and amount of material used.	(Lu et al. 2003; Serino et al. 2003)
	polyanhydride	Polyanhydrides and their degradation products have not been found to cause significant harmful responses and are considered to be biocompatible. *In vivo*, polyanhydrides degrade into non-toxic diacid monomers that can be metabolized and eliminated from the body.	(Tamada and Langer 1992; Kumar et al. 2002)
	polyorthoester	This polymer degrades at its surface and becomes thinner with time rather than crumbling. It can cause minor moderate inflammation reaction, compared with PLA.	(Ekholm et al. 1997)

Table 2. Carrier materials for bone growth factors.

5. Conclusion

The literature has shown that early bone loss can be significantly reduced by socket grafting. The process of socket grafting requires an understanding of wound healing and an appreciation of the biological properties of the products available for socket grafting. Various types of alloplastic bone substitution materials have been created and showed ossification and new bone formation. The huge variety of biomaterials makes it difficult to decide which material is adequate for which indication. To date, tissue engineered bone is far from a routine clinical application. Clinical investigations using alloplastic bone substitution materials are very rare in the literature but, because of similar bone remodelling processes in pigs and humans, we found the same details about usage of alloplasts in dentistry. The most alloplastic materials are not popular in dentistry and, because of this, further studies are necessary.

6. Acknowledgment

The authors would like to thank Dr. Dagmar Richter (University of Rostock) for cell culture experiments with primary osteoblasts and electron scanning microscopy, Dr. Silke Lucke (University of Greifswald) for the analysis of muscle and bone histology as well as Ingrid Pieper (University of Greifswald) for excellent technical assistance.

7. References

Aahmat, Y., Chen, T., Chen, Z., Liu, D. and Wang, Z. (2005). [An experimental study on repairing bone defect with the biodegradable polycaprolactone material]. *Zhongguo Xiu Fu Chong Jian Wai Ke Za Zhi*, Vol.19, No.6, pp. 439-442

Abdallah, B.M. and Kassem, M. (2008). Human mesenchymal stem cells: from basic biology to clinical applications. *Gene Ther*, Vol.15, No.2, pp. 109-116

Aberg, M., Ljungberg, C., Edin, E., Millqvist, H., Nordh, E., Theorin, A., Terenghi, G. and Wiberg, M. (2009). Clinical evaluation of a resorbable wrap-around implant as an alternative to nerve repair: a prospective, assessor-blinded, randomised clinical study of sensory, motor and functional recovery after peripheral nerve repair. *J Plast Reconstr Aesthet Surg*, Vol.62, No.11, pp. 1503-1509

Abshagen, K., Schrodi, I., Gerber, T. and Vollmar, B. (2009). In vivo analysis of biocompatibility and vascularization of the synthetic bone grafting substitute NanoBone. *J Biomed Mater Res A*, Vol.91, No.2, pp. 557-566

Abukawa, H., Papadaki, M., Abulikemu, M., Leaf, J., Vacanti, J.P., Kaban, L.B. and Troulis, M.J. (2006). The engineering of craniofacial tissues in the laboratory: a review of biomaterials for scaffolds and implant coatings. *Dent. Clin. North. Am.*, Vol.50, No.2, pp. 205-216, viii

Ahn, J.J., Cho, S.A., Byrne, G., Kim, J.H. and Shin, H.I. (2011). New bone formation following sinus membrane elevation without bone grafting: histologic findings in humans. *Int J Oral Maxillofac Implants*, Vol.26, No.1, pp. 83-90

Albrektsson, T. and Johansson, C. (2001). Osteoinduction, osteoconduction and osseointegration. *Eur Spine J*, Vol.10 Suppl 2, pp. S96-101

Ashammakhi, N., Suuronen, R., Tiainen, J., Tormala, P. and Waris, T. (2003). Spotlight on naturally absorbable osteofixation devices. *J Craniofac Surg*, Vol.14, No.2, pp. 247-259

Bansal, S., Chauhan, V., Sharma, S., Maheshwari, R., Juyal, A. and Raghuvanshi, S. (2009). Evaluation of hydroxyapatite and beta-tricalcium phosphate mixed with bone marrow aspirate as a bone graft substitute for posterolateral spinal fusion. *Indian J Orthop*, Vol.43, No.3, pp. 234-239

Bax, B. and Müssig, J. (2008). Impact and tensile properties of PLA/Cordenka and PLA/flax composites *Composites science and technology*, Vol.68, No.7-8, pp. 1601-1607

Behravesh, E., Yasko, A.W., Engel, P.S. and Mikos, A.G. (1999). Synthetic biodegradable polymers for orthopaedic applications. *Clin Orthop Relat Res*, Vol.No.367 Suppl, pp. S118-129

Bernd, H.E., Kunze, C., Freier, T., Sternberg, K., Kramer, S., Behrend, D., Prall, F., Donat, M. and Kramp, B. (2009). Poly(3-hydroxybutyrate) (PHB) patches for covering anterior skull base defects - an animal study with minipigs. *Acta Otolaryngol*, Vol.129, No.9, pp. 1010-1017

Bernhardt, A., Lode, A., Peters, F. and Gelinsky, M. (2010). Novel ceramic bone replacement material Osbone((R)) in a comparative in vitro study with osteoblasts. *Clin Oral Implants Res*, Vol.

Bertelloni, S., Baroncelli, G.I. and Mora, S. (2010). Bone health in disorders of sex differentiation. *Sex Dev*, Vol.4, No.4-5, pp. 270-284

Bikle, D.D. (2008). Integrins, insulin like growth factors, and the skeletal response to load. *Osteoporos Int*, Vol.19, No.9, pp. 1237-1246

Bostrom, M.P. and Asnis, P. (1998). Transforming growth factor beta in fracture repair. *Clin Orthop Relat Res*, Vol.No.355 Suppl, pp. S124-131

Breithaupt-Faloppa, A.C., Kleinheinz, J. and Crivello, O., Jr. (2006). Endothelial cell reaction on a biological material. *J Biomed Mater Res B Appl Biomater*, Vol.76, No.1, pp. 49-55

Browaeys, H., Bouvry, P. and De Bruyn, H. (2007). A literature review on biomaterials in sinus augmentation procedures. *Clin Implant Dent Relat Res*, Vol.9, No.3, pp. 166-177

Burg, K.J., Porter, S. and Kellam, J.F. (2000). Biomaterial developments for bone tissue engineering. *Biomaterials*, Vol.21, No.23, pp. 2347-2359

Burgeson, R.E. and Nimni, M.E. (1992). Collagen types. Molecular structure and tissue distribution. *Clin Orthop Relat Res*, Vol.No.282, pp. 250-272

Calvo-Guirado, J.L., Mate-Sanchez, J., Delgado-Ruiz, R., Ramirez-Fernandez, M.P., Cutando-Soriano, A. and Pena, M. (2011). Effects of growth hormone on initial bone formation around dental implants: a dog study. *Clin Oral Implants Res*, Vol.22, No.6, pp. 587-593

Canalis, E. (1983). The hormonal and local regulation of bone formation. *Endocr Rev*, Vol.4, No.1, pp. 62-77

Ceravolo, F.J., Famili, P. and Li, S.T. (1987). Alveolar ridge augmentation utilizing collagen wound dressing. *Int J Oral Implantol*, Vol.4, No.2, pp. 15-18

Cheng, H., Jiang, W., Phillips, F.M., Haydon, R.C., Peng, Y., Zhou, L., Luu, H.H., An, N., Breyer, B., Vanichakarn, P., Szatkowski, J.P., Park, J.Y. and He, T.C. (2003). Osteogenic activity of the fourteen types of human bone morphogenetic proteins (BMPs). *J Bone Joint Surg Am*, Vol.85-A, No.8, pp. 1544-1552

Chuenjitkuntaworn, B., Inrung, W., Damrongsri, D., Mekaapiruk, K., Supaphol, P. and Pavasant, P. (2010). Polycaprolactone/hydroxyapatite composite scaffolds: preparation, characterization, and in vitro and in vivo biological responses of human primary bone cells. *J Biomed Mater Res A*, Vol.94, No.1, pp. 241-251

Clarke, S.A., Brooks, R.A., Lee, P.T. and Rushton, N. (2004). The effect of osteogenic growth factors on bone growth into a ceramic filled defect around an implant. *J Orthop Res*, Vol.22, No.5, pp. 1016-1024

Clarotti, G., Schue, F., Sledz, J., Ait Ben Aoumar, A., Geckeler, K.E., Orsetti, A. and Paleirac, G. (1992). Modification of the biocompatible and haemocompatible properties of polymer substrates by plasma-deposited fluorocarbon coatings. *Biomaterials*, Vol.13, No.12, pp. 832-840

Cornish, J., Callon, K.E. and Reid, I.R. (1996). Insulin increases histomorphometric indices of bone formation In vivo. *Calcif Tissue Int*, Vol.59, No.6, pp. 492-495

Damien, E., Hing, K., Saeed, S. and Revell, P.A. (2003). A preliminary study on the enhancement of the osteointegration of a novel synthetic hydroxyapatite scaffold in vivo. *J Biomed Mater Res A*, Vol.66, No.2, pp. 241-246

De Souza Nunes, L.S., De Oliveira, R.V., Holgado, L.A., Nary Filho, H., Ribeiro, D.A. and Matsumoto, M.A. (2010) Immunoexpression of Cbfa-1/Runx2 and VEGF in sinus lift procedures using bone substitutes in rabbits. *Clin. Oral. Implants Res.*, Vol.21, No.6, pp. 584-590

de Tayrac, R., Chentouf, S., Garreau, H., Braud, C., Guiraud, I., Boudeville, P. and Vert, M. (2008). In vitro degradation and in vivo biocompatibility of poly(lactic acid) mesh for soft tissue reinforcement in vaginal surgery. *J Biomed Mater Res B Appl Biomater*, Vol.85, No.2, pp. 529-536

del Real, R.P., Wolke, J.G., Vallet-Regi, M. and Jansen, J.A. (2002). A new method to produce macropores in calcium phosphate cements. *Biomaterials*, Vol.23, No.17, pp. 3673-3680

den Boer, F.C., Wippermann, B.W., Blokhuis, T.J., Patka, P., Bakker, F.C. and Haarman, H.J. (2003). Healing of segmental bone defects with granular porous hydroxyapatite augmented with recombinant human osteogenic protein-1 or autologous bone marrow. *J Orthop Res*, Vol.21, No.3, pp. 521-528

Deng, Y., Zhao, K., Zhang, X.F., Hu, P. and Chen, G.Q. (2002). Study on the three-dimensional proliferation of rabbit articular cartilage-derived chondrocytes on polyhydroxyalkanoate scaffolds. *Biomaterials*, Vol.23, No.20, pp. 4049-4056

Dezawa, M., Kanno, H., Hoshino, M., Cho, H., Matsumoto, N., Itokazu, Y., Tajima, N., Yamada, H., Sawada, H., Ishikawa, H., Mimura, T., Kitada, M., Suzuki, Y. and Ide, C. (2004). Specific induction of neuronal cells from bone marrow stromal cells and application for autologous transplantation. *J Clin Invest*, Vol.113, No.12, pp. 1701-1710

Dominiak, M., Lysiak-Drwal, K., Gedrange, T., Zietek, M. and Gerber, H. (2009). Efficacy of healing process of bone defects after apicectomy: results after 6 and 12 months. *J Physiol Pharmacol*, Vol.60 Suppl 8, pp. 51-55

Donzelli, E., Salvade, A., Mimo, P., Vigano, M., Morrone, M., Papagna, R., Carini, F., Zaopo, A., Miloso, M., Baldoni, M. and Tredici, G. (2007). Mesenchymal stem cells cultured on a collagen scaffold: In vitro osteogenic differentiation. *Arch Oral Biol*, Vol.52, No.1, pp. 64-73

Drury, J.L. and Mooney, D.J. (2003). Hydrogels for tissue engineering: scaffold design variables and applications. *Biomaterials*, Vol.24, No.24, pp. 4337-4351

Duneas, N., Crooks, J. and Ripamonti, U. (1998). Transforming growth factor-beta 1: induction of bone morphogenetic protein genes expression during endochondral bone formation in the baboon, and synergistic interaction with osteogenic protein-1 (BMP-7). *Growth Factors*, Vol.15, No.4, pp. 259-277

Eckardt, H., Ding, M., Lind, M., Hansen, E.S., Christensen, K.S. and Hvid, I. (2005). Recombinant human vascular endothelial growth factor enhances bone healing in an experimental nonunion model. *J Bone Joint Surg Br*, Vol.87, No.10, pp. 1434-1438

Ekholm, M., Salo, A., Syrjanen, S., Laine, P., Lindqvist, C., Kellomaki, M., Virtanen, I. and Suuronen, R. (1997). Biocompatibility of solid poly (ortho ester). *J Mater Sci Mater Med*, Vol.8, No.5, pp. 265-269

Fei, W., Yang, X.M., Li, Z., Yin, M.P., Shen, Z.H. and Liao, C.H. (2008). [Experimental study of the bioresorbable collagen membrane used for guided bone regeneration around dental implants]. *Hua Xi Kou Qiang Yi Xue Za Zhi*, Vol.26, No.5, pp. 494-498

Frost, H. (1964). Dynamics of bone remodelling. Boston, Little Brown.

Frost, H. (1991). A new direction for osteoporosis research: a review and proposal. *Bone Biodynamics*, Vol.12, pp. 429-437

Fuse, M., Hayakawa, T., Kozaki, M., Ishikura, K., Ichimura, M., Tsuzukibashi, O., Fukatsu, A., Fukumoto, M. and Makimura, M. (2009). Attachment of human gingival fibroblasts onto collagen PLA porous scaffold. *J Jpn Assoc Regenerative Dent*, Vol.7, No.1, pp. 1-9

Garric, X., Moles, J.P., Garreau, H., Guilhou, J.J. and Vert, M. (2005). Human skin cell cultures onto PLA50 (PDLLA) bioresorbable polymers: influence of chemical and morphological surface modifications. *J Biomed Mater Res A*, Vol.72, No.2, pp. 180-189

Gedrange, T., Mai, R., Weingaertner, J., Hietschold, V., Bourauel, C., Pradel, W., Lauer, G. and Proff, P. (2008). Finite element representation of bone substitute remodelling in the jaw bone. *Biomed Tech (Berl)*, Vol.53, No.5, pp. 220-223

Gerber, T., Holzhuter, G., Gotz, W., Bienengraber, V., Henkel, K.O. and Rumpel, E. (2006). Nanostructuring of biomaterials - a pathway to bone grafting substitute. *Eur. J. Trauma*, Vol.32, pp. 132-140

Gerstenfeld, L.C., Cullinane, D.M., Barnes, G.L., Graves, D.T. and Einhorn, T.A. (2003). Fracture healing as a post-natal developmental process: molecular, spatial, and temporal aspects of its regulation. *J Cell Biochem*, Vol.88, No.5, pp. 873-884

Ghanaati, S., Orth, C., Barbeck, M., Willershausen, I., Thimm, B.W., Booms, P., Stubinger, S., Landes, C., Sader, R.A. and Kirkpatrick, C.J. (2010). Histological and histomorphometrical analysis of a silica matrix embedded nanocrystalline hydroxyapatite bone substitute using the subcutaneous implantation model in Wistar rats. *Biomed Mater*, Vol.5, No.3, pp. 035005

Giannoudis, P.V., Dinopoulos, H. and Tsiridis, E. (2005). Bone substitutes: an update. *Injury*, Vol.36 Suppl 3, pp. S20-27

Gogolewski, S., Jovanovic, M., Perren, S.M., Dillon, J.G. and Hughes, M.K. (1993). Tissue response and in vivo degradation of selected polyhydroxyacids: polylactides (PLA), poly(3-hydroxybutyrate) (PHB), and poly(3-hydroxybutyrate-co-3-hydroxyvalerate) (PHB/VA). *J Biomed Mater Res*, Vol.27, No.9, pp. 1135-1148

Gotz, W., Gerber, T., Michel, B., Lossdorfer, S., Henkel, K.O. and Heinemann, F. (2008). Immunohistochemical characterization of nanocrystalline hydroxyapatite silica gel (NanoBone(r)) osteogenesis: a study on biopsies from human jaws. *Clin. Oral. Implants Res.*, Vol.19, No.10, pp. 1016-1026

Gough, J.E., Christian, P., Scotchford, C.A. and Jones, I.A. (2003). Craniofacial osteoblast responses to polycaprolactone produced using a novel boron polymerisation technique and potassium fluoride post-treatment. *Biomaterials*, Vol.24, No.27, pp. 4905-4912

Gredes, T., Gedrange, T., Spassov, A. and Kunert-Keil, C. (2010a). Bone substitution materials on the basis of BONITmatrix® up-regulate expression of IGF1 and Col1a1. *Ann. Anat.*, Vol.submitted,

Gredes, T., Kunert-Keil, C., Dominiak, M., Gedrange, T., Wrobel-Kwiatkowska, M. and Szopa, J. (2010b). The influence of biocomposites containing genetically modified flax fibers on gene expression in rat skeletal muscle. *Biomed Tech (Berl)*, Vol.55, No.6, pp. 323-329

Gredes, T., Spassov, A., Mai, R., Mack, H., Loster, B.W., Mazurkiewicz-Janik, M., Kubein-Meesenburg, D., Fanghanel, J. and Gedrange, T. (2009). Changes in insulin like growth factors, myostatin and vascular endothelial growth factor in rat musculus latissimus dorsi by poly-3-hydroxybutyrate implants. *J Physiol Pharmacol*, Vol.60 Suppl 3, pp. 77-81

Gunatillake, P.A. and Adhikari, R. (2003). Biodegradable synthetic polymers for tissue engineering. *Eur Cell Mater*, Vol.5, pp. 1-16; discussion 16

Habibovic, P., Kruyt, M.C., Juhl, M.V., Clyens, S., Martinetti, R., Dolcini, L., Theilgaard, N. and van Blitterswijk, C.A. (2008). Comparative in vivo study of six hydroxyapatite-based bone graft substitutes. *J. Orthop. Res.*, Vol.26, No.10, pp. 1363-1370

Harris, C.T. and Cooper, L.F. (2004). Comparison of bone graft matrices for human mesenchymal stem cell-directed osteogenesis. *J Biomed Mater Res A*, Vol.68, No.4, pp. 747-755

Hayashi, T., Kawai, T., Ishikawa, A., Kawai, H., Nakano, K., Takei, Y. and Kuroki, K. (2008). Histological analysis of induced cartilage on the biodegradable or nonbiodegradable membranes from immature muscular tissue in vitro. *J Biomed Mater Res A*, Vol.86, No.4, pp. 1048-1054

Heckmann, L., Schlenker, H.J., Fiedler, J., Brenner, R., Dauner, M., Bergenthal, G., Mattes, T., Claes, L. and Ignatius, A. (2007). Human mesenchymal progenitor cell responses to a novel textured poly(L-lactide) scaffold for ligament tissue engineering. *J Biomed Mater Res B Appl Biomater*, Vol.81, No.1, pp. 82-90

Heinemann, F., Mundt, T., Biffar, R., Gedrange, T. and Goetz, W. (2009). A 3-year clinical and radiographic study of implants placed simultaneously with maxillary sinus floor augmentations using a new nanocrystalline hydroxyapatite. *J Physiol Pharmacol*, Vol.60 Suppl 8, pp. 91-97

Heino, T.J. and Hentunen, T.A. (2008). Differentiation of osteoblasts and osteocytes from mesenchymal stem cells. *Curr Stem Cell Res Ther*, Vol.3, No.2, pp. 131-145

Helm, G.A. and Gazit, Z. (2005). Future uses of mesenchymal stem cells in spine surgery. *Neurosurg Focus*, Vol.19, No.6, pp. E13

Hermann, J.S. and Buser, D. (1996). Guided bone regeneration for dental implants. *Curr Opin Periodontol*, Vol.3, pp. 168-177

High, W.B., Capen, C.C. and Black, H.E. (1981). Effects of thyroxine on cortical bone remodeling in adult dogs: a histomorphometric study. *Am J Pathol*, Vol.102, No.3, pp. 438-446

Hill, P.A. (1998). Bone remodelling. *Br J Orthod*, Vol.25, No.2, pp. 101-107

Hollinger, J.O. and Battistone, G.C. (1986). Biodegradable bone repair materials. Synthetic polymers and ceramics. *Clin Orthop Relat Res*, Vol.No.207, pp. 290-305

Hollinger, J.O., Hart, C.E., Hirsch, S.N., Lynch, S. and Friedlaender, G.E. (2008). Recombinant human platelet-derived growth factor: biology and clinical applications. *J Bone Joint Surg Am*, Vol.90 Suppl 1, pp. 48-54

Hollinger, J.O. and Schmitz, J.P. (1997). Macrophysiologic roles of a delivery system for vulnerary factors needed for bone regeneration. *Ann N Y Acad Sci*, Vol.831, pp. 427-437

Holzl, F., Pfannschmidt, O., Manegold, E., Rohrmann, D., Jakse, G. and Brauers, A. (2000). [In vitro analysis and animal experiment study of surface modified biodegradable polylactide ureteral stents]. *Urologe A*, Vol.39, No.6, pp. 557-564

Hutmacher, D.W., Goh, J.C. and Teoh, S.H. (2001a). An introduction to biodegradable materials for tissue engineering applications. *Ann Acad Med Singapore*, Vol.30, No.2, pp. 183-191

Hutmacher, D.W., Schantz, T., Zein, I., Ng, K.W., Teoh, S.H. and Tan, K.C. (2001b). Mechanical properties and cell cultural response of polycaprolactone scaffolds designed and fabricated via fused deposition modeling. *J Biomed Mater Res*, Vol.55, No.2, pp. 203-216

Ishaug, S.L., Yaszemski, M.J., Bizios, R. and Mikos, A.G. (1994). Osteoblast function on synthetic biodegradable polymers. *J Biomed Mater Res*, Vol.28, No.12, pp. 1445-1453

Ishii, D., Ying, T.H., Mahara, A., Murakami, S., Yamaoka, T., Lee, W.K. and Iwata, T. (2009). In vivo tissue response and degradation behavior of PLLA and stereocomplexed PLA nanofibers. *Biomacromolecules*, Vol.10, No.2, pp. 237-242

Ishikawa, K., Miyamoto, Y., Yuasa, T., Ito, A., Nagayama, M. and Suzuki, K. (2002). Fabrication of Zn containing apatite cement and its initial evaluation using human osteoblastic cells. *Biomaterials*, Vol.23, No.2, pp. 423-428

Isobe, M., Yamazaki, Y., Mori, M., Ishihara, K., Nakabayashi, N. and Amagasa, T. (1999). The role of recombinant human bone morphogenetic protein-2 in PLGA capsules at an extraskeletal site of the rat. *J Biomed Mater Res*, Vol.45, No.1, pp. 36-41

Iwamatsu-Kobayashi, Y., Nishihara, D., Hirata, M., Kindaichi, K. and Komatsu, M. (2005). Effects of biomaterials on cell adhesion of human peridontal ligament fibroblasts and fibronectin absorption. *International Congress Series*, Vol.1284, pp. 334-335

Janssens, K., ten Dijke, P., Janssens, S. and Van Hul, W. (2005). Transforming growth factor-beta1 to the bone. *Endocr Rev*, Vol.26, No.6, pp. 743-774

Jarosz-Cichulska, H. (1988). [Studies on perfecting Polish-made linen threads for surgical use]. *Polim Med*, Vol.18, No.1-2, pp. 3-49

Jayakumar, A., Rajababu, P., Rohini, S., Butchibabu, K., Naveen, A., Reddy, P.K., Vidyasagar, S., Satyanarayana, D. and Pavan Kumar, S. (2011). Multi-centre, randomized clinical trial on the efficacy and safety of recombinant human platelet-derived growth factor with beta-tricalcium phosphate in human intra-osseous periodontal defects. *J Clin Periodontol*, Vol.38, No.2, pp. 163-172

Jurgens, W.J., Kroeze, R.J., Bank, R.A., Ritt, M.J. and Helder, M.N. (2011). Rapid attachment of adipose stromal cells on resorbable polymeric scaffolds facilitates the one-step surgical procedure for cartilage and bone tissue engineering purposes. *J Orthop Res*, Vol.

Kato, T., Kawaguchi, H., Hanada, K., Aoyama, I., Hiyama, Y., Nakamura, T., Kuzutani, K., Tamura, M., Kurokawa, T. and Nakamura, K. (1998). Single local injection of recombinant fibroblast growth factor-2 stimulates healing of segmental bone defects in rabbits. *J Orthop Res*, Vol.16, No.6, pp. 654-659

Kaufmann, E.A., Ducheyne, P. and Shapiro, I.M. (2000). Effect of varying physical properties of porous, surface modified bioactive glass 45S5 on osteoblast proliferation and maturation. *J. Biomed. Mater. Res.*, Vol.52, No.4, pp. 783-796

Kauschke, E., Rumpel, E., Fanghanel, J., Bayerlein, T., Gedrange, T. and Proff, P. (2006). The in vitro viability and growth of fibroblasts cultured in the presence of different bone grafting materials (NanoBone and Straumann Bone Ceramic). *Folia Morphol (Warsz)*, Vol.65, No.1, pp. 37-42

Khor, H.L., Ng, K.W., Htay, A.S., Schantz, J.T., Teoh, S.H. and Hutmacher, D.W. (2003). Preliminary study of a polycaprolactone membrane utilized as epidermal substrate. *J Mater Sci Mater Med*, Vol.14, No.2, pp. 113-120

Kim, J.H., Kim, C.H. and Kim, K.W. (2008). Bone healing capacity of the collagen bone filler (TERUPLUG(R)) and rhBMP-2 in the rabbit cranium defect. *J Korean Assoc Oral Maxillofac Surg*, Vol.34, No.2, pp. 119-130

Kiremitci, M. and Piskin, E. (1990). Cell adhesion to the surfaces of polymeric beads. *Biomater Artif Cells Artif Organs*, Vol.18, No.5, pp. 599-603

Kobayashi, H., Turner, A.S., Seim, H.B., 3rd, Kawamoto, T. and Bauer, T.W. (2010). Evaluation of a silica-containing bone graft substitute in a vertebral defect model. *J Biomed Mater Res A*, Vol.92, No.2, pp. 596-603

Komori, T., Yagi, H., Nomura, S., Yamaguchi, A., Sasaki, K., Deguchi, K., Shimizu, Y., Bronson, R.T., Gao, Y.H., Inada, M., Sato, M., Okamoto, R., Kitamura, Y., Yoshiki, S. and Kishimoto, T. (1997). Targeted disruption of Cbfa1 results in a complete lack of bone formation owing to maturational arrest of osteoblasts. *Cell*, Vol.89, No.5, pp. 755-764

Kroese-Deutman, H.C., Ruhe, P.Q., Spauwen, P.H. and Jansen, J.A. (2005). Bone inductive properties of rhBMP-2 loaded porous calcium phosphate cement implants inserted at an ectopic site in rabbits. *Biomaterials*, Vol.26, No.10, pp. 1131-1138

Kruyt, M.C., Dhert, W.J., Oner, C., van Blitterswijk, C.A., Verbout, A.J. and de Bruijn, J.D. (2004). Optimization of bone-tissue engineering in goats. *J Biomed Mater Res B Appl Biomater*, Vol.69, No.2, pp. 113-120

Kubler, A., Neugebauer, J., Oh, J.H., Scheer, M. and Zoller, J.E. (2004). Growth and proliferation of human osteoblasts on different bone graft substitutes: an in vitro study. *Implant Dent*, Vol.13, No.2, pp. 171-179

Kulkarni, R.K., Moore, E.G., Hegyeli, A.F. and Leonard, F. (1971). Biodegradable poly(lactic acid) polymers. *J Biomed Mater Res*, Vol.5, No.3, pp. 169-181

Kumar, N., Langer, R.S. and Domb, A.J. (2002). Polyanhydrides: an overview. *Adv Drug Deliv Rev*, Vol.54, No.7, pp. 889-910

Kundu, B., Lemos, A., Soundrapandian, C., Sen, P.S., Datta, S., Ferreira, J.M. and Basu, D. (2010). Development of porous HAp and beta-TCP scaffolds by starch consolidation with foaming method and drug-chitosan bilayered scaffold based drug delivery system. *J Mater Sci Mater Med*, Vol.21, No.11, pp. 2955-2969

Kunert-Keil, C., Gredrange, T., Mai, R., Spassov, A., Lucke, S., Klinke, T., Kalukin, J., Loster, B.W. and Gredes, T. (2009). Morphological evaluation of bone defect regeneration after treatment with two different forms of bone substitution materials on the basis of BONITmatrix. *J. Physiol. Pharmacol.*, Vol.60 Suppl 8, pp. 57-60

Lauer, G., Wiedmann-Al-Ahmad, M., Otten, J.E., Hubner, U., Schmelzeisen, R. and Schilli, W. (2001). The titanium surface texture effects adherence and growth of human gingival keratinocytes and human maxillar osteoblast-like cells in vitro. *Biomaterials*, Vol.22, No.20, pp. 2799-2809

Lean, J.M., Mackay, A.G., Chow, J.W. and Chambers, T.J. (1996). Osteocytic expression of mRNA for c-fos and IGF-I: an immediate early gene response to an osteogenic stimulus. *Am J Physiol*, Vol.270, No.6 Pt 1, pp. E937-945

Lee, S.J., Khang, G., Lee, Y.M. and Lee, H.B. (2002). Interaction of human chondrocytes and NIH/3T3 fibroblasts on chloric acid-treated biodegradable polymer surfaces. *J Biomater Sci Polym Ed*, Vol.13, No.2, pp. 197-212

Lindsey, W.H., Ogle, R.C., Morgan, R.F., Cantrell, R.W. and Sweeney, T.M. (1996). Nasal reconstruction using an osteoconductive collagen gel matrix. *Arch Otolaryngol Head Neck Surg*, Vol.122, No.1, pp. 37-40

Lu, H.H., El-Amin, S.F., Scott, K.D. and Laurencin, C.T. (2003). Three-dimensional, bioactive, biodegradable, polymer-bioactive glass composite scaffolds with improved mechanical properties support collagen synthesis and mineralization of human osteoblast-like cells in vitro. *J Biomed Mater Res A*, Vol.64, No.3, pp. 465-474

Lucas, P.A., Laurencin, C., Syftestad, G.T., Domb, A., Goldberg, V.M., Caplan, A.I. and Langer, R. (1990). Ectopic induction of cartilage and bone by water-soluble proteins from bovine bone using a polyanhydride delivery vehicle. *J Biomed Mater Res*, Vol.24, No.7, pp. 901-911

Luk, J.M., Wang, P.P., Lee, C.K., Wang, J.H. and Fan, S.T. (2005). Hepatic potential of bone marrow stromal cells: development of in vitro co-culture and intra-portal transplantation models. *J Immunol Methods*, Vol.305, No.1, pp. 39-47

Luu, H.H., Song, W.X., Luo, X., Manning, D., Luo, J., Deng, Z.L., Sharff, K.A., Montag, A.G., Haydon, R.C. and He, T.C. (2007). Distinct roles of bone morphogenetic proteins in osteogenic differentiation of mesenchymal stem cells. *J Orthop Res*, Vol.25, No.5, pp. 665-677

Macedo, N.L., Matuda, F., Macedo, L., Gonzales, M. and Carvalho, Y. (2005). Bone defect regeneration with bioactive glass implantation in rats.

Macedo, N.L., Matuda Fda, S., Macedo, L.G., Gonzales, M.B., Ouchi, S.M. and Carvalho, Y.R. (2004). Bone defect regeneration with bioactive glass implantation in rats. *J Appl Oral Sci*, Vol.12, No.2, pp. 137-143

Mack, H.B., Mai, R., Lauer, G., Mack, F., Gedrange, T., Franke, R. and Gredes, T. (2008). Adaptation of myosin heavy chain mRNA expression after implantation of poly(3)hydroxybutyrate scaffolds in rat m. latissimus dorsi. *J Physiol Pharmacol*, Vol.59 Suppl 5, pp. 95-103

Madhavan Nampoothiri, K., Nair, N.R. and John, R.P. (2010). An overview of the recent developments in polylactide (PLA) research. *Bioresour Technol*, Vol.101, No.22, pp. 8493-8501

Maenpaa, K., Ella, V., Mauno, J., Kellomaki, M., Suuronen, R., Ylikomi, T. and Miettinen, S. (2010). Use of adipose stem cells and polylactide discs for tissue engineering of the temporomandibular joint disc. *J R Soc Interface*, Vol.7, No.42, pp. 177-188

Mai, R., Hagedorn, M.G., Gelinsky, M., Werner, C., Turhani, D., Spath, H., Gedrange, T. and Lauer, G. (2006). Ectopic bone formation in nude rats using human osteoblasts seeded poly(3)hydroxybutyrate embroidery and hydroxyapatite-collagen tapes constructs. *J Craniomaxillofac Surg*, Vol.34 Suppl 2, pp. 101-109

Malm, T., Bowald, S., Karacagil, S., Bylock, A. and Busch, C. (1992). A new biodegradable patch for closure of atrial septal defect. An experimental study. *Scand J Thorac Cardiovasc Surg*, Vol.26, No.1, pp. 9-14

Manolagas, S.C., Kousteni, S. and Jilka, R.L. (2002). Sex steroids and bone. *Recent Prog Horm Res*, Vol.57, pp. 385-409

Marie, P.J. (2003). Fibroblast growth factor signaling controlling osteoblast differentiation. *Gene*, Vol.316, pp. 23-32

Marukawa, K., Ueki, K., Okabe, K., Nakagawa, K. and Yamamoto, E. (2011). Use of self-setting alpha-tricalcium phosphate for maxillary sinus augmentation in rabbit. *Clin Oral Implants Res*, Vol.22, No.6, pp. 606-612

Miller, N.D. and Williams, D.F. (1987). On the biodegradation of poly-beta-hydroxybutyrate (PHB) homopolymer and poly-beta-hydroxybutyrate-hydroxyvalerate copolymers. *Biomaterials*, Vol.8, No.2, pp. 129-137

Milosevski, M., Bossert, J., Milosevski, D. and Gruevska, A. (1999). Preparation and properties of dense and porous calcium phosphate *Ceramics International*, Vol.25, No.8, pp. 693-696

Misra, S.K., Valappil, S.P., Roy, I. and Boccaccini, A.R. (2006). Polyhydroxyalkanoate (PHA)/inorganic phase composites for tissue engineering applications. *Biomacromolecules*, Vol.7, No.8, pp. 2249-2258

Miyamoto, S., Takaoka, K., Okada, T., Yoshikawa, H., Hashimoto, J., Suzuki, S. and Ono, K. (1992). Evaluation of polylactic acid homopolymers as carriers for bone morphogenetic protein. *Clin Orthop Relat Res*, Vol.No.278, pp. 274-285

Mohanty, A.K., Misra, M. and Drzal, L.T. (2005). Natural Fibers, Biopolymers, and Biocomposites Boca Raton, CRC Press.

Muller, P., Bulnheim, U., Diener, A., Luthen, F., Teller, M., Klinkenberg, E.D., Neumann, H.G., Nebe, B., Liebold, A., Steinhoff, G. and Rychly, J. (2008). Calcium phosphate surfaces promote osteogenic differentiation of mesenchymal stem cells. *J. Cell. Mol. Med.*, Vol.12, No.1, pp. 281-291

Mundy, G.R. (1994). Peptides and growth regulatory factors in bone. *Rheum Dis Clin North Am*, Vol.20, No.3, pp. 577-588

Nakamura, T., Hara, Y., Tagawa, M., Tamura, M., Yuge, T., Fukuda, H. and Nigi, H. (1998). Recombinant human basic fibroblast growth factor accelerates fracture healing by enhancing callus remodeling in experimental dog tibial fracture. *J Bone Miner Res*, Vol.13, No.6, pp. 942-949

Neer, R.M., Arnaud, C.D., Zanchetta, J.R., Prince, R., Gaich, G.A., Reginster, J.Y., Hodsman, A.B., Eriksen, E.F., Ish-Shalom, S., Genant, H.K., Wang, O. and Mitlak, B.H. (2001). Effect of parathyroid hormone (1-34) on fractures and bone mineral density in postmenopausal women with osteoporosis. *N Engl J Med*, Vol.344, No.19, pp. 1434-1441

Nesic, D., Whiteside, R., Brittberg, M., Wendt, D., Martin, I. and Mainil-Varlet, P. (2006). Cartilage tissue engineering for degenerative joint disease. *Adv Drug Deliv Rev*, Vol.58, No.2, pp. 300-322

Niehaus, A.J., Anderson, D.E., Samii, V.F., Weisbrode, S.E., Johnson, J.K., Noon, M.S., Tomasko, D.L. and Lannutti, J.J. (2009). Effects of orthopedic implants with a polycaprolactone polymer coating containing bone morphogenetic protein-2 on osseointegration in bones of sheep. *Am J Vet Res*, Vol.70, No.11, pp. 1416-1425

Niu, T. and Rosen, C.J. (2005). The insulin-like growth factor-I gene and osteoporosis: a critical appraisal. *Gene*, Vol.361, pp. 38-56

Noetzel, J. and Kielbassa, A.M. (2005). [Calcium phosphate cements in medicine and dentistry--a review of literature]. *Schweiz Monatsschr Zahnmed*, Vol.115, No.12, pp. 1148-1156

Ohlsson, C., Bengtsson, B.A., Isaksson, O.G., Andreassen, T.T. and Slootweg, M.C. (1998). Growth hormone and bone. *Endocr Rev*, Vol.19, No.1, pp. 55-79

Okumura, M., Ohgushi, H., Dohi, Y., Katuda, T., Tamai, S., Koerten, H.K. and Tabata, S. (1997). Osteoblastic phenotype expression on the surface of hydroxyapatite ceramics. *J. Biomed. Mater. Res.*, Vol.37, No.1, pp. 122-129

Otto, F., Thornell, A.P., Crompton, T., Denzel, A., Gilmour, K.C., Rosewell, I.R., Stamp, G.W., Beddington, R.S., Mundlos, S., Olsen, B.R., Selby, P.B. and Owen, M.J. (1997). Cbfa1, a candidate gene for cleidocranial dysplasia syndrome, is essential for osteoblast differentiation and bone development. *Cell*, Vol.89, No.5, pp. 765-771

Papachroni, K.K., Karatzas, D.N., Papavassiliou, K.A., Basdra, E.K. and Papavassiliou, A.G. (2009). Mechanotransduction in osteoblast regulation and bone disease. *Trends Mol Med*, Vol.15, No.5, pp. 208-216

Payer, M., Lohberger, B., Stadelmeyer, E., Bartmann, C., Windhager, R. and Jakse, N. (2010). Behaviour of multipotent maxillary bone-derived cells on beta-tricalcium phosphate and highly porous bovine bone mineral. *Clin Oral Implants Res*, Vol.21, No.7, pp. 699-708

Pecora, G., Andreana, S., Margarone, J.E., 3rd, Covani, U. and Sottosanti, J.S. (1997). Bone regeneration with a calcium sulfate barrier. *Oral Surg Oral Med Oral Pathol Oral Radiol Endod*, Vol.84, No.4, pp. 424-429

Peter, S.J., Miller, M.J., Yasko, A.W., Yaszemski, M.J. and Mikos, A.G. (1998). Polymer concepts in tissue engineering. *J Biomed Mater Res*, Vol.43, No.4, pp. 422-427

Punke, C., Zehlicke, T., Boltze, C. and Pau, H.W. (2008). Experimental studies on a new highly porous hydroxyapatite matrix for obliterating open mastoid cavities. *Otol Neurotol*, Vol.29, No.6, pp. 807-811

Radomsky, M.L., Thompson, A.Y., Spiro, R.C. and Poser, J.W. (1998). Potential role of fibroblast growth factor in enhancement of fracture healing. *Clin Orthop Relat Res*, Vol.No.355 Suppl, pp. S283-293

Rai, B., Ho, K.H., Lei, Y., Si-Hoe, K.M., Jeremy Teo, C.M., Yacob, K.B., Chen, F., Ng, F.C. and Teoh, S.H. (2007a). Polycaprolactone-20% tricalcium phosphate scaffolds in combination with platelet-rich plasma for the treatment of critical-sized defects of the mandible: a pilot study. *J Oral Maxillofac Surg*, Vol.65, No.11, pp. 2195-2205

Rai, B., Oest, M.E., Dupont, K.M., Ho, K.H., Teoh, S.H. and Guldberg, R.E. (2007b). Combination of platelet-rich plasma with polycaprolactone-tricalcium phosphate scaffolds for segmental bone defect repair. *J Biomed Mater Res A*, Vol.81, No.4, pp. 888-899

Redey, S.A., Nardin, M., Bernache-Assolant, D., Rey, C., Delannoy, P., Sedel, L. and Marie, P.J. (2000). Behavior of human osteoblastic cells on stoichiometric hydroxyapatite and type A carbonate apatite: role of surface energy. *J Biomed Mater Res*, Vol.50, No.3, pp. 353-364

Reichert, C., Al-Nawas, B., Smeets, R., Kasaj, A., Gotz, W. and Klein, M.O. (2009). In vitro proliferation of human osteogenic cells in presence of different commercial bone substitute materials combined with enamel matrix derivatives. *Head Face Med*, Vol.5, pp. 23

Renier, M.L. and Kohn, D.H. (1997). Development and characterization of a biodegradable polyphosphate. *J Biomed Mater Res*, Vol.34, No.1, pp. 95-104

Rentsch, C., Rentsch, B., Breier, A., Hoffmann, A., Manthey, S., Scharnweber, D., Biewener, A. and Zwipp, H. (2009). Evaluation of the osteogenic potential and vascularization of 3D poly(3)hydroxybutyrate scaffolds subcutaneously implanted in nude rats. *Journal of Biomedical Materials Research Part A*, Vol.pp. 185-195

Reusch, R.N. and Sadoff, H.L. (1983). D-(-)-poly-beta-hydroxybutyrate in membranes of genetically competent bacteria. *J Bacteriol*, Vol.156, No.2, pp. 778-788

Rimondini, L., Nicoli-Aldini, N., Fini, M., Guzzardella, G., Tschon, M. and Giardino, R. (2005). In vivo experimental study on bone regeneration in critical bone defects using an injectable biodegradable PLA/PGA copolymer. *Oral Surg Oral Med Oral Pathol Oral Radiol Endod*, Vol.99, No.2, pp. 148-154

Ripamonti, U., Duneas, N., Van Den Heever, B., Bosch, C. and Crooks, J. (1997). Recombinant transforming growth factor-beta1 induces endochondral bone in the baboon and synergizes with recombinant osteogenic protein-1 (bone morphogenetic protein-7) to initiate rapid bone formation. *J Bone Miner Res*, Vol.12, No.10, pp. 1584-1595

Rosen, C.J. (2004). Insulin-like growth factor I and bone mineral density: experience from animal models and human observational studies. *Best Pract Res Clin Endocrinol Metab*, Vol.18, No.3, pp. 423-435

Ruhé, P.Q., Wolke, J.G., Spauwen, P.H. and Jansen, J.A. Calcium phosphate ceramics for bone tissue engineering. Engineering and artificial organs (The biomedical engineering handbook). J. D. Bronzino. Boca Raton, London, New York, Taylor and Francis: 38.31 - 38.18.

Rumpel, E., Wolf, E., Kauschke, E., Bienengraber, V., Bayerlein, T., Gedrange, T. and Proff, P. (2006). The biodegradation of hydroxyapatite bone graft substitutes in vivo. *Folia Morphol. (Warsz.)*, Vol.65, No.1, pp. 43-48

Saito, T., Tomita, K., Juni, K. and Ooba, K. (1991). In vivo and in vitro degradation of poly(3-hydroxybutyrate) in rat. *Biomaterials*, Vol.12, No.3, pp. 309-312

Schantz, J.T., Hutmacher, D.W., Ng, K.W., Khor, H.L., Lim, M.T. and Teoh, S.H. (2002). Evaluation of a tissue-engineered membrane-cell construct for guided bone regeneration. *Int J Oral Maxillofac Implants*, Vol.17, No.2, pp. 161-174

Schmack, G., Jehnichen, D., Vogel, R. and Tandler, B. (2000). Biodegradable fibres of Poly (3-hydroxybutyrate) produced by high-speed melt spinning and spindrawing. *Polymer Physics*, Vol.38, pp. 2841-2850

Schneider, R.K., Puellen, A., Kramann, R., Raupach, K., Bornemann, J., Knuechel, R., Perez-Bouza, A. and Neuss, S. (2010). The osteogenic differentiation of adult bone marrow and perinatal umbilical mesenchymal stem cells and matrix remodelling in three-dimensional collagen scaffolds. *Biomaterials*, Vol.31, No.3, pp. 467-480

Schofer, M., Fuchs-Winkelmann, S., Wack, C., Rudisile, M., Dersch, R., Leifeld, I., Wendorff, J., Greiner, A., Paletta, J.R. and Boudriot, U. (2009). Lack of obvious influence of PLLA nanofibers on the gene expression of BMP-2 and VEGF during growth and differentiation of human mesenchymal stem cells. *ScientificWorldJournal*, Vol.9, pp. 313-319

Schuckert, K.H., Jopp, S. and Teoh, S.H. (2009). Mandibular defect reconstruction using three-dimensional polycaprolactone scaffold in combination with platelet-rich plasma and recombinant human bone morphogenetic protein-2: de novo synthesis of bone in a single case. *Tissue Eng Part A*, Vol.15, No.3, pp. 493-499

Sciadini, M.F., Dawson, J.M. and Johnson, K.D. (1997). Evaluation of bovine-derived bone protein with a natural coral carrier as a bone-graft substitute in a canine segmental defect model. *J Orthop Res*, Vol.15, No.6, pp. 844-857

Sculean, A., Nikolidakis, D. and Schwarz, F. (2008). Regeneration of periodontal tissues: combinations of barrier membranes and grafting materials - biological foundation and preclinical evidence: a systematic review. *J Clin Periodontol*, Vol.35, No.8 Suppl, pp. 106-116

Serino, G., Biancu, S., Iezzi, G. and Piattelli, A. (2003). Ridge preservation following tooth extraction using a polylactide and polyglycolide sponge as space filler: a clinical and histological study in humans. *Clin Oral Implants Res*, Vol.14, No.5, pp. 651-658

Shinji, K., Kazuhisa, B., Kazuma, F., Yasunori, O., Jun´Ya, S., Kenji, K. and Tadahiko, I. (2003). Expreimental study of bone inducing ability of recombinant human bone morphogenetic protein-2 with atelo-collagen sponge (TERUPLUG) as a carrier-Comparison with atelo-peptide collagen (Cellmatrix LA) as a carrier-. *Japanese J Oral Maxillofac Surg*, Vol.49, No.4, pp. 241-245

Shishatskaya, E.I. and Volova, T.G. (2004). A comparative investigation of biodegradable polyhydroxyalkanoate films as matrices for in vitro cell cultures. *J Mater Sci Mater Med*, Vol.15, No.8, pp. 915-923

Shishatskaya, E.I., Volova, T.G., Puzyr, A.P., Mogilnaya, O.A. and Efremov, S.N. (2004). Tissue response to the implantation of biodegradable polyhydroxyalkanoate sutures. *J Mater Sci Mater Med*, Vol.15, No.6, pp. 719-728

Skorkowska-Telichowska, K., Zuk, M., Kulma, A., Bugajska-Prusak, A., Ratajczak, K., Gasiorowski, K., Kostyn, K. and Szopa, J. (2010). New dressing materials derived from transgenic flax products to treat long-standing venuos ulcers-a pilot study. *Wound Repair and Regeneration*, Vol.578, pp. 1-11

Street, J., Bao, M., deGuzman, L., Bunting, S., Peale, F.V., Jr., Ferrara, N., Steinmetz, H., Hoeffel, J., Cleland, J.L., Daugherty, A., van Bruggen, N., Redmond, H.P., Carano, R.A. and Filvaroff, E.H. (2002). Vascular endothelial growth factor stimulates bone repair by promoting angiogenesis and bone turnover. *Proc Natl Acad Sci U S A*, Vol.99, No.15, pp. 9656-9661

Sun, H., Ye, F., Wang, J., Shi, Y., Tu, Z., Bao, J., Qin, M., Bu, H. and Li, Y. (2008). The upregulation of osteoblast marker genes in mesenchymal stem cells prove the osteoinductivity of hydroxyapatite/tricalcium phosphate biomaterial. *Transplant. Proc.*, Vol.40, No.8, pp. 2645-2648

Suwantong, O., Waleetorncheepsawat, S., Sanchavanakit, N., Pavasant, P., Cheepsunthorn, P., Bunaprasert, T. and Supaphol, P. (2007). In vitro biocompatibility of electrospun poly(3-hydroxybutyrate) and poly(3-hydroxybutyrate-co-3-hydroxyvalerate) fiber mats. *Int J Biol Macromol*, Vol.40, No.3, pp. 217-223

Szopa, J., Wrobel-Kwiatkowska, M., Kulma, A., Zuk, M., Skorkowska-Telichowska, K., Dyminska, L., Maczka, M., Hanusa, J., Zebrowski, J. and Preisner, M. (2009). Chemical composition and molecular structure of fibers from transgenic flax producing polyhydroxybutyrate, and mechanical properties and platelet aggregation of composite materials containing these fibers. *Composites science and technology*, Vol.69, No.14, pp. 2438-2446

Tamada, J. and Langer, R. (1992). The development of polyanhydrides for drug delivery applications. *J Biomater Sci Polym Ed*, Vol.3, No.4, pp. 315-353

Theisen, C., Fuchs-Winkelmann, S., Knappstein, K., Efe, T., Schmitt, J., Paletta, J.R. and Schofer, M.D. (2010). Influence of nanofibers on growth and gene expression of human tendon derived fibroblast. *Biomed Eng Online*, Vol.9, pp. 9

Thian, E.S., Huang, J., Best, S.M., Barber, Z.H. and Bonfield, W. (2005). Magnetron co-sputtered silicon-containing hydroxyapatite thin films--an in vitro study. *Biomaterials*, Vol.26, No.16, pp. 2947-2956

Thimm, B.W., Unger, R.E., Neumann, H.G. and Kirkpatrick, C.J. (2008). Biocompatibility studies of endothelial cells on a novel calcium phosphate/SiO2-xerogel composite for bone tissue engineering. *Biomed Mater*, Vol.3, No.1, pp. 015007

Toung, J.S., Ogle, R.C., Morgan, R.F. and Lindsey, W.H. (1999). Repair of a rodent nasal critical-size osseous defect with osteoblast augmented collagen gel. *Laryngoscope*, Vol.109, No.10, pp. 1580-1584

Twardowski, T., Fertala, A., Orgel, J.P. and San Antonio, J.D. (2007). Type I collagen and collagen mimetics as angiogenesis promoting superpolymers. *Curr Pharm Des*, Vol.13, No.35, pp. 3608-3621

Tzaphlidou, M. (2005). The role of collagen in bone structure: an image processing approach. *Micron*, Vol.36, No.7-8, pp. 593-601

van Dam, J.E.G., van Vilsteren, G.E.T., Zomers, F.H.A., Shannon, W.E. and Hamilton, I.T. (1996). Increased application of domestically produced plant fibres in textile, pulp and paper production, and composite materials. *Industrial Fiber Crops, European Commission Directorate-General XII*, Vol.

Vance, R.J., Miller, D.C., Thapa, A., Haberstroh, K.M. and Webster, T.J. (2004). Decreased fibroblast cell density on chemically degraded poly-lactic-co-glycolic acid, polyurethane, and polycaprolactone. *Biomaterials*, Vol.25, No.11, pp. 2095-2103

Vunjak-Novakovic, G., Obradovic, B., Martin, I., Bursac, P.M., Langer, R. and Freed, L.E. (1998). Dynamic cell seeding of polymer scaffolds for cartilage tissue engineering. *Biotechnol Prog*, Vol.14, No.2, pp. 193-202

Wallach, S., Farley, J.R., Baylink, D.J. and Brenner-Gati, L. (1993). Effects of calcitonin on bone quality and osteoblastic function. *Calcif Tissue Int*, Vol.52, No.5, pp. 335-339

Weinand, C., Pomerantseva, I., Neville, C.M., Gupta, R., Weinberg, E., Madisch, I., Shapiro, F., Abukawa, H., Troulis, M.J. and Vacanti, J.P. (2006). Hydrogel-beta-TCP scaffolds and stem cells for tissue engineering bone. *Bone*, Vol.38, No.4, pp. 555-563

Weiss, R.E., Singer, F.R., Gorn, A.H., Hofer, D.P. and Nimni, M.E. (1981). Calcitonin stimulates bone formation when administered prior to initiation of osteogenesis. *J Clin Invest*, Vol.68, No.3, pp. 815-818

Wettenhall, R.E., Schwartz, P.L. and Bornstein, J. (1969). Actions of insulin and growth hormone on colagen and chondroitin sulfate synthesis in bone organ cultures. *Diabetes*, Vol.18, No.5, pp. 280-284

Williams, S.F. and Martin, D.P. (2002). Biopolymers for Medicinal and Pharmaceutical Applications. Weinheim, Wiley-VCH.

Wilson, J. and Low, S.B. (1992). Bioactive ceramics for periodontal treatment: comparative studies in the Patus monkey. *J Appl Biomater*, Vol.3, No.2, pp. 123-129

Wollendorfer, M. and Bader, H. (1998). Influence of natural fibers on the machanical properties of biodegradable polymers. *Ind Crop Prod*, Vol.8, pp. 105-112

Wozney, J.M. (2002). Overview of bone morphogenetic proteins. *Spine (Phila Pa 1976)*, Vol.27, No.16 Suppl 1, pp. S2-8

Wrobel-Kwiatkowska, M., Skorkowska-Telichowska, K., Dyminska, L., Maczka, M., Hanuza, J. and Szopa, J. (2009). Biochemical, mechanical, and spectroscopic analyses of genetically engineered flax fibers producing bioplastic (poly-beta-hydroxybutyrate). *Biotechnol Prog*, Vol.25, No.5, pp. 1489-1498

Wrobel-Kwiatkowska, M., Zebrowski, J., Starzycki, M., Oszmianski, J. and Szopa, J. (2007). Engineering of PHB synthesis causes improved elastic properties of flax fibers. *Biotechnol Prog*, Vol.23, No.1, pp. 269-277

Wrobel, M., Zebrowski, J. and Szopa, J. (2004). Polyhydroxybutyrate synthesis in transgenic flax. *J Biotechnol*, Vol.107, No.1, pp. 41-54

Xu, J.L., Khor, K.A., Sui, J.J., Zhang, J.H. and Chen, W.N. (2009). Protein expression profiles in osteoblasts in response to differentially shaped hydroxyapatite nanoparticles. *Biomaterials*, Vol.30, No.29, pp. 5385-5391

Xu, S., Lin, K., Wang, Z., Chang, J., Wang, L., Lu, J. and Ning, C. (2008). Reconstruction of calvarial defect of rabbits using porous calcium silicate bioactive ceramics. *Biomaterials*, Vol.29, No.17, pp. 2588-2596

Xynos, I.D., Edgar, A.J., Buttery, L.D., Hench, L.L. and Polak, J.M. (2000a). Ionic products of bioactive glass dissolution increase proliferation of human osteoblasts and induce insulin-like growth factor II mRNA expression and protein synthesis. *Biochem Biophys Res Commun*, Vol.276, No.2, pp. 461-465

Xynos, I.D., Hukkanen, M.V., Batten, J.J., Buttery, L.D., Hench, L.L. and Polak, J.M. (2000b). Bioglass 45S5 stimulates osteoblast turnover and enhances bone formation In vitro: implications and applications for bone tissue engineering. *Calcif Tissue Int*, Vol.67, No.4, pp. 321-329

Yamada, M., Kubo, K., Ueno, T., Iwasa, F., Att, W., Hori, N. and Ogawa, T. (2010). Alleviation of commercial collagen sponge- and membrane-induced apoptosis and dysfunction in cultured osteoblasts by an amino acid derivative. *Int J Oral Maxillofac Implants*, Vol.25, No.5, pp. 939-946

Yang, X., Zhao, K. and Chen, G.Q. (2002). Effect of surface treatment on the biocompatibility of microbial polyhydroxyalkanoates. *Biomaterials*, Vol.23, No.5, pp. 1391-1397

Yarosh, E.B., Dmitrevskii, B.A., Naryzhnyi, V.P. and Tsvetkov, S.K. (2001). Some Characteristics of Synthetic Hydroxyapatite *Russian Journal of Applied Chemistry*, Vol.74, No.6, pp. 1058-1060

Ye, Q., Zund, G., Benedikt, P., Jockenhoevel, S., Hoerstrup, S.P., Sakyama, S., Hubbell, J.A. and Turina, M. (2000). Fibrin gel as a three dimensional matrix in cardiovascular tissue engineering. *Eur J Cardiothorac Surg*, Vol.17, No.5, pp. 587-591

Yilgor, P., Sousa, R.A., Reis, R.L., Hasirci, N. and Hasirci, V. (2010). Effect of scaffold architecture and BMP-2/BMP-7 delivery on in vitro bone regeneration. *J Mater Sci Mater Med*, Vol.21, No.11, pp. 2999-3008

Zhao, K., Deng, Y. and Chen, G. (2003). Effect of surface morphology on the biocompatibility of polyhydroxyalkanoates. *Biochem Eng J*, Vol.16, pp. 115-123

Zhao, S., Pinholt, E.M., Madsen, J.E. and Donath, K. (2000). Histological evaluation of different biodegradable and non-biodegradable membranes implanted subcutaneously in rats. *J Craniomaxillofac Surg*, Vol.28, No.2, pp. 116-122

Zhao, Y.M., Wang, Z.Y., Wang, J., Mai, H.Z., Yan, B. and Yang, F. (2004). Direct Synthesis of Poly(D,L-lactic acid) by Melt Polycondensation and Its Application in Drug Delivery. *J Appl Polym Sci*, Vol.91, pp. 2143-2150

Zhou, H., Hammonds, R.G., Jr., Findlay, D.M., Martin, T.J. and Ng, K.W. (1993). Differential effects of transforming growth factor-beta 1 and bone morphogenetic protein 4 on gene expression and differentiated function of preosteoblasts. *J Cell Physiol*, Vol.155, No.1, pp. 112-119

Zhu, Y., Gao, C. and Shen, J. (2002). Surface modification of polycaprolactone with poly(methacrylic acid) and gelatin covalent immobilization for promoting its cytocompatibility. *Biomaterials*, Vol.23, No.24, pp. 4889-4895

8

Immediate Dental Implants and Bone Graft

Khalid S. Hassan[1] and Adel S. Alagl[2],
[1]Department of Preventive Dental Sciences, Division of Periodontics,
College of Dentistry, University of Dammam,
Faculty of Dental Medicine, Al-Azhar University, Assiut Branch,
[2]Chairman of Department of Preventive Dental Sciences,
College of Dentistry, University of Dammam,
[1]Egypt

1. Introduction

Dental implants were initiated in 1922 by Branemark, who and associates described the relationship between titanium implant and bone which termed osteointegration, defined as the direct structural and functional connection between living bone and the surface of an implant (Albrektsson et al., 1981). Immediate implant placement, defined as the placement of dental implant immediately into fresh extraction socket site after tooth extraction , has been considered a predictable and acceptable procedure (Schwartz et al., 2000). In addition, with immediate implant placement there is minimal use of surgical drills because the socket is already found except for slight increase of the socket length in an attempt to improve primary stability (Barzilay et al., 1991). The decreased surgical trauma of immediate placement type will decrease the risk of bone necrosis and permit bone remodeling process to occur, i.e. the healing period is rapid and allows the woven bone to be transformed into lamellar bone (Hansson et al., 1983, Ericsson, 2000). Moreover, the natural socket is rich in periodontal cells and matrix, which makes the healing faster and more predictable.
Based on the review article by Penarrocha et al., 2004 and the time elapsed between tooth extraction and implantation, the following classification has been established relating the receptor zone to the required therapeutic approach. (a) Immediate implantation, when the remnant bone sufficient to ensure primary stability of the implant, which is inserted in the course of surgical extraction of the tooth to be, replaced (primary immediate implants). (b) Recent implantation, when approximately 6-8 weeks have elapsed from extraction to implantation – a time during which the soft tissues heal, allowing adequate mucogingival covering of the alveolus (secondary immediate implants). (c) Delayed implantation, when the receptor zone is not optimum for either immediate or recent implantation. Bone promotion first carried out with bone grafts and/or barrier membranes, followed approximately six months later by implant positioning (delayed implants). (d) Mature implantation, when over nine months have elapsed from extraction to implantation. Mature bone is found in such situations.

Block and Kent, 1991 described indications and contraindications for immediate dental implants placement into the extraction sites. Summarized in the following indications; 1) traumatic loss of teeth with a small amount of bone loss;2) tooth lost because of gross decay without purulent exudates or cellulites; 3) inability to complete endodontic therapy;4) presence of severe periodontal bone loss without purulent exudates; 5) adequate soft tissue health to obtain primary wound closure. Contraindications, include; 1) presence of purulent exudates at the time of extraction; 2) adjacent soft tissue cellulites and granulation tissue;3) lack of an adequate bone apical to the socket; 4) adverse location of the mandibular neurovascular bundle, maxillary sinus and nasal cavity; 5) poor anatomical configuration of remaining bone.

In order to achieve good osseiointegrated dental implant with a high degree of predictability, the implant must be1) sterile; 2) made of a highly bio-compatible material, e.g. titanium; 3) inserted with/an a traumatic surgical procedure that avoids overheating; 4) placed with initial stability; and 5) not functionally loaded during healing period of 4-6 months (Branemark et al., 1989).

It is important to note that, after tooth extraction there are four stages of healing. In the initial angiogenic stage, blood clotting occurs with capillary formation within the first five days after tooth extraction. In the second stage (new-bone formation stage) the entire socket transforming into granulation tissues. In the third stage (bone-growth stage) immature woven bone forms within four to five weeks. In the last stage (bone-reorganization stage), which occurs after six weeks and continues for six months. In addition, bone can take up to 52 weeks to fully mature (Block et al., 2002). Moreover, the periosteum has an important role to alveolar bone formation. Cells from the inner layer of the periosteum are responsible for bone remodeling, and the cortical bone receives 80% of its arterial blood supply from the periosteum. Therefore, careful a traumatic tooth extraction and maintenance of the periosteum helps in preservation of alveolar bone (Misch, 1999).

Regarding bone remodeling after tooth extraction, in the anterior maxilla the facial bone will resorb up to 25% within the first year after tooth extraction and up to 40% to 60% over the next three years. In the posterior region, the rate of bone loss is greater reaching up to 50% within the first year after extraction, especially if a portion of the buccal plate is lost during extraction resulting in limited bucco-lingual dimension, which reducing the available bone for placement of implants (Misch and Judy, 2000).

Several clinical as well as animal studies (Babbush et al., 1986, Whhrle et al., 1992, Sagaral et al., 1993, Piattelli et al., 1997, Levine et al., 1998 and Piattelli et al., 1998) demonstrated that when the implants are loaded immediately after placement, the osseintegration could occur under specific circumstances. The clinical success is dependent on a number of factors summarized in the following: 1) bone quality in the insertion site; 2) surface pattern of the implant material; 3) design of the implant; 4) amount of loading, e.g. the occlusal condition; and 5) immobilization of the implants immediately after surgery.

2. Bone-grafting materials and immediate dental implant

Following an extraction, there is a 25% decrease in the width of the alveolar bone during the first year, and an average 4mm decrease in height during the first year following multiple extractions (Carlson & Persson,1967). Misch (1999) have observed a 40%-60% decrease in alveolar bone width after the first two to three years post extraction, and Christensen (1996) reports an annual resorption rate of at least 0.5% to 1% during the remainder for the rest of a Patient's life. Preservation of bone contour for dental implants, pontic design, denture stability, soft tissue aesthetics, and maintaining the periodontal status of adjacent teeth are important considerations following an extraction.

The natural pattern of resorption of the alveolar ridge after tooth extraction would result in a different ridge that could be problematic for future of implant placement. To achieve both functional and aesthetic requirements, it might be necessary to plan implant placement after tooth extraction and socket grafting/ridge preservation. Bone graft materials have played on important role in periodontal regeneration for many years (Hoexter, 2002). To preserve alveolar bone width and height for implant placement or for prosthetic concerns, allografts, xenografts and alloplasts have been used to graft extraction sites.

Additionally,in an effort to preserve and create sufficient bone for implant placement after tooth extraction, Michael et al., 2002 used human mineralized cancellous bone as a graft material. Their results indicate that restoration of extraction sites using human mineralized bone has potential. It can preserve or recreate an extraction site's bone bulk in preparation for implant placement.

2.1 Autografts

The gold standard of bone grafting materials is autografts. Autografts are obtained from the same patient, taken from one site and placed in another site and forms bone by the process of osteogenesis and osteoinduction. Osteogenesis is defined as bone growth from viable bone cells known as osteoblasts, osteoinduction is the process that involves materials that are capable of inducing cells to differentiate into osteoblasts. Autograft materials are obtained intraorally form edentulous areas, tuberosity mandibular symphysis and mandibualr ramus. Extra oral autografts are obtained from iliac crest, rib, tibia and calvarium. The advantages of autograft bone material is that it maintains bone structures such as minerals, collagen and viable osteoblasts and bone morphogenic proteins (BMPs), while the main disadvantage is the morbidity of a second surgical site (Hoextor, 2002). Authors such as Brugnami et al., 1996 and Dealemans et al., 1997 recommended the use of autografts instead of allografts, due to the absence of immune reactions associated with the former. In this sense, the general impression appears to be that autologous grafts are the best choice for osseoinductive purposes. Recently, Hassan et al., 2008 demonstrated a comparative evaluation of immediate dental implant with autogenous versus synthetic guided bone regeneration. The major aim of this clinical and radiographic study was to compare autogenous and synthetic bone grafting with dental implant placement. The results showed that the autogenous bone graft appeared to be superior and the graft of choice because it maintained bone structure and has activated the osteogenesis process (Fig.1, 2&Table1).

One region that has not been previously described as a potential donor site is the mandibular torus, defined as hyperostosis or enlargement of the lingual aspect of the mandible. The mandibular tori generally occur bilaterally in the premolar region, but the hyperostoses may extend distally to the third molar and mesially to the lateral incisor. The lingual tori are unnecessary bony extensions, which may limit tongue space and create phonetic difficulties. When considering any type of prosthetic reconstruction, the tori can become an obstacle. In the study of Scott D and Ganz DMD,1997 utilizing mandibular tori as a source for onlay bone augmentation with immediate implant placement. The author postulates that an ideal site to harvest bone for augmentation procedures would be a local area of excess bone (exostosis) that offers no structural or aesthetic benefits to the patient. In addition, When local bone augmentation is required, and the mandibular tori are present, they can be considered as excellent potential donor sites. However, these hyperostoses will be exhibited by only a minute segment of the patient population. When the donor site and recipient site are located within the same half of the mandibular arch, the surgical procedure is reduced to one mutually inclusive incision, which gains access to the donor bone on the lingual aspect and the recipient site on the buccal aspect. The removal of the tori can be accomplished with minimal trauma and low postoperative morbidity. Therefore, the cortical and cancellous nature of the bone, with a thickened outer cortical plate of haversian bone, makes it an excellent choice as a donor site for onlay grafting procedures.

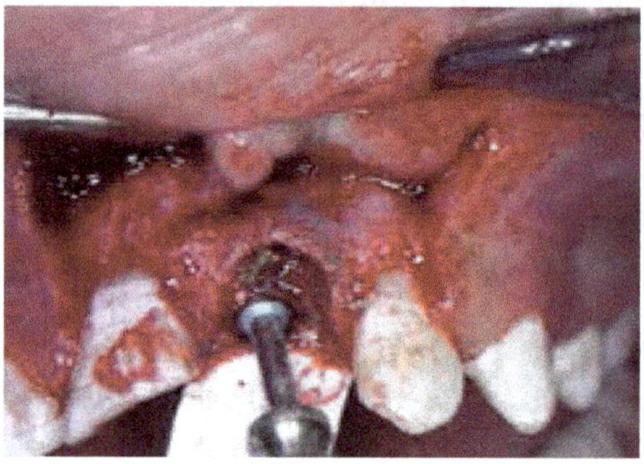

Fig. 1. Immediate dental implant placement into fresh socket augmented with autogenous bone graft.

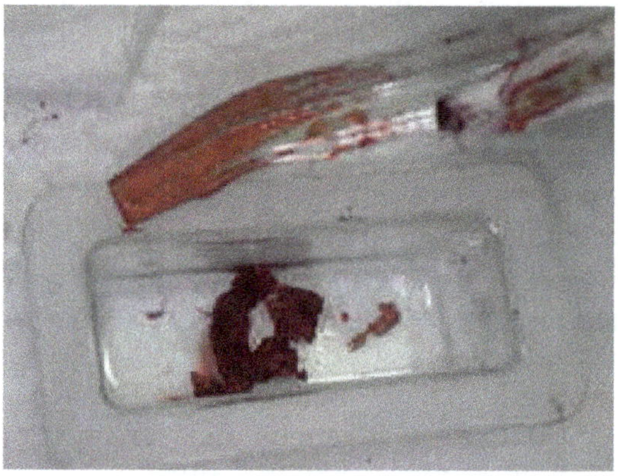

Fig. 2. Autogenous bone graft collected from the same surgical site by safe scraper.

	Bone density			Marginal bone loss		
	GI	GII	P-value	GI	GII	P-value
3M	102.49 ±10.20	99.89 ±14.32	0.470	3.56 ±0.21	3.87 ±0.43	0.067
6M	110.06 ±7.67	102.54 ±13.44	0.185	3.20 ±0.23	3.70 ±0.30	0.001 **
9M	120.93 ±8.66	105.11 ±11.81	0.013	2.73 ±0.21	3.41 ±032	0.0001 **
12M	134.56 ±11.29	109.66 ±12.13	0.0009 **	2.50 ±0.21	3.27 ±0.24	0.000 **

Table 1. Bone density (in pixels) and marginal bone loss (in mm) in the Autogenous grafted group (I) and the synthetic grafted group (II) during different observation periods.

2.2 Allografts

Allograft bone is obtained from individuals of the same species, derived from human-cadaver bone that has been selected and tested to be free of HIV and transmitted diseases. The most common allograft used is dematerialized freeze-dried bone allograft (DFDBA), provide type I collagen, which comprises most of the organic component of bone (Scahalhorn, 1972). In addition, allograft contains BMPs, which stimulate osteoinduction. There are thirteen proteins have been identified (BMP1-BMP13) which are osteoinductive compounds and stimulate new bone formation (Hoexter, 2002). Fugazzatto (2004) demonstrated that, a combination of osseous coagulum collected during preparation and freeze-dried bone allograft placed at immediate implant insertion and loading. After six months from surgery, there was a clinically immobile implant and healthy surrounding soft tissues; no postoperative gingival recession. Moreover; there was no probing depth exceed than 3mm an any aspect of the implant; no bleeding on probing; no sensitivity to pressure; and does not exculpate around the implant.

2.3 Xenografts

Xenografts are graft materials derived from the inorganic portion of animal bones; the most common source is bovine the removal of the organic component are processed to remove their antigenicity, while the remaining inorganic components provide a natural matrix as well as an excellent source of calcium. The disadvantage of xenografts is that they are only osteoconductive and the resorption rate of bovine cortical bone is slow. In addition, patients may have anxiety to mad cow disease or bovine spongiform encephalitis (Berlungh and Lindhe, 1997). Cornelini et al.,evaluated the use of a porous bone mineral matrix xenograft (Bio-Oss) as an adjunct to a biodegradable barrier membrane (Bio-Gide) to support healing following the immediate placement of transmucosal implants into extraction sockets. Their results revealed that, the radiographic bone level remained unchanged compared to baseline in the test and control groups. No differences were observed between test and control groups in terms of mean probing attachment level. At proximal sites, the soft tissue margin was located 2.6 mm more coronal than the shoulder of the implant in the test group, compared to 1.3 mm in the control group. They concluded that the use of deproteinized bovine bone mineral as a membrane support at immediately placed transmucosal implants may offer an advantage in areas with high esthetic demands in terms of soft tissue support.

2.4 Alloplasts

Alloplastic bone grafts are synthetic materials that have developed to replace human bone to avoid transmitted diseases such as HIV, bovine spongiform encephalitis (BSE), or hepatitis. They are biocompatible and osteoconductive materials. The most common types of alloplasts used are calcium phosphates, bioactive glasses and biocompatible composite polymers. Moreover, the main disadvantage of alloplasts is that they are unpredictable in allowing bone formation; therefore, particles can be uncounted within the grafted site (Knapp et al., 2003). Furthermore, the natural biocorals are calcium carbonate materials, with similar to the natural bone hydroxyapatite structure.

Advanced synthetic bioactive resorbable bone graft materials having similar chemical and mechanical properties as the host bone, can provide the means to modify existing bone topography. In the study performed by Scott and Maurice, 2002 using a synthetic bioactive restorable bone graft of low-temperature HA material mixed with autogenous bone graft for implant reconstruction. The implants were allowed to osseointegrate for four months, at this time the site was re-entered and examined. The results were showed that, the underlying implants were found to be covered with a thick layer of mature bone. In addition, the histological section revealed that mature bone was seen surrounding the remaining crystals of bioactive restorable particulates.

Paulino Castellon et al., 2004 demonstrated that immediate implant placement in sockets augmented with HTR synthetic bone. The restorative phase was initiated after six months from implant placement. The results of this study recorded that, the gingival contour was excellent in 61% and good in 35% of cares. They concluded that, immediate implant placement in combination with HTR synthetic bone graft is a predictable procedure and provides a good bone for successful prosthetic reconstruction.

In a study performed by Stanley et al., 1997 using bioglass cones as endosseous ridge maintenance implants to prevent ridge resorption. A bioactive glass can be regarded as a three-dimensional silica network, which is modified by incorporating oxides such as sodium oxide, calcium oxide, phosphorus pentoxide, aluminum oxides and barium oxide or halides such as calcium fluoride. The results of this study showed that a loss of 14.3% of the implants was seen and 7.7% of the implants requiring re-contouring (dehiscence) when the cones are placed into fresh extraction sockets during a 5-years, suggest that favorable clinical results can be obtained with this materials.

3. Combined bone-grafts and immediate dental implant

Bone defects can originate from infections, periodontal diseases or during the placement of implants, which can provoke a vestibular or lingual dehiscence due to the reduced buccal lingual dimension of the crest associated with the presence of fistula, root fractures, endodontic complications or from atrophies that developed after previous extractions.

A variety of regenerative techniques using combinations of bone grafts and barrier membranes have been suggested promoting bone regeneration in localized defects at implants placed into extraction sockets (Schwartz and Chaushu, 1997, Mayfield, 1999).

It is important to note that autogenous bone graft appeared to be the graft of choice in treatment of intrabony defects and defects around dental implants. The ability of bone replacement graft to bind with bone and enhance both osteoinduction and osteoconduction are important. In the study of Hassan, 2009 used a combined technique of using autogenous bone graft and polyglaycolic polylactic acid polymer in an attempt to obtain osteoinductive as well as the osteoconductive actions. The grafting materials used in this study included both autogenous bone graft and synthetic graft. They are safe materials because there is no disease transmission. The synthetic co-polymer used in these cases proved to be extremely easy to handle because of the various forms available (sponge, powder, and gel) which easily adapt to the various cases requiring use of a filler with subsequent formation of new bone. In addition, due to its synthetic origin, there is a complete absence of biologic risk. The histological findings showed that the co-polymer remained in the site of the graft until completion of the natural healing processes. At the same time, it is penetrated and gradually and totally replaced by trabecular bone.

In this study, the Safe-Scraper was used for autogenous bone collection from the intact area with good crestal bone in the same surgical field to avoid patient morbidity. Moreover, this work attempted also to avoid the common donor sites that are usually submitted to autogenous bone grafting, such as maxillary tuberosity and mental and mandibular retromolar areas, to preserve the tissues and to avoid morbidity of the donor area.

In this study using, a full-thickness mucoperiosteal flap with vertical releasing incisions where necessary. Teeth carefully luxated and removed with forceps. Extraction sockets were debrided with hand instruments to remove granulation tissue and prepared for implantation. Various sizes of titanium plasma spray implants (diameters 3.25 and 3.75 mm, lengths 14-16 mm) then placed according to standard protocol. Implants were then placed with the collar of the implant at the level of the bone crest on the labial aspect. Where the labial plate was damaged or absent, the level of the labial crest before loss was estimated in the following way. A periodontal probe was placed horizontally at the bone crest of intact portions of the labial plate on either side of the dehiscence defect. Then, the implant was placed with the collar positioned at this level. All implants were placed with primary stability and were completely housed within the extraction socket. After implant placement, the following measurements (bone sounding) were taken using the same William's color-coded periodontal probe (Hu-Friedy, USA). 1) Vertical height of the defect, measured from the most apical extent of the defect to the coronal aspect of the implant collar. 2) Horizontal depth of the defect, estimated by measuring the horizontal distance from the implant collar to a periodontal probe placed against the intact portions of the labial plate at the level of the implant collar. After local anesthesia, these measurements were taken again after six and nine months. Group I patients received autogenous bone grafts collected during preparation using a Safe-Scraper (Micross, Reggio Emilia, Italy) for cortical bone collectionand mixed with a synthetic bioabsorbable polylactic polyglycolic acid polymer (Fisiograft). Group II patients received autogenous bone grafts alone.
Furthermore, the results of this study showed a significant gain in clinical attachment levels, as well as reduction in PPD after the composite graft. There was a statistical significant difference between both groups regarding horizontal bone sounding suggesting that the use of Fisiograft combined with autogenous bone graft in this study was found to give optimum regenerative results (Fig.3, 4&Table.2).

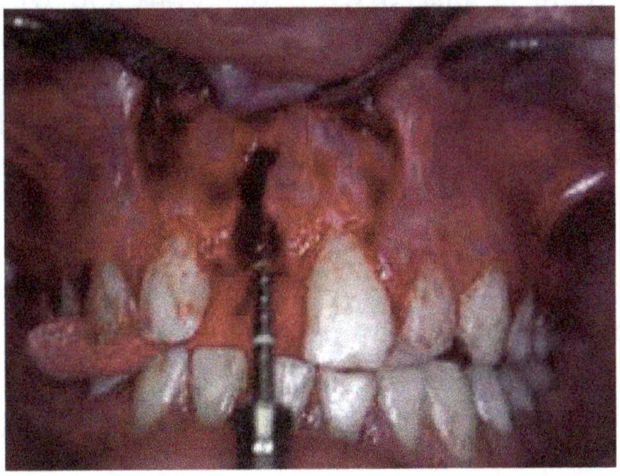

Fig. 3. Labial dehiscence at maxillary central incisor.

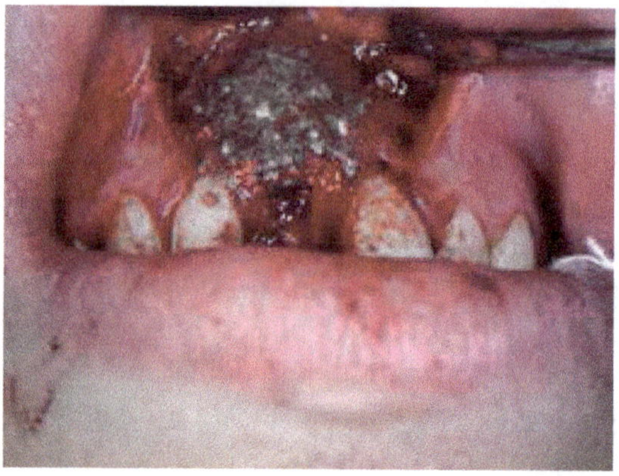

Fig. 4. Immediate dental implant placement into fresh socket and augmented with combined bone graft.

	GI n=10		GII n=10	
	VDH	HDD	VDH	HDD
Baseline	11.0±0.05	3.1±0.2	11.1±0.04	2.7±0.2
6m	5.3±0.04	1.9±0.3	5.6±0.04	1.7±0.2
9m	5.2±0.04	1.8±0.3	5.4±0.04	1.7±0.2
p-value	0.001	0.01	0.001	0.01

VDH= Vertical height of the defect HDD= Horizontal depth of the defect

Table 2. Vertical and horizontal bone sounding (Probing bone level measurements) at the base line and different postoperative periods in the tested groups.

4. Conclusion

1. To achieve a good osseointegrated implant with a high degree of predictability, the immediate implant might be placed with bone graft and without immediate loading. For aesthetic needs, can be used provisional restoration and free from occlusion.
2. The immediate dental implant placement with autogenous bone graft was significantly superior to synthetic bone graft. In addition, the immediate placement- delayed loaded dental implant remains the procedure of choice for predictably achieving osseointegration.
3. The combination of autogenous bone and synthetic grafts showed a slight superiority to autogenous bone graft alone, suggesting that it could be an optimum bone substitute for treatment of dehiscence around immediate dental implant.

5. Acknowledgment

The authors would like to express many thanks for assistant staff in College of Dentistry, University of Dammam, Kingdom of Saudi Arabia and Prof. Ahmed Kassim, Professor of Oral Medicine and Periodontology, Dean of Faculty of Dental Medicine, Al-Azhar University, Assiut Branch, Egypt.

6. References

Albrektsson T, Branemark P, Hansson H & Lindstrom J. (1981). Osteointegration titanium implants. Acta Orthop Scand 52: 155-159

Babbush CA, Kent JN & Misliek DJ. (1986). Titanium plasma sprayed screw implants for the reconstruction of the edentulous mandible. J Oral Maxillofac Surg 44: 274- 282

Barzilay, I, Graser, GN, & Iranpour, B. (1991). Immediate implantation of pure titanium implant into an extraction socket: Report of a pilot procedure. Int J Oral Maxillofac Implants 6: 277-284

Berlungh TM & Lindhe J. (1997). Healing around impalnts palced in bone defects treated with Bio-Oss: an experimental study in the dog. Clin Oral Impaltns Res 8: 117-124

Block MS & Kent JN. (1991). Placement of endosseaus implants, into tooth extraction sites. J Oral Maxillofac Surg 49: 1269-1276

Block MS, Finger I,& Lytle R. (2002). Human mineralized bone in extraction sites before implant placement-perliminary results. J Am Dent Assoc 133: 1631-1638

Branemark P, Zarb GA &Albrektsson T.(1989). Tissue integration prosthese. Berlin Quintessence Publishing

Brugnami F, Then P, & Moproi H. (1996). Histological evaluation of human extraction sockets treated with demineralized freeze-dried bone allograft and cell occlusive membrane. J Periodontol 67:821-5

Carlson G &Persson G. (1967). Morphologic changes of the mandible after extraction and wearing of dentures: a longitudinal clinical and x-ray cephalometric study covering 5 years Odont Rev; 18:27-54

Christensen GJ. (1996).Ridge Preservation:Why Not? J Am Dent Assoc. 127:669-670

Cornelini R, Cangini F, Martuscelli G, Wennström J.(2004). Deproteinized bovine bone and biodegradable barrier membranes to support healing following immediate placement of transmucosal implants: a short-term controlled clinical trial. Int J Periodontics Restorative Dent 24(6):555-63

Dealemans P, Hermanns M, & Godet F. (1997).Autologous bone graft to augment the maxillary sinus in conjunction with immediate endosseous implants: a retrospective study up to 5 years. Int J Periodontics Restorative Dent 17: 27-39

Ericsson, I. (2000). Early functional loading of branemark dental implants: 5-years clinical follow up study. Clin Implant Dent Relat Res 2 (2): 70-77

Fugazzotto PA. (2004). Guided bone regeneration at immediate implant insertion and loading: A care report. Implant Dent 13: 223-227

Hansson, HA, Albrektsson, T, & Branemark, PI. (1983). Structural aspects of the interface between tissue and titanium implants. J Prosth Dent 50:108-113

Hassan K S, Kassim A, & Al Ogaly A. (2008). A comparative evaluation of immediate dental implant with autogenous versus synthetic guided bone regeneration. Oral Surg Oral Med Oral Pathol Oral Radiol Endod 106:e8-e15

Hassan KS. (2009). Autogenous bone graft combined with polylactic polyglycolic acid polymer for treatment of dehiscence around immediate dental implants. Oral Surg Oral Med Oral Pathol Oral Radiol Endod 108:e19-e25

Hoexter D. (2002). Bone regeneration graft materials. J Oral Implant 26: 290-294 Knapp CI, Feuillev, Cochran D& Melloning JT. (2003). Clinical and histological evaluation of bone replacement grafts in the treatment of localized alveolar ridge defects. Part II: bioactive glass particulates. Int J Periodontics Rest Dent 23: (2) 129-137

Levine RA, Rose L & Salama H. (1998). Immediate loading of root-shaped implants: Two clinical case reports three years after loading. Int J Periodontics Restorative Dent 18: 307-317

Mayfield LJ. (1999). Immediate, delayed and late submerged and transmucosal implants. In: Lang NP, Karring T, Lindhe J, editors. Proceedings of the 3rd European Workshop on Periodontology: Implant Dentistry. Berlin: Quintessenz, p. 520-34

Michael S, Israel F, & Robert L. (2002). Human mineralized bone in extraction sites before implant placement Preliminary results. J Am Dent Assoc 133:1631-1638

Mish CE & Judy KWM. (2000). Classification of partially edentulous arches for implant dentistry. Int J Oral Implantol 26: 127-128

Misch CE. (1999).Contemporary Implant Dentistry. 2nd ed. St Louis: Mosby Inc: 455-464

Paulino Castellon D, Raymond A & Yukna DMD. (2004). Immediate dental implant placement in sockets augmented with HTR synthetic bone. Implant Dent 13: 42-48

Peñarrocha M, Uribe R, & Balaguer J. (2004). Immediate implants after extraction. a review of the current situation Med Oral 9:234-42

Piatteli A, Paolantonio M, Corigliano M & Scarano A.(1997). Immediate loading of titanium plasma-spayed screw-shaped implants in man: A clinical and histological report of two cases. J Periodontol 68: 591-597

Piattelli A, Corigliano M, Costiggliola G & Paolantionio M. (1998). Immediate loading of titanium plasma-sprayed implants: An histologic analysis in monkeys. J Periodontol 69: 321-327

Sagara M, Akagawa Y, Nikai H & Tsuru H. (1993). The effects of early occlusal loading on one-stage titanium alloy implants in beagle doss. J Prosthet Dent 69: 281-288

Scahalhorn RG. (1972). Human alografts of iliac concellous bone and marow in periodontal osseous defects II. Clinical observation. J Periodontol 43: 67-81

Schwart ZA., Gulayev N & Choushu G. (2000). Immediate versus non-immediate implantation for full arch fixed reconstruction following extraction of all residual teeth. A retrospective comparative study. J Periodontol 71: 923-9

Schwartz-Arad D, & Chaushu G. (1997).The ways and wherefores of immediate placement of implants into fresh extraction sites: a literature review. J Periodontol 68:915-23

Scott DG & Maurice V. (2002). Predictable synthetic bone grafting procedures for implant reconstruction: Pant two. J Oral Implant 8 (4): 178-183

Scott D. Ganz, DMD.(1997) . Mandibular Tori as a Source for Onlay Bone Graft Augmentation: A Surgical Procedure. The Implant Report 9:973 982.

Stanley HR, Mathew BH, Clark AE, King CJ & Hench L. (1997). Using 4555 bioglass cones as endosseous ridge maintenance implants prevent alveolar ridge reserption: A 5-year evaluation. Int J Oral Maxillofac Implants 12: 95-105

Wohrle Ps, Schnitman PA, DaSilva JD, Wang NH, & Koch GG. (1992). Branemark implants palced into immediate function: 5-year results. J Oral Implantol 18: 382

9

Bone Quality Assessment for Dental Implants

Ayse Gulsahi
Baskent University Faculty of Dentistry, Ankara, Turkey

1. Introduction

Dental implants have become a predictable treatment option for restoring missing teeth. The purpose of tooth replacement with implants is to restore adequate function and esthetics without affecting adjacent hard and/or soft tissue structures. The use of dental implants in oral rehabilitation has currently been increasing since clinical studies with dental implant treatment have revealed successful outcomes (Turkyilmaz et al., 2008a). The successful outcome of any implant procedure depends on a series of patient-related and procedure-dependent parameters, including general health conditions, biocompatability of the implant material, the feature of the implant surface, the surgical procedure, and the quality and quantity of the local bone. (Turkyilmaz et al., 2007)

Successfully providing dental implants to patients who have lost teeth and frequently the surrounding bone relies on the careful gathering of clinical and radiological information, on interdisciplinary communication and on detailed planning. One of the most important factors in determining implant success is proper treatment planning. In the past, periapical radiographs along with panoramic images were used as the sole determinants of implant diagnosis and treatment planning. With the advancement of radiographic technology, Computed tomography (CT), as well as cone-beam computed tomography (CBCT) is increasingly considered essential for optimal implant placement, especially in the case of complex reconstructions (Benson & Shetty, 2009; Chan et al., 2010; Resnik et al., 2008).

2. Radiologic examination

The objectives of diagnostic imaging depend on a number of factors, including the amount and type of information required and the period of the treatment rendered. The desicion to image the patient is based on the patient's clinical needs. After a desicion has been made to obtain images, the imaging modality is used that yields the necessary diagnostic information related to the patient's clinical needs and results in the least radiologic risk (Resnik et al., 2008). The ideal imaging technique for dental implant care should have several essential characteristics, including the ability to visualize the implant site in the mesiodistal, bucco-lingual and superioinferior dimensions; the ability to allow reliable, accurate measurements; a capacity to evaluate trabecular bone density and cortical thickness; reasonable access and cost to the patient and minimal radiation risk (Benson & Shetty, 2009). Diagnostic imaging is an integral part of dental implant therapy for preoperative planning, intraoperative assessment, and postoperative assessment by use of a variety of imaging techniques.

2.1 Selecting imaging technique for preoperative implant planning

The objectives of the preoperative implant imaging include all necessary surgical and prosthetic information to determine the quantity, quality and angulations of bone; selection of the potential implant sites, and to verify absence of pathology. However, there is no ideal imaging technique in the field of oral implantology that would be acceptable for all patients. All imaging techniques have inherent advantages and disadvantages (Resnik et al. 2008).

In dental and medical radiology, a recommended principle when selecting the appropriate radiographic modality is based on radiologic dosage. Obviously, the goal is to choose a radiographic method providing sufficient diagnostic information for treatment planning with the least possible radiation dose (ALARA principle: as low as reasonably achievable) and costs for the patient. The preferred imaging procedure for this purpose seems to vary much among different parts of the world as well as among individual dentists.

2.1.1 Intraoral radiography

Traditionally, conventional radiographic images e.g., periapical and panoramic images have been used to assist practitioners in planning implant treatment. Periapical radiographs commonly are used to evaluate the status of adjacent teeth and remaining alveolar bone in the mesiodistal dimension. In addition they have been used for determining vertical height, architecture and bone quality (bone density, amount of cortical bone and amount of trabecular bone). Although readily available and relatively inexpensive, periapical radiography has geometric and anatomic limitations. If the paralleling technique is not used, periapical radiographs create an image with foreshortening and elongation (Benson & Shetty, 2009; Chan et al., 2010). When the x-ray beam is perpendicular to the film, but the object is not parallel to the film, foreshortening will occur. If the x-ray beam is oriented perpendicular to the object but not the film, elongation will occur. The most accurate intraoral radiographic technique used for implant planning is the paralleling technique. These principles in positioning will allow for an intraoral image with minimal distortion and magnification. Therefore, standardized periapical radiographs with bite-blocks by using paralling technique should be perform to the longitudinal studies (Benson & Shetty, 2009; Resnik et al., 2008).

Because the periapical radiographs are unable to provide any cross-sectional information, occlusal radiographs are used to determine bucco-lingual dimensions of the mandibular alveolar ridge. However, the occlusal image records only the widest portion of the mandible, which typically is located inferior to the alveolar ridge. This may give the clinician the impression that more bone is available in the cross-sectional dimension than actually exists. The occlusal technique is not useful for the maxillary arch because of the anatomic limitations (Benson & Shetty, 2009).

2.1.2 Panoramic radiography

Panoramic radiographs have been used frequently as a radiographic method for preimplant evaluation and the preparation of treatment protocols. Although the resolution and sharpness of panoramic radiographs are less than those of intraoral radiographs, panoramic radiographs is an excellent tool for the overview of the maxillofacial area, including many of the vital structures, such as maxillary sinus, inferior alveolar nerve and nasal fossa. Panoramic radiography units are widely available, making this imaging technique very useful and popular as a screening (Benson & Shetty, 2009; Chan et al., 2010). (Figure 1)

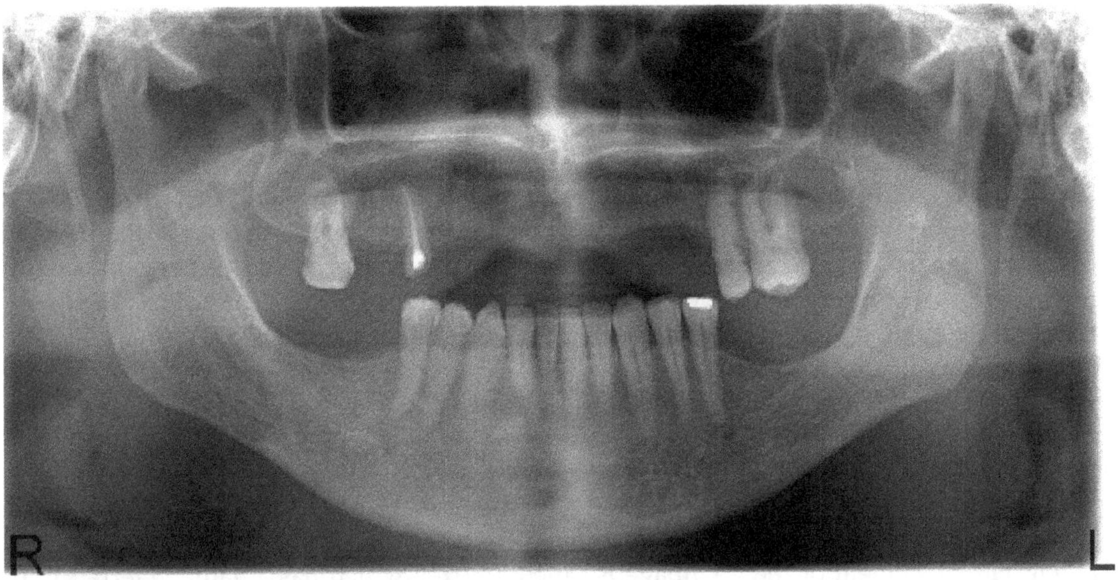

Fig. 1. Panoramic radiography before implant placement

Information acquired from panoramic radiographs must be applied judiciously because this technique has significant limitations as a definitive preoperative planning tool. With regard to panoramic radiographs, the lack of image sharpness and resolution, coupled with nonuniform distortion often leads to inaccurate interpretation and measurements (Benson & Shetty, 2009; Chan et al., 2010). The magnification of panoramic radiographs can be >30%, especially when patients are not in the optimal position. Angular measurements on panoramic radiographs tend to be accurate, but linear measurements are not. Vertical measurements are unreliable because of foreshortening and elongation of the anatomic structures because the x-ray beam is not perpendicular to the long axis of the anatomic structures or to plane of the image receptor. Similarly, dimensional accuracy in the horizontal plane of panoramic radiographs is highly dependent on the position of the structures of interest relative to the central plane of the image layer (Benson & Shetty, 2009). However, the magnification factor can be calculated at the given site by dividing the actual diameter of the object by the diameter measured on the radiographs. Diagnostic templates that have ball bearings or wires incorporated around the curvature of the dental arch and worn by the patient during the panoramic examination enable the dentist to determine the amounts of magnification in the radiograph (Resnik et al., 2008).

2.1.3 Computed tomography

Clinicians have been diagnosing, treatment planning, placing and restoring dental implants using periapical and panoramic radiographs to assess bone anatomy for several decades. Two dimensional images have been found to have limitations because of inherent distortion factors and the non-interactive nature of film itself provides. With the advent of technology, CT has lead to a new era of implant imaging.

CT enables the evaluation of proposed implant sites and provides diagnostic information that other imaging or combinations of imaging techniques cannot provide. CT has several advantages over conventional radiography. First, CT eliminates the superimposition of images of structures outside the area of interest. Second, because of the inherent high-contrast resolution of CT, differences between tissues that differ in physical density bt less than 1% can be distinguished; conventional radiography requires a 10% difference in physical density to distinguish between tissues. Third, data from a single CT imaging procedure, consisting of either multiple contiguous or one helical scan, can be viewed as images in the axial, coronal or sagittal planes or in any arbitrary plane depending on the diagnostik task. This is referred to as multiplanar reformatted imaging (Frederiksen, 2009). (Figure 2) Direct images are problematic in the coronal plane because of difficulties in positioning the patient and metallic artifacts from dental materials. For this reason, special software programs have been developed to reformat the data from axial CT scans into the sagittal and coronal planes or any other arbitrary plane (Benson & Shetty, 2009; Chan et al., 2010; Resnik et al., 2008). DentaScan provides programmed reformation, organization and display of the imaging study. The radiologist simply indicates the curvature of the maxillary and mandibular arch, and the computer is programmed to generate referenced cross-sectional and tangential or panoramic images of the alveolus along with three-dimensional images of the arch. The cross-sectional and panoramic images are spaced 1 mm apart and enable accurate preoperative treatment planning (Resnik et al., 2008).

The individual element of the CT image is called a voxel, which has a value, referred to in Hounsfield units (HU), that describes the density of the CT image at that point. HU also known CT numbers, range from -1000 (air) to +3000 (enamel), each corresponding to a different level of beam attenuation (Benson & Shetty, 2009; Frederiksen, 2009; Resnik et al., 2008). The density of structures within the image is absolute and quantitative and can be used to differentiate tissues in the region (i.e., muscle, 35–70 HU; fibrous tissue, 60–90 HU, cartilage, 80–130 HU; bone 150–1800 HU) and characterize bone quality (D1 bone, >1250 HU; D2 bone, 750–1250 HU; D3 bone, 375–750 HU; D4 bone, <375 HU) (Misch, 2008).

The utility of CT for dental implant treatment planning was evident, but the access to these imaging techniques is limited. Nevertheless, CT scans are not without their limitations/concerns and radiation exposure and cost are the major two (Benson & Shetty, 2009; Chan et al., 2010, Scarfe & Farman, 2008).

2.1.4 Cone-beam computed tomography

Because of higher radiation exposure, higher cost, huge footprint, and difficulty in accessibility associated with CT, CBCT was developed. As the name implies, CBCT generates cone-shaped beams and the images are acquired in one rotation by an image intensifier of flat panel detector, resulting in reasonably low levels of radiation dosage (Arai et al., 1999; Chan et al., 2010; Scarfe & Farman, 2008). During the rotation, multiple (from 150 to more than 600) sequential planar projection images of the field of view (FOV) are acquired in a complete, or sometimes partial arch. Obvious advantages of such a system, which provides a shorter examination time, include the reduction of image unsharpness caused by the translation of the patient, reduced image distortion due to internal patient movements, and increased x-ray tube efficiency. However, its main disadvantage, especially with larger FOVs, is a limitation in image quality related to noise and contrast resolution because of the detection of large amounts of scattered radiation (Scarfe & Farman, 2008).

The resolution and therefore detail of CBCT imaging is determined by the individual volume elements or voxels produced from the volumetric data set. In CBCT imaging, voxel dimensions primarily depend on the pixel size on the area detector, unlike those in CT, which depend on slice thickness. The resolution of the area detector is submillimeter.

Therefore, the theoretical resolution of CBCT is higher than CT (Scarfe & Farman, 2008; 2009). In the literature, the accuracy of CT and CBCT in the assessment of implant site dimensions were compared and CBCT measurements found more accurate than CT measurements (Al-Ekrish & Ekram, 2011; Kobayashi et al., 2004; Loubele et al., 2008; Suomalainen et al., 2008).

The reformetted images of CBCT data result in three basic image types; axial images with a computer generated superimposed curve of the alveolar process and the associated reformatted alveolar cross-sectional images and panoramic-like images. Such reformatted images provide the clinician with accurate two dimensional diagnostic information in all three dimensions. Both CT and CBCT images provide information on the continuity of the cortical bone plates, residual bone in the mandible and maxilla, the relative location of adjoining vital structures and the contour of soft tissues covering the osseos structures (Benson & Shetty, 2009; Scarfe & Farman, 2008).

Voxel values obtained from CBCT images are not absolute values, like HU values obtained using CT, various methods have been proposed to evaluate the bone density (Naitoh et al. 2009; 2010; Mah et al., 2010). HU provide a quantitative assessment of bone density as measured by its ability to attenuate an x-ray beam. To date, there was not any standard system for scaling the grey levels representing the reconstructed values. In a study, (Katsumata et al., 2007), the authors found that calculated HU on a CBCT scan varied widely from a range of -1500 to over +3000 for different types of bone. However, after a correction has been applied to grey levels with the CBCT, the HU values are much similar to those one would expect in a medical CT device than to the original grey levels obtained from the CBCT scanners (Naitoh et al. 2009; 2010; Nomura et al., 2010, Mah et al., 2010).

The clinical utility of preoperative implant planning by use of in imaging stent that helps relate the radiographic image and its information to a precise anatomic location or a potential implant site. The intended implant sites are identified by radiopaque markers retained within an acrylic stent which the patient wears during the imaging procedure so that images of the markers will b created in the diagnostic images. The imaging stent subsequently may be used as a surgical guide to Orient the insertion angle of the guide bur and hence the angle of the implant. Generally, nonmetallic radiopaque markers are used in CT and CBCT imaging (Benson & Shetty, 2009).

The availability of CBCT is also expanding the use of additional diagnostic and treatment software applications. CBCT permits more than diagnosis, it facilitates image-guided surgery. Diagnostic and planning software are available to assist in implant planning to fabricate surgical models (eg, Biomedical Modeling Inc., USA); to facilitate virtual implant placement,; to create diagnostic and surgical implant guidance stents (eg, Virtual Implant Placement, Implant Logic Systems, Cedarhurst, USA; Simplant, Materialise, Belgium; Easy Guide, Keystone Dental, USA) and even to assist in the computer-aided design and manufacture of implant prosthetics (NobelGuide/Procera software, Nobel Care AG, Sweden) (Scarfe & Farman, 2008). When those programs are applied, different diameters and length of implants can be 'tried in' before the most optimal one is selected. Furthermore, the placed implant can be assessed from several different viewpoints as well as from three dimensional view. Moreover, once treatment planning is determined in the computer, it can be saved and applied to surgical sites by means of image-aided template production or image-aided navigation. It is important to note that although computer aided implant placement is a promising technique, the unexpected linear and anguler deviation can be a major concern (Chan et al., 2010; Ganz, 2008).

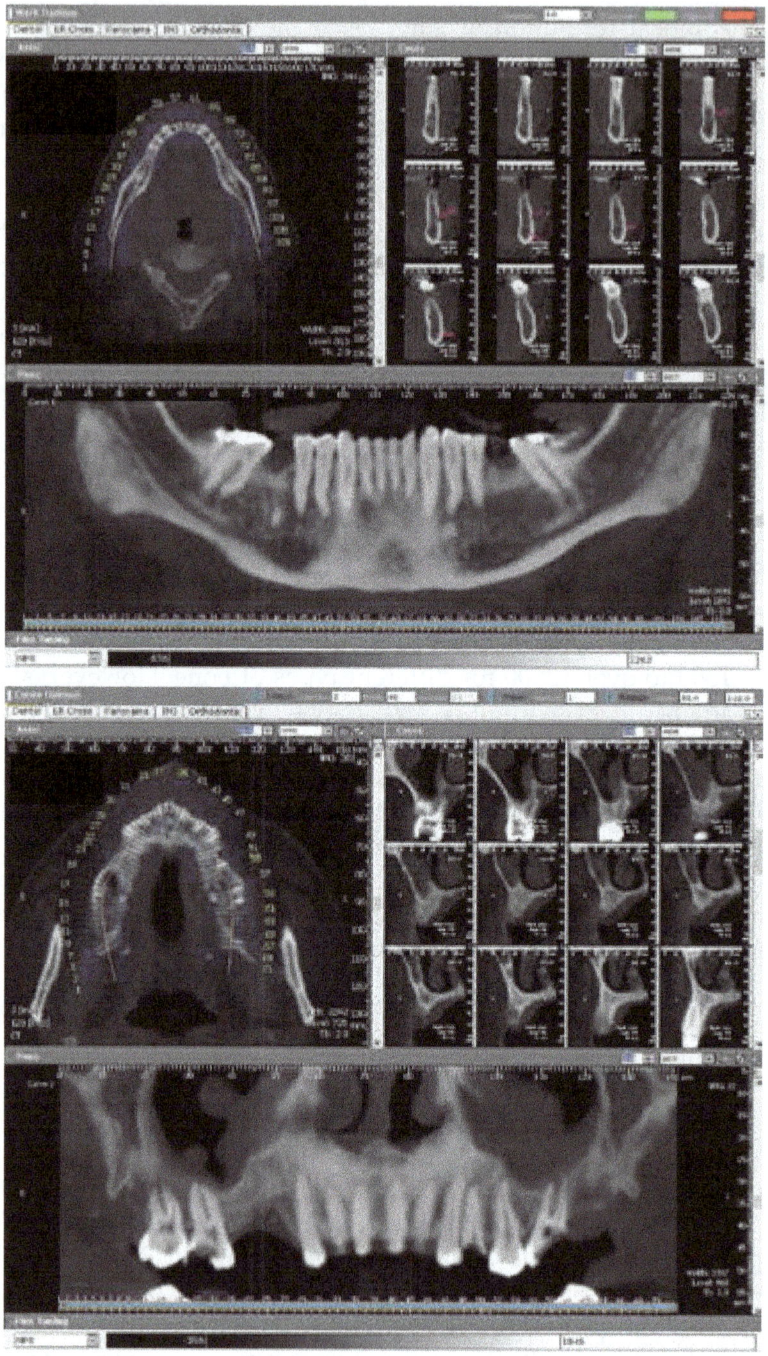

Fig. 2. CT images of preoperative implant site.

2.2 Bone quality assessment of implant sites

Several factors, such as implant geometry, preparation technique, and quality and quantity of local bone influence primary stability, and primary implant stability is one of the main factors influencing implant survival rates. (Friberg et al., 1991; Meredith, 1998, Turkyilmaz & McGlumphy, 2008a).

2.2.1 Implant stability measurements

Implant stability can be measured by non-invasive clinical test methods (i.e., insertion torque, the periotest, resonance frequency analysis). One of these quantitative methods is the *insertion torque* described by Johansson and Strid (1994). This method records the torque required to place the implant and provides valuable information about local bone quality.

Another method, named *Periotest*, has been developed to measure the degree of the periodontal integration of teeth and the stiffness of the bone/implant interface (Olive & Aparicio, 1990; Turkyilmaz & McGlumphy, 2008b). The Periotest instrument measures the deflection/deceleration of a tooth or implant that has been struck by a small pistil from inside the instrument's hand piece. The contact time of the accelerated pistil to the implant, which moves according to the strike, is calculated into a value called the Periotest value. However, Periotest values include only a narrow range over the scale of the instrument and thus, provide relatively less sensitive information about implant stability. Therefore, its benefit on detection of osseointegration is a matter of debate.

Another method, *resonance frequency analysis* (RFA) has been introduced by Meredith and coworkers (1996). In RFA, the stiffness of the bone/ implant interface is calculated from a resonance frequency as a reaction to oscillations exerted onto the implant/bone system. The implant is excited with an oscillating transducer screwed onto the implant and the resonance specific to the resonance system 'implant/bone' is captured electronically over a range of 5 to 15 kHz. RF values have clinically been correlated with changes in implant stability during osseous healing, failure of implants to integrate and the supracrestal dimensions of the implant. The results of a histomorphometric study suggested that RFA values correlated well with the amount of bone-to-implant contact. These findings support the use of RFA in evaluating changes in the bone healing and osseointegration process following implant placement (Turkyilmaz & McGlumphy, 2008b).

2.2.2 Bone quality and quantity

The term *bone quality* is commonly used in implant treatment and in reports on implant success and failure. Lindh et al. (2004) emphasized that *bone density (Bone Mineral Density, BMD)* and *bone quality* are not synonymous. Bone quality encompasses factors other than bone density such as skeletal size, the architecture and 3-dimensional orientation of the trabeculea, and matrix properties. Bone quality is not only a matter of mineral content, but also of structure. It has been shown that the quality and quantity of bone available at the implant site are very important local patient factors in determining the success of dental implants (Drage et al., 2007; Lindh et al., 2004).

The success rate obtained with dental implants depends to a great extent on the volume and quality of the surrounding bone. Therefore, it is important to know the bone quantity and quality of the jaws when planning implant treatment. Bone quantity of jawbone is broken down into five groups (from minimal to severe, A- E), based on residual jaw shape different rates of bone resorption following tooth extraction (Ribeiro-Rotta et al., 2010). During all stages of atrophy of the alveolar ridge, characteristic shapes result from the resorptive process. It is difficult to obtain implant anchorage in bone that is not very dense. Sufficient bone density and volume are therefore crucial factors for ensuring implant success (Lekholm & Zarb, 1985).

Bone quality is broken down into four groups according to the proportion and stucture of compact and trabecular bone tissue (Ribeiro-Rotta et al., 2010). Bone quality is categorized into four groups: groups 1-4 or type I to IV (Bone Quality Index-BQI) (Figure 3).

Type I: homogeneous cortical bone;
Type II: thick cortical bone with marrow cavity;
Type III: thin cortical bone with dense trabecular bone of good strength;
Type IV: very thin cortical bone with low density trabecular bone of poor strength.

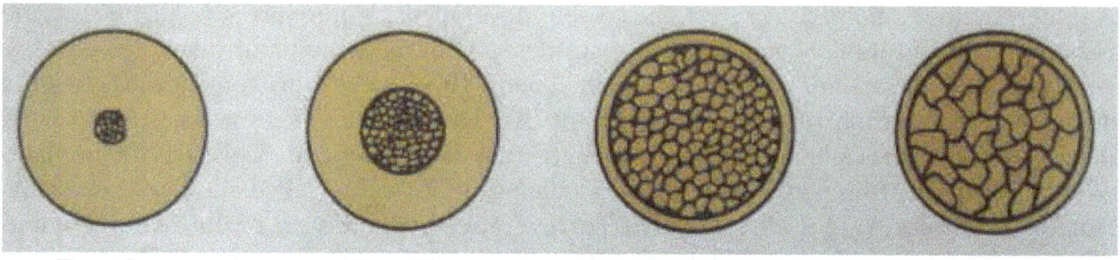

Type I Type II Type III Type IV

Fig. 3. Bone Quality Index

In the jaws, an implant placed in poor-quality bone with thin cortex and low-density trabeculae (Type IV bone) has a higher chance of failure compared with the other types of bones. This low density bone is often found in the posterior maxilla and several studies report higher implant failure rates in this region (Bryant, 1998; Drage et al., 2007; Penarrocha et al., 2004). When compared to the maxilla, clinical reports have indicated a higher survival rate for dental implants in the mandible, particularly in the anterior region of the mandible, which has been associated with better volume and density of the bone (Turkyilmaz et al., 2008). Histomorphometric studies show that the posterior maxilla has a lower trabecular volume, with a reduction in the thickness and number of trabeculae (Drage et al., 2007). Regional differences in jaw anatomy and bone structure may explain some of the variation in clinical success rate of implant therapy in the maxilla and the increased rate of residual ridge resorption reported in the mandible. Surveys have shown that implant therapy in the maxilla has a significantly higher clinical failure rate than that in the mandible, and regional differences in maxillary BMD may be partly responsible (Devlin et al., 2008).
Mish (2008) defined four bone density groups (D1 to D4) in all regions of the jaws that vary in both macroscopic cortical and trabecular bone types. The homogeneous, dense D1 bone type presents several advantages for implant dentistry. The cortical lameller bone may heal with little interim woven bone formation, ensuring excellent bone strength while healing next to the implant. D1 bone is more often found in anterior mandibles with moderate to severe resorption. The percentages of light microscopic contact of bone at the implant interface is greatest in D1 bone type and greater than 80%. In addition, this bone density exhibits greater strength than any other type. The strongest bone also benefits from the greatest bone-implant contact. Less stresess are transmitted to the apical third of the implants than other bone types. D1 bone has fewer blood vessels than the other three types, and therefore it is more dependent on the periosteum for its nutrion. The cortical bone receives the outer one third of all its arterial and venous supply from the periosteum. This bone density is almost all cortical and the capacity of regeneration is impaired because of the poor blood circulation. Also, greater heat is often generated at the apical portion of the D1 bone. D2 is a combination of of dense-to-porous cortical bone on the crest and coarse trabecular bone on the inside. The D2 bone trabeculae are 40% to 60% stronger than D3

tarbeculae. This bone type occurs most frequently in the anterior mandible, followed by the posterior mandible. On occasion it is observed in the anterior maxilla, especially for a single missing tooth. D2 bone provides excellent implant interface healing, and osseointegration is very predictable. The intrabony blood supply allows bleeding during the osteotomy, which helps control overheating during preparation and is most beneficial for bone-implant interface healing. D3 is composed of thinner porous cortical bone on the crest and fine trabecular bone within the ridge. The trabecula are approximtely 50% weaker than those in D2 bone. D3 bone is found most often in the anterior maxilla and posterior regions of the mouth in either arch. The D3 anterior maxilla is usually of less width than its mandibular D3 counterpart. The D3 bone is not only 50% weaker than D2 bone, the bone-implant contact is also less favorable in D3 bone. The additive factors can increase the risk of implant failure. D4 bone has very little density and little or no cortical crestal bone. It is the opposite spectrum of D1 (dense cortical bone). The most commen locations for this type of bone are the posterior region of the maxilla. It is rarely observed in mandible. The bone trabeculae may be up to 10 times weaker than the cortical bone of D1. The bone-implant contact after initial loading is often less than 25%. Bone trabeculae are sparse and, as a result, initial fixation of any implant design presents a surgical challenge (Misch, 2008).

2.2.3 Bone mineral density measurements

BMD is the amount of bone tissue in a certain volume of bone. Assessment of jaw BMD may be considered useful in implant planning (Gulsahi et al., 2010). Several approaches have been introduced to measure jawbones and skeletal bones density. Densitometric measurements of panoramic and periapical radiographs have been used, as have more advanced methods such as Dual Energy X-Ray Absorptiometry (DEXA), CT and CBCT.

By including and referencing an aluminum step-wedge standard image with each exposure, densitometric evaluation of periapical or panoramic radiographs can be performed (Figure 4). Equal thicknesses of mineralized tissue and aluminum produce similar radiographic densities. The optical density of the jawbone site, and each step of the stepwedge is measured on the reference radiograph, and the values are plotted against the corresponding thickness of aluminum. The curve is obtained provided the corresponding aluminum equivalents in millimeters to the measured mean optical density of the jawbone (Gulsahi et al., 2007).

DEXA is a technique that enables fast, noninvasive, and highly precise measurement of BMD). In daily clinical practice, DEXA is the most useful method for BMD assessment in the vertebrae, femoral neck, and forearms. This technique was introduced in 1987. Its operation is based on the principle that bone and soft tissue exhibit different properties of attenuation as a function of photon energy. Therefore, DEXA uses an x-ray source to produce a beam of discrete energies that is attenuated as it travels through the patient. The radiation dose is low enough to allow BMD measurements in different skeletal sites and in longitudinal studies (Devlin et al. 1998; Hildebolt, 1997; Hildebolt et al., 1993; von Wovern, 2001). Most studies have examined mandibular or maxillary BMD by DEXA (Drage et al., 2007; Drozdzowska et al., 2002; Gulsahi et al., 2007; Gulsahi et al., 2010; Horner & Devlin, 1998a, 1998b; Pluskiewicz et al., 2000). Studies revaled that maxillary BMD is lower than mandibular BMD (Devlin et al., 1998; Drage et al., 2007; Gulsahi et al., 2010). However, the relation between the jawbone BMD and other skeletal sites BMD is still controversy (Figure 5).

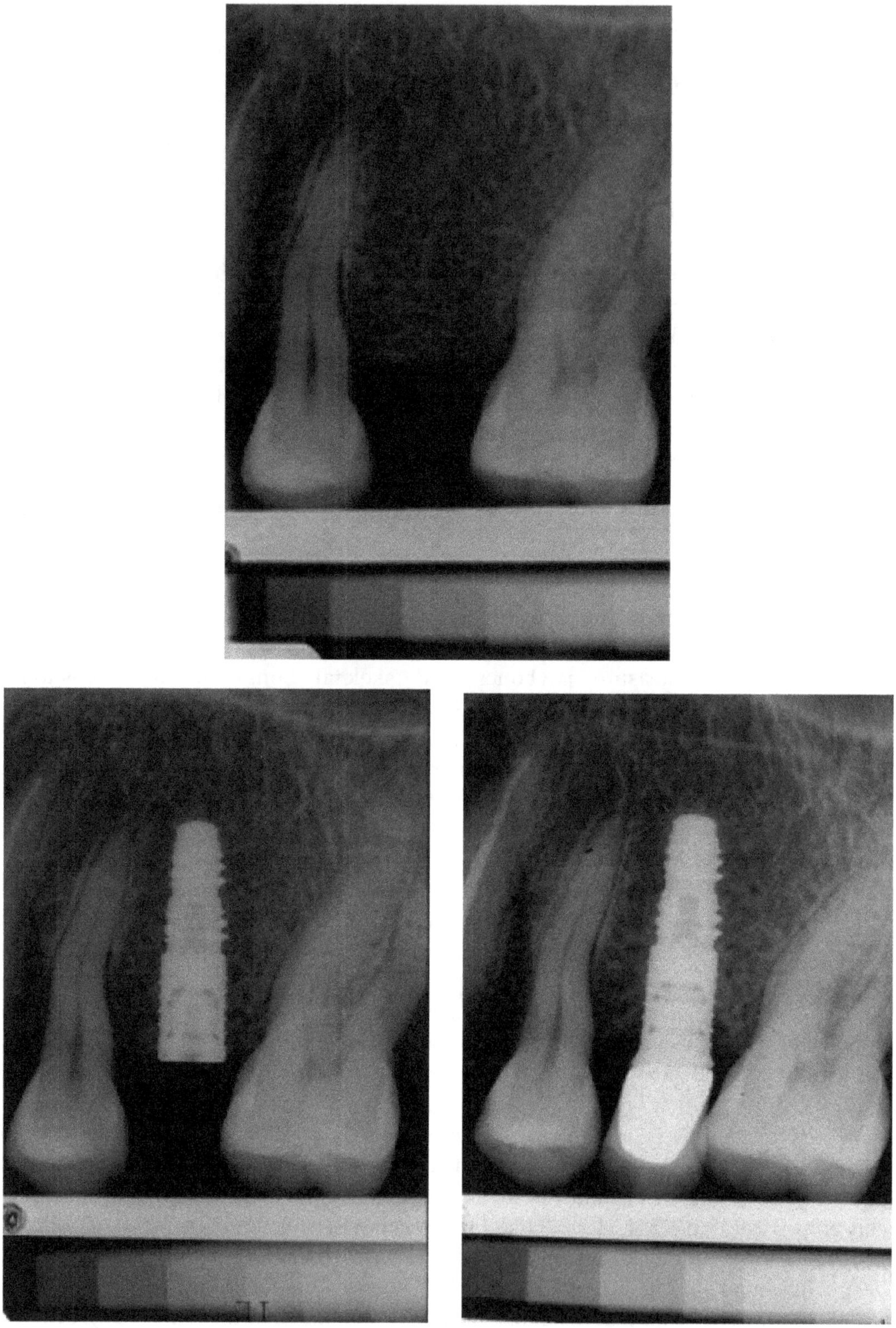

Fig. 4. Periapical radiographs obtained with aluminum stepwedge for densitometric evaluation before and after implant placement.

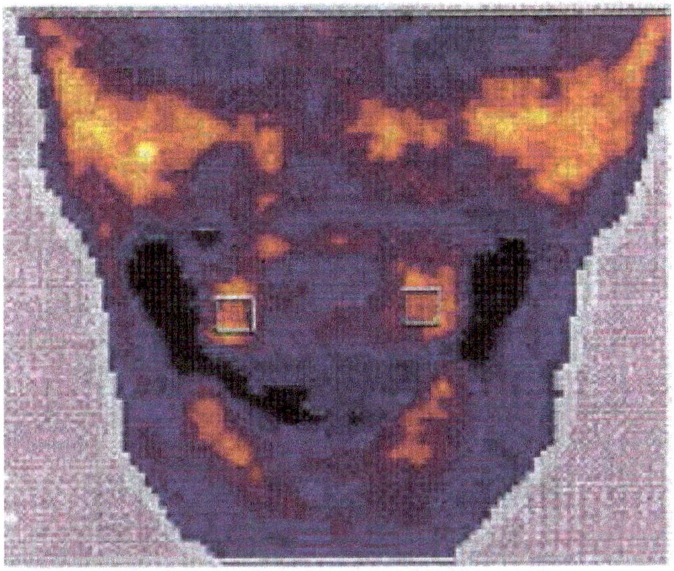

Fig. 5. DEXA measurement before implant placement.

Qualitative and quantitative indexes, including the mandibular cortical index (MCI), mental index (MI) or panoramic mandibular index (PMI) have also been used for panoramic radiographs to assess the bone quality. MCI is the appearance of the inferior mandibular cortical thickness as follows; C1; the endosteal margin of the cortex is even and sharp on both sides, C2; the endosteal margin shows semilunar defects (lacunar resorption) and/or seems to form endosteal cortical residues on one or both sides, C3; the cortical layer forms heavy endosteal cortical residues and clearly porous (Klemetti et al., 1994) (Figure 6).
MI is measurement of the cortical width at the mental foramen region (Ledgerton et al., 1999).

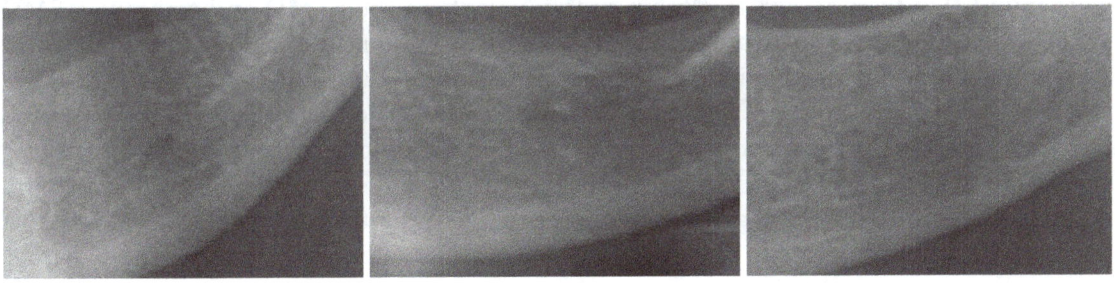

Fig. 6. Shows the C1, C2 and C3 classification of mandibular cortex index.

The inferior PMI is the ratio of the thickness of mandibular cortex to the distance between the inferior margin of mental foramen and the inferior mandibular cortex (Benson et al., 1991) (Figure 7). Some authors concluded that panoramic radiomorphometric indices significantly correlated with mandibular BMD (Horner & Devlin 1998a, 1998b; Drozdzowska et al. 2002). However in a study, there was no found such a correlation (Gulsahi et al. 2010).

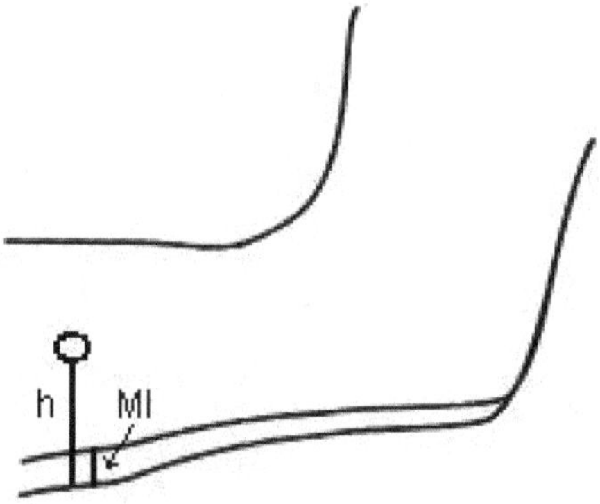

Fig. 7. Shows the MI and PMI (MI/h) measurements.

Assessments have primarily been made of the bone tissue status of the entire jaw, and site-specific variations have been ignored, as have the consequences of differences between the compact and trabecular parts of jawbone tissue. CT is the only method that allows the components of trabecular and compact bone tissue to be investigated separately (Lindh et al., 2004). With CT, it is possible to measure bone density that its effect on the survival of the implant can be estimated. Norton & Gamble (2001) suggested an objective scale of bone density that was besed on mean HU values taken from CT and could be used for bone tissue classification before implant treatment. They reported the mean bone density from CT was 682 HU for 139 sites. They recorded that the mean bone densities in the anterior mandible, the posterior mandible, the anterior maxilla, the posterior maxilla were 970, 669, 696, and 417 HU respectively. Shapurian et al. (2006) reported that the average bone density values in the anterior mandible, the anterior maxilla, the posterior maxilla, the posterior mandible were 559, 517, 333 and 321 HU for 219 implant sites. When considering all implant sites, the mean bone density was 887±180 HU in the other study (Turkyilmaz & McGlumphy, 2008a), which is higher than those reported earlier (Norton & Gamble, 2001; Shapurian et al., 2006). However, in the other study, variations in bone density between different regions of maxilla were found (Lindh et al., 2004). Within individuals, both total BMD and trabecular BMD values were higher in the cuspid-frontal regions than in the posterior region of maxilla. In addition, a significant correlation was found between the total BMD and trabecular BMD and between the mean BMD values and mean HU values. The large variations between the BMD of the different region in the maxilla or mandible emphasize the importance of the site-specific measurements of tissue before implant placement. In the study, the authors noted that it is important that an objective tool for the evaluation of bone tissue is found so that clinicians can more easily determine whether to load the implant immediately, earlier or later (Ericsson et al., 2002).

2.3 Intraoperative and postoperative assessments

Intraoral and panoramic radiographs usually are adequate for both intraoperative and postoperative assessments. Intraoperative imaging may be required to confirm correct placement of the implant or to locate a lost implant. The two aspects that are usually assessed with time after implant placement are the alveolar bone height around the implant and the appearance of the bone immediately adjacent to and surrounding the implant. In general, periapical radiographs are appropriate for longitudinal assessments. The angulation of the x-ray beam must be within 9 degrees of the long axis of the fixture to open the threads on the image on most threaded fixtures (Benson & Shetty, 2009).

In evaluating the the bone height around an implant, an effort should be made to reproduce the vertical angulation of the central ray of the x-ray beam as closely as possible between radiographs. Distal and mesial marginal bone height is measured from a collar of the implant, or in tha case of threaded implants by use of known interthreaded measurements and compared with bone levels in previous periapical radiographs. The presence of relatively distinct bone margins with a constant height relative to the implant suggests successful osseos integration. Any resorptive changes, if present, are evidenced by apical migration of the alveolar bone or distinct osseos margins. Radiographic studies suggest that the rate of marginal bone loss after successful implantation is approximately 1.2 mm in the first year, subsequently tapering off to about 0.1 mm in succeeding years (Benson & Shetty, 2009).

The success of an implant can also be evaluated by the appearance of normal bone surrounding it and its apposition to the surface of the implant body. The development of a thin radiolucent area that closely follows the outline of the implant usually correlates to clinically detectable implant mobility, it is an important indicator of failed osseointegration. Changes in the periodontal ligament space of associated teeth are also useful in monitoring the functional competence of the implant-prostheses composite. Any widening of the periodontal ligament space compared with baseline radiographs indicates poor stress distribution and forecasts implant failure (Benson & Shetty, 2009).

After successful implantation, radiographs may be made at regular intervals to assess the success or failure of the implant fixture (Benson & Shetty, 2009).

3. Conclusion

In summary, diagnostic imaging is an integral part of dental implant therapy for preoperative planning, intraoperative and posoperative assessment by use of variety of techniques. In general, good starting point would be proceed with panoramic radiograph and possibly intraoral radiographs if greater image detail is required. If images are required of all of the maxilla and mandible to evaluate possible implant sites, cross-sectional images assists to clinician. Today, CBCT is the best modality for the ease of acquisition and relatively low radiation risk even for single implants.

4. Acknowledgement

Special thanks to Dr İlker Cebeci for the CBCT images from his archieve.

5. References

Al-Ekrish, A.A., Ekram, M. (2011). A comparative study of the aacuracy and reliability of multidetector computed tomography and cone beam computed tomography in the assessment of dental implant site dimension. *Dentomaxillofac Radiol*, 40, 67-75.

Arai, Y., Tammisalo, E., Iwai, K. (1999). Development of a compact computed tomographic apparatus for dental use. *Dentomaxillofac Radiol*, 28, 245-8.

Benson BW, Prihoda TJ, Glass BJ. (1991). Variations in adult cortical bone mass as measured by a panoramic mandibular index. *Oral Surg Oral Med Oral Pathol*, 71, 349-356.

Benson, B.W. & Shetty, V (2009). Dental Implants, In: *Oral Radiology Principles and Interpretation*, S.C. White & M. J. Pharoah, pp. 597-612, Mosby, Elsevier, ISBN 978-0-323-04983-2, St. Louis, Missouri.

Bryant, S.R. (1998). The effects of age, jaw site, and bone condition on oral implant outcomes. *Int J Prosth*, 11, 470-90.

Chan H-L., Misch K., Wang H-L. (2010). Dental Imaging in Implant Treatment Planning. *Implant Dent*, 19, 288-298.

Devlin H, Horner K, Ledgerton D. (1998). A comparison of maxillary and mandibular bone mineral densities. *J Prosthet Dent*, 79, 323-7.

Drage NA, Palmer RM, Blake G, Wilson R, Crane F, Fogelman I. (2007). A comparison of bone mineral density in the spine, hip and jaws of edentulous subjects. *Clin Oral Impl Res*, 18, 496-500.

Drozdzowska B., Pluskiewicz W., Tarnawska B. (2002). Panoramic based mandibular indices in relation to mandibular bone mineral density and skeletal status assessed by dual energy X-ray absorptiometry and quantitative ultrasound. *Dentomaxillofac Radiol*, 31, 361-7.

Ericsson, I., Nilner, K. (2002). Early functional loading using Branemark dental implants. *J Periodont Restor Dent*, 22, 9-19.

Frederiksen, N., L. (2009). Advanced Imaging, In: *Oral Radiology Principles and Interpretation*, S.C. White & M. J. Pharoah, pp. 207-224, Mosby, Elsevier, ISBN 978-0-323-04983-2, St. Louis, Missouri.

Friberg B, Jemt T, Lekholm U. (1991). Early failures in 4641 consecutively placed Branemark dental implants: a study from stage I surgery to the connection of completed prostheses. *Int J Oral Maxillofac Implants*, 6, 142–6.

Johansson, P., Strid K.G. (1994). Assessment of bone quality from placement resistance during implant surgery. *Int J Oral Maxillofac Implants*, 9, 279-88.

Ganz, S. (2008). Computer-aided Design/Computer-aided Manufacturing Applications Using CT and Cone Beam CT Scanning Technology. *Dent Clin N Am*, 52, 777-808.

Gulsahi A., Paksoy C.S., Yazicioglu N., Arpak N., Kucuk NO, Terzioglu H. The Assessment of Bone Density Differences between Conventional and Bone-Condensing Techniques using Dual Energy X-Ray Absorptiometry and Radiography. (2007). *Oral Surg Oral Med Oral Pathol Oral Radiol Endod*, 104, 692-98.

Gulsahi, A., Ozden, S., Paksoy, C.S., Kucuk, O., Cebeci, A.R.I, Genc Y. (2010). Assessment of Bone Mineral Density in The Jaws and Its Relationship to radiomorphometric Indices. *Dentomaxillofac Radiol*, 39, 284-89.

Hildebolt CF (1997). Osteoporosis and oral bone loss. *Dentomaxillofac Radiol*, ;26, 3-15.

Hildebolt CF, Rupich RC, Vannier MW, Zerbolio DJ Jr, Shrout MK, Cohen S, et al. (1993). Inter relationships between bone mineral content measures. Dual energy radiography (DER) and bitewing radiographs (BWX). *J Clin Periodontol*, 20, 739-45.

Horner K, Devlin H. (1998a). The relationship between mandibular bone mineral density and panoramic radiographic measurements. *J Dent*, 26, 337-343.

Horner K, Devlin H. (1998b). The relationships between two indices of mandibular bone quality and bone mineral density measured by dual energy x-ray absorptiometry. *Dentomaxillofac Radiol*, 27, 17-21.

Johansson, P., Strid, K.G. (1994). Assessment of bone quality from placement resistance during implant surgery. *Int J Oral Maxillofac Implants*, 9, 279-88.

Katsumata, A., Hirukawa, A., Okumura, S., Naitoh, M., Fujishita, M., Ariji, E., et al. (2007). Effects of image artifacts on gray-value density in limited-volume-cone-beam Computerized tomography. *Oral Surg Oral Med Oral Pathol Oral Radiol Endod,* 104, 829-36.

Klemetti E, Kolmakov S, Kroger H. (1994). Pantomography in assessment of the osteoporosis risk group. *Scand J Dent Res,* 102, 68-72.

Kobayashi, K., Shimoda, S.,Nakagawa, Y., Yamamoto, A. (2004). Accuracy in measurement of distance using limited cone beam computerized tomography. *Int J Oral Maxillofac Implants,* 19, 228-31.

Ledgerton D, Horner K, Devlin H, Worthington H. (1999). Radiomorphometric indices of the mandible in a British female population. *Dentomaxillofac Radiol,* 28,173-181.

Lekholm U, Zarb G.A, (1985). Patient selection and preparation. In: Branemark PI, Zarb GA, Albrektsson T, editors. Tissue-integrated prostheses: osseointegration in clinical dentistry. pp. 199-209, Chicago: Quintessence.

Lindh C, Obrant K, Petersson A. (2004). Maxillary bone mineral density and its relationship to the bone mineral density of the lumbar spine and hip. *Oral Surg Oral Med Oral Pathol Oral Radiol Endod,* 98, 102-109.

Loubele, M., Van Assche, N., Carpentier, K., Maes, F., Jacobsi R., van Steenberghe, D., et al. (2008). Comparative localized linear accuracy of small-field cone beam CT and multislice CT for alveolar bone measurements. *Oral Surg Oral Med Oral Pathol Oral Radiol Endod,* 105, 512-18.

Mah, P., Reeves, T.E., McDavid, W.D. (2010). Deriving Hounsfield units using grey levels in cone-beam computed tomography. *Dentomaxillofac Radiol,* 39, 323-35.

Meredith N. Assessment of implant stability as a prognostic determinant. (1998). *Int J Proshodont,* 11, 491–501.

Meredith, N., Alleyne, D., Cawley P. (1996). Quantitative determination of the stability of the implant-tissue interface using resonance frequency analysis. *Clin Oral Implants Res,* 7, 261–7.

Misch C.,E. (2008). Density of Bone: Effects on surgical approach and healing, In: *Contemporary Implant Dentistry,* C.E. Misch (ed), pp. 645-667, Mosby, Elsevier, ISBN 978-0-323-04373-1, Canada.

Naitoh, M., Hirukawa, A., Katsumata, A., Ariji, E. (2009). Evaluation of voxel values in mandibular cancellous bone: Relationship between cone-beam computed tomography and multislice helical computed tomography. *Clin Oral Implants Res,* 20, 503-6.

Naitoh, M., Hirukawa, A., Katsumata, A., Ariji, E. (2010). Prospective study to estimate mandibular cancellous bone density using large-volume cone-beam computed tomography. *Clin Oral Implants Res,* 21, 1309-13.

Nomura, Y., Watanabe, H., Honda, E., Kurabayashi, T. (2010). Reliability of voxel values from cone-beam computed tomography for Dental use in evaluating bone mineral density. *Clin Oral Implants Res,* 21, 558-62.

Norton, M.R., Gamble, C. (2001). Bone classification: an objective scale of bone density using the computerized tomography scan. *Clin Oral Impl Res,* 12, 79-84.

Olive, J., Aparicio, C. (1990). Periotest method as a measure of osseointegrated oral implant stability. *Int J Oral Maxillofac Implants,* 5, 390-400.

Penarrocha, M., Palomar, M., Sanchis, J.,M., Guarinos, J., Balaguer, J. (2004). Radiologic study of marginal bone loss around 108 dental implants and its relationship to smoking, implant location and morphology. *Int J Oral Maxillofac Impl* 19, 861-7.

Pluskiewicz W., Tarnawska B., Drozdzowska B. (2000). Mandibular bone mineral density measured using dual-energy X-ray absorptiometry: relationship to hip bone mineral density and quantitative ultrasound at calcaneus and hand phalanges. *Br J Radiol,* 73, 288-292.

Resnik, R.R., Kircos, L. and Misch C.,E. (2008). Diagnostic Imaging and Techniques, In: *Contemporary Implant Dentistry,* C.E. Misch (ed), pp. 38-67, Mosby, Elsevier, ISBN 978-0-323-04373-1, Canada.

Ribeiro-Rotta, R.F., Lindh, C., Pereira, A.C., Rohlin, M. Ambiguity in bone tissue characteristics as presentes in studies on dental implant planning and placement: a systematic review. *Clin Oral Impl Res, (in-press)*

Scarfe, W.C., Farman, A.G. (2008). What is Cone-Beam CT and How Does it Work? *Dent Clin N Am,* 52, 707-730.

Scarfe, W.C., Farman, A.G. (2009). Cone-Beam Computed Tomography, In: *Oral Radiology Principles and Interpretation,* S.C. White & M. J. Pharoah, pp. 225-243, Mosby, Elsevier, ISBN 978-0-323-04983-2, St. Louis, Missouri.

Shapurian, T., Damoulis, P.D., Reiser, G.M., Griffin, T.J., Rand. W.M. (2006). Quantitative evaluation of bone density using the Hounsfield Index. *Int J Oral Maxillofac Implants,* 21, 290–97.

Suomalainen, A., Vehmas, T., Kortesniemi, M., Robinson, S., Peltola, J. (2008). Accuracy of linear measurements using Dental cone beam and conventional multislice computed tomography. *Oral Surg Oral Med Oral Pathol Oral Radiol Endod,* 37, 10-17.

Turkyilmaz, I., McGlumphy, E.A. (2008a). Is there a lower threshold value of bone density for early loading protocols of dental implants? *Journal of Oral Rehabilitation,* 35, 775–81.

Turkyilmaz, I., McGlumphy, E.A. (2008b). Influence of bone density on implant stability parameters and implant success: a retrospective clinical study. *BMC Oral Health,* 8, 32.

Turkyilmaz, I., Tözüm, T.F., Tümer, C. (2007). Bone density assessments of oral implant sites using computerized tomography. *J Oral Rehabil,* 34, 267–72.

Turkyilmaz, I., Ozan, O., Yilmaz, B., Ersoy, A.E. (2008). Determination of Bone Quality of 372 Implant Recipient Sites Using Hounsfield Unit from Computerized Tomography: A Clinical Study. *Clin Implant Dent Relat Res,*10, 238-44.

von Wowern N. (2001). General and oral aspects of osteoporosis: a review. *Clin Oral Investig,* 5, 71-82.

10

Various Ways to Enhance the Results of Maxillary Sinus Augmentation Procedures

Jun-Beom Park
Department of Molecular Medicine and Biopharmaceutical Sciences,
Graduate School of Convergence Science and Technology,
Seoul National University, Seoul,
Korea

1. Introduction

The placement of dental implants in the distal edentulous maxillary region is challengin due to the significant resorption following tooth extraction and the pneumatization of th maxillary sinus (Tadjoedin et al., 2003). Maxillary sinus augmentation is a well-establishe procedure for functional rehabilitation of partially or completely edentulous patients, a demonstrated by Boyne and James (1980) (Boyne and James 1980) (Figures 1-4). The surviva rate for implants placed in graft sinuses showed comparable results to those generall reported for implants placed in pristine bone in the non-grafted posterior maxilla (Wallac and Froum 2003).

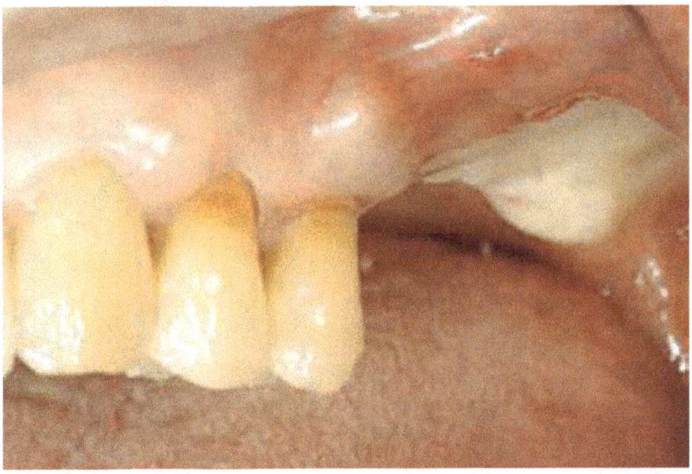

Fig. 1. Preoperative clinical view.

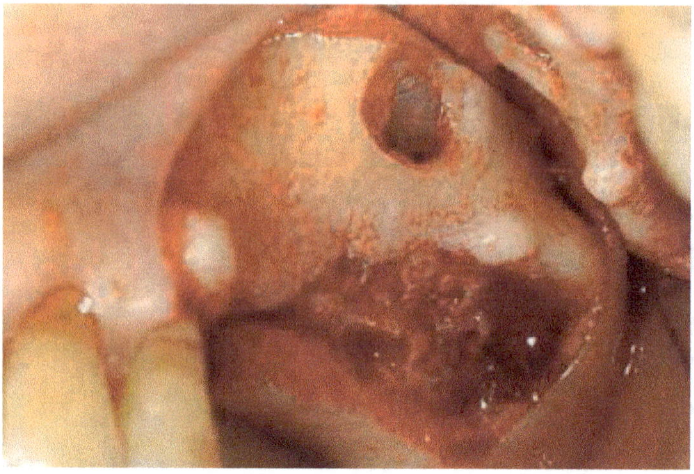

Fig. 2. Buccal view after elevation of sinus membrane.

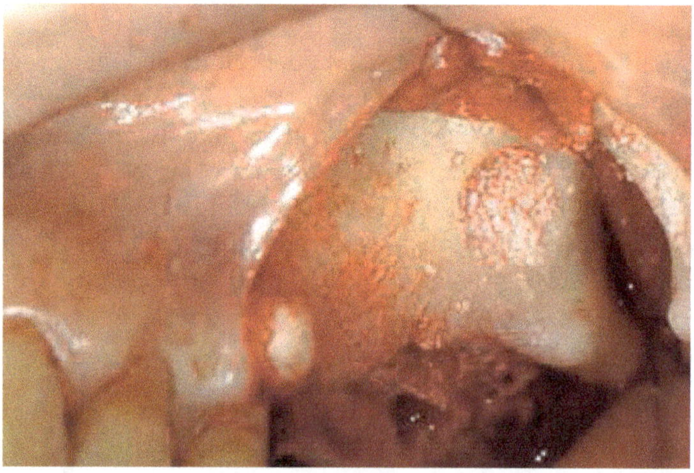

Fig. 3. Clinical view after application of graft material.

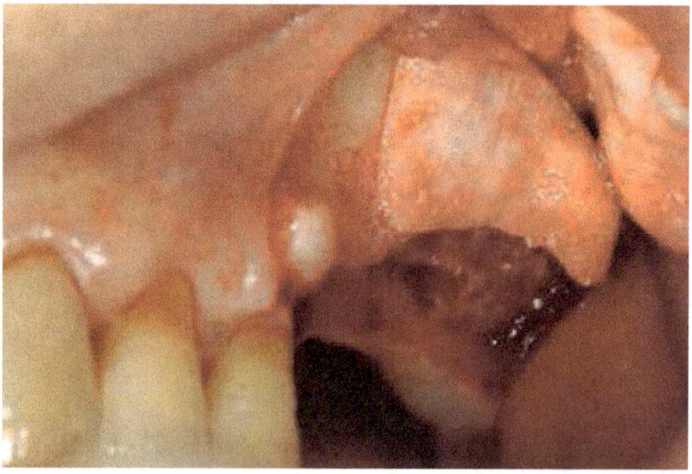

Fig. 4. The lateral wall is covered with a membrane.

Autogenous bone obtained from various donor sites from the patients performed with good results in bone regeneration and served as the gold standard (Tadjoedin et al., 2003). Various bone-grafting materials are being used in sinus augmentation including freeze-dried bone allograft (Avila et al., 2010), bovine xenograft (Chaushu et al., 2009), and alloplastic material (Bae et al., 2010) as an alternative or supplement to autogenous bone. Sinus augmentation procedures are highly predictable, with many studies reporting over 95% success (Del Fabbro et al., 2008). However, sinus augmentation may be influenced by the choice of graft material and implant surface micromorphology (Del Fabbro et al., 2008), and controversies still exist related to the most suitable way to perform sinus augmentation.

2. Type of graft

2.1 Autogenous graft

Although autogenous bone grafting is still the gold standard, according to the clinical results (Nkenke and Stelzle 2009), it is considered to have osteoinductive and osteoconductive properties, and it is known to contain growth factors (Turhani et al., 2005). Autogenous corticocancellous bone cores can be obtained intraorally or extraorally (Galindo-Moreno et al., 2007), however, this requires an additional second surgical donor site and additional morbidity (Park 2010).

A bone trap may be used to harvest bone debris during implant preparation, with additional bone collected by further drilling adjacent to the implant sites or by using a bone scraper to harvest cortical bone chips from the zygomatic buttress and from the lateral sinus wall before opening a bony window (Johansson et al., 2010). By using this approach, the autogenous bone can be achieved adjacent to the surgical site without the need for a remote second surgical donor site and additional morbidity (Park 2010). Furthermore, the amount of autogenous bone graft available for harvesting is limited and may be insufficient to fill large osseous defects (Mirzayan et al., 2001). Due to the complications associated with harvesting autogenous bone and its limited supply, many surgeons have sought bone-graft-substitute materials (Mirzayan et al., 2001).

2.2 Allograft

Allograft has been used for grafting in multiple intraoral applications such as periodontics (infrabony defects), oral surgery (extraction sites), and implant dentistry (ridge augmentation) (Froum et al., 2006). Allografts are bony tissue from a donor of the same species and they are known to contain no viable cells (Hallman and Thor 2008). This allograft may be prepared by demineralization of the bone in hydrochloric acid to expose bone morphogenetic protein and this demineralized freeze-dried bone allograft may be considered to have osteoconductivity and osteoinductivitiy (Kalish et al., 2008).

Atrophic maxillary floor augmentations were performed by mineralized human bone allograft in sinuses of different size, and the results showed that this material produced satisfactory bone formation (Maria Soardi et al., 2010). Histologic evaluation using mineralized freeze-dried bone allografts for sinus augmentation revealed a mean of 29.1% newly formed bone and graft particles were mainly in close contact with newly formed bone, primarily with features of mature bone with numerous osteocytes (Kolerman et al., 2008). Similar results were achieved with other reports that most of the specimens presented newly formed bone, and the interface areas between new and old bone were not discernible (Stacchi et al., 2008). There was no evidence of an acute inflammatory infiltrate in both studies (Kolerman et al., 2008; Stacchi et al., 2008).

However, histological evaluation revealed a chronic inflammatory reaction when demineralized freeze-dried bone was used in sinus augmentation, and the authors suggested that demineralized freeze-dried bone homografts may not be recommended to be used alone (Haas et al., 2002).

2.3 Xenograft

Deproteinized bovine bone is one of the most widely researched grafting materials and is used in the maxillofacial region because of its similarity to human (Hallman and Thor 2008). The complete absence of protein has been demonstrated, and its safety with respect to transmission of disease has been confirmed (Norton et al., 2003). Deproteinized cancellous bovine bone was placed as a grafting material for sinus floor elevation and histologic evaluation was performed after 6 months of healing (Valentini et al., 1998). Histologic evaluation showed that, in the grafted area and the previously existing area of the sinus floor, the bone was primarily of lamellar structure and intimate contact between newly formed bone and the particles of the graft was present (Valentini et al., 1998).

Dental implants installed in sinuses augmented with xenograft showed bone-to-implant contact of 27% to 63%, and xenograft was shown to be very slowly restored and seemed to behave as a semipermanent grafting material (Wallace and Froum 2003). If xenograft is used with autogenous bone, this may give additional advantages such as an increase in the volume of the graft and longer space-maintaining effects due to prolonged resorption (Galindo-Moreno et al., 2007).

2.4 Alloplastic materials

Alloplastic materials consist of a large group of chemically diverse synthetic calcium-based biomaterials, including calcium sulfate, calcium phosphate, bioactive glasses, and polymers (Hallman and Thor 2008), and these bone substitutes possess osteoconductive properties (Moore et al., 2001).

A study by Zijderveld, Zerbo, et al. showed that sinus augmentation using a limited volume of beta-tricalcium phosphate appeared to be a clinically reliable procedure, although autogenous bone grafting is still the gold standard (2005) (Zijderveld et al., 2005). This material is reported to act as an osteoconductive material and it allows osteoprogenitor cells to grow on its surface or into its porosity and differentiate into osteoblasts, thus bringing about bone deposition (Zerbo et al., 2005).

Calcium sulfate hemihydrate has been proposed as a grafting material for sinus augmentation, and this resulted in good, new tissue formation within the sinuses when clinically and radiographically evaluated. The histomorphometiric analysis revealed bone density of 34.3% to 55.54% (De Leonardis and Pecora 2000). Similar results were achieved by other investigators (Pecora et al., 1998), and the study done at two years revealed new irregular trabecular design was seen radiographically and revealed normal, vital trabecular bone with woven and lamellar structure in all the histollogically examined sections (Guarnieri et al., 2006).

2.5 Titanium granule

Resorption of grafting material may lead to unpredictable long-term results when rehabilitating the resorbed posterior maxilla. Nonresorbable, osteoconductive bone substitutes may therefore be an advantage over autogenous bone grafts. Titanium granules were used as bone substitute in patients scheduled to receive augmentation of the sinus floor prior to or in conjunction with placement of dental implants (Bystedt and Rasmusson 2009).

3. Growth factors and the cell-based approach

3.1 Platelet-rich plasma

The use of platelet-rich plasma to enhance bone regeneration has been documented in periodontal defects, in extraction sockets, during implant placement, and in guided bone regeneration procedures around implants, including sinus augmentation (Kim et al., 2002). The use of platelet-rich plasma in conjunction with autogenous bone graft materials has been advocated for use in sinus augmentation surgery as a means of enhancing both quantity and quality of newly forming bone (Danesh-Meyer et al., 2001). The use of platelet-rich plasma is based on the premise that autogenous plasma, rich in platelets, contributes large quantities of mitogenic polypeptides such as platelet-derived growth factor, transforming growth factor-beta and insulin-like growth factor-I, thereby enhancing osteogenesis, improving soft tissue healing, and reducing postoperative morbidity (Danesh-Meyer et al., 2001; Boyapati and Wang 2006; Browaeys et al., 2007). The handling of the particulate bone grafts is reported to be improved due to the adhesive capacity of platelet-rich plasma via its hemostatic capacity of fibrin (Galindo-Moreno et al., 2007; Arora et al., 2010).

In some reports, sinus augmentations were performed successfully with greater bone maturation when using a composite graft of cortical autogenous bone, bovine bone, and platelet-rich plasma (Galindo-Moreno et al., 2007). A randomized clinical trial was performed to test the efficacy of platelet-rich plasma in sinus augmentation procedures (Badr et al., 2010). No appreciable clinical effect could be observed when using platelet-rich plasma with autologous iliac crest bone graft in the maxilla. No statistically significant differences were observed for soft tissue healing indices ($P=0.4$) and mean graft resorption ($P=0.5$) between groups (autogenous bone only vs. bone + platelet-rich plasma). The findings suggest that the addition of platelet-rich plasma to bone derivative/substitute materials may not significantly enhance bone formation in the maxillary sinus area (Danesh-Meyer et al., 2001).

The results from the other study showed that the marginal bone level measurements showed no significant differences, although there was a tendency toward less resorption on platelet-rich plasma sides. Resonance frequency analysis measurements showed statistically significantly higher implant stability quotient values for platelet-rich plasma sites at abutment connectios in the anterior but not in the posterior regions (Thor et al., 2005).

Theoretically, it seems to have significant beneficial effects on the soft and hard tissue healing; however, the disparity in study design, surgical techniques, and different outcome assessment variables used makes it difficult to assess the practical benefit of its clinical use (Arora et al., 2010). Although platelet-rich plasma has been extensively studied for over a decade, there are no definitive reports proving the benefit of using platelet-rich plasma in sinus augmentation procedures (Arora et al., 2010). Therefore, the use of platelet-rich plasma may not be recommended as a standard method to support bone regeneration for maxillary sinus augmentation (Schaaf et al., 2008).

3.2 Platelet rich fibrin

Platelet-rich fibrin, a second-generation platelet concentrate, is a leucocyte- and platelet-rich fibrin biomaterial (Dohan Ehrenfest et al., 2009). Platelet-rich fibrin belongs to a new generation of platelet concentrates characterized by simplified processing and without biochemical blood handling (Dohan et al., 2006). Platelets are activated during platelet-rich fibrin processing by centrifugation, and massive degranulation allows the release of cytokine (Mazor et al., 2009). Platelet-rich fibrin is reported to release transforming growth factor-beta1, platelet-derived growth factor-AB and vascular endothelial growth factor up to the whole experimental time (Dohan Ehrenfest et al., 2009). Slow fibrin polymerization during platelet-rich fibrin processing leads to the intrinsic incorporation of platelet cytokines and glycanic chains in the fibrin meshes (Mazor et al., 2009). Thus, results showed that platelet-rich fibrin, unlike the other platelet concentrates, would be able to progressively release cytokines during fibrin matrix remodeling, leading enhanced healing properties in experimental and clinical situations (Dohan et al., 2006).

Platelet-rich fibrin was used in sinus augmentation procedures both in lateral and crestal approaches. In the lateral approach, platelet-rich fibrin was applied with or without the graft material, and the use of autogenous bone in combination with platelet-rich fibrin glue as a grafting material for maxillary sinus augmentation with simultaneous implant placement was tested in dogs (Lee et al., 2007). The results showed that the use of autogenous bone mixed with platelet-enriched fibrin glue can achieve results superior to those for grafts of autogenous bone alone in terms of enhanced osseointegration of dental implants (40.5±14.4% vs. 32.3±12.0%) and increased height of new bone (12.0±1.0% vs. 10.7±1.0%) (Lee et al., 2007).

Other studies used no bone substitutes, and the biopsies were taken in the center of the regenerated osteotomy window of the sinus lift. Therefore, all of the observed bone must be considered new bone built starting from the sole platelet-rich fibrin matrix (Mazor et al., 2009). All biopsies showed well-organized and vital bone, often with more than 30% bone matrix (33% ± 5%).

Osteotome-mediated sinus floor elevation was performed using only platelet-rich fibrin, and of the 138 implants that had been placed, 97 have been restored function for an average loading time of 5.2 months with a survival rate of 97.8% (Toffler et al., 2010). Early review of the osteotome-mediated sinus floor elevation with platelet-rich fibrin technique presented for localized sinus floor elevation and implant placement demonstrates a high degree of safety and success at sites with 5- to 8-mm residual subantral bone height (Toffler et al., 2010).

3.3 Bone morphogenetic protein

Growth factors are present at low concentrations in bone matrix and plasma, but they execute important biologic functions (Hallman and Thor 2008). The growth factors are believed to have an osseous regenerative effect on the mesenchymal stem cells and contribute to cellular proliferation, matrix formation, collagen synthesis, and osteoid production (Yamada et al., 2008). Bone morphogenetic proteins are multi-functional growth factors belonging to the transforming growth factor-beta superfamily, and bone morphogenetic proteins are reported to have a variety of functions (Wang et al., 1990; Xiao et al., 2007). Bone morphogenetic protein molecules not only induce the formation of both cartilage and bone but also play a role in a number of non-osteogenic developmental processes (Xiao et al., 2007), and they are capable of inducing ectopic cartilage and bone formation, a process that mimics embryonic endochondral bone formation (Xiao et al., 2007). Bone morphogenetic protein 2, 4 and 7, in particular, are reported to be the most effective growth factors in terms of osteogenesis and osseous defect repair (Schilephake 2002), and three bone morphogenetic proteins— bone morphogenetic protein 2, 7, and 14—have been applied in sinus augmentation procedures (Park 2009). The efficacy of Bone morphogenetic proteins for defect repair is strongly dependent on the type of carrier and has been subject to unknown factors in clinical feasibility trials resulting in ambiguous results.

Autogenous bone graft demonstrated greater increases in mineralization and probably angiogenesis of bone than the other bioimplants in rabbit sinus augmentation models when bone morphogenetic protein was delivered at the same time (Hu et al., 2010).

The effectiveness of recombinant human bone morphogenetic protein-2 on an absorbable collagen sponge was compared with an autogenous bone graft when used for two-stage maxillary sinus floor augmentation (Triplett et al., 2009). No marked differences were found in the histologic parameters evaluated between the two groups, but the induced bone in the recombinant human bone morphogenetic protein-2/absorbable collagen sponge group was significantly denser than that in the bone graft group (Triplett et al., 2009). Additionally, collagen sponge was shown to induce new bone equally as well as the other composite material when loaded with bone morphogenetic protein (Pekkarinen et al., 2005). The effects of mineralized bone replacement grafts (e.g., xenografts and allografts) on recombinant human bone morphogenetic protein-2/absorbable collagen sponge were tested, and bone graft densities tended to increase more with the xenograft than with the allograft (Tarnow et al., 2010). The increased density in allograft cases was likely the result of both compression of the mineralized bone replacement graft and vital bone formation, seen histologically (Tarnow, Wallace, et al., 2010). Loss of volume was greater with the four-sponge dose than the two-sponge dose because of compression, and resorption of the sponges and vital bone formation in the allograft cases ranged from 36% to 53% (Tarnow et al., 2010). Hydroxyapatite, biphasic tri-calcium phosphate-hydroxyapatite, and natural coral are reported to be equally good as framing material for bone morphogenetic protein (Pekkarinen et al., 2005).

Deproteinized bovine bone mineral is known to show excellent osteoconductive properties, and it has been used for sinus augmentation clinically (Terheyden et al., 1999). The bovine xenograft composite promotes formation of new bone in a similar fashion to autogenous bone when bone morphogenetic proteins were bound to the graft material, and could therefore be considered a biomaterial with potential applications as a bone substitute in maxillary sinus floor augmentation (Sicca et al., 2008).

It has been shown that beta-tricalcium phosphate is suitable as a biodegradable, highly biocompatible, and osteoconductive carrier for bone morphogenetic proteins in sinus augmentation procedures (Gruber et al., 2008). Both experimentally and clinically, recombinant human bone morphogenetic protein-14/beta-tricalcium phosphate was found to be effective and safe as the control treatment with autologous bone mixed with beta-tricalcium phosphate in sinus floor augmentation (Koch et al., 2010). Self-setting alpha-tricalcium phosphate was used in maxillary sinus augmentation, and it was shown to have bone-conductive activity and shown to maintain the rigidity of implanted bone screws (Marukawa et al., 2010).

Composite material has been used for bone morphogenetic protein-2 release in mandibular defect areas (Wen, Karl, et al., 2011). While in-vitro bone morphogenetic protein-2 release was highest for the polyethylene glycol hydrogel, the scaffold most successful in vivo was the collagen-hydroxyapatite composite infused with polyethylene glycol-hydrogel scaffold because it had the necessary mechanical strength to perform well in the mandibular bone environment (Wen et al., 2011). The in vitro release studies suggested a threshold dose of 5 μg that was confirmed by the in vivo dose response studies (Wen, Karl, et al., 2011). Many studies have demonstrated the potential for the bone morphogenetic proteins to increase bone formation in sinus augmentation procedures and further studies are warranted to find an appropriate carrier scaffold for the optimal release of bone morphogenetic proteins (Park 2009).

Bone morphogenetic protein-7 was loaded onto a poloxamer carrier or demineralized bone matrix in a poloxamer carrier (Ho et al., 2010). These bioimplants had more rapid initial bone production than all other materials, including autogenous bone, and these bone morphogenetic protein-containing bioimplants demonstrated promise as alternatives to autogenous bone grafts for sinus-augmentation procedures (Ho et al., 2010).

In the future, such biomaterials may enable earlier placement of dental implants into augmented maxillary sinuses.

3.4 Platelet-derived growth factor

Platelet-derived growth factor plays an important role in inducing proliferation of undifferentiated mesenchymal cells (Schilephake 2002); it is a stimulator of the proliferation and recruitment of both bone cells and periodontal ligaments (Nevins et al., 2003). It is an important mediator for bone healing and remodeling during trauma and infection, and it is reported to enhance bone regeneration in conjunction with other growth factors (Schilephake 2002).

Recombinant human platelet-derived growth factor-BB was used in simultaneous vertical guided bone regeneration and guided tissue regeneration in the posterior maxilla (Urban et al., 2009). The results demonstrated successful use of recombinant human platelet-derived growth factor-BB in conjunction with autogenous bone, anorganic bone mineral, and barrier membranes to reconstruct severe alveolar bone defects (Urban et al., 2009). A significant amount of periodontal bone gain was achieved in close apposition to a previously denuded root surface, giving the possibility of vertical periodontal regeneration (Urban et al., 2009). The use of purified recombinant human platelet-derived growth factor-BB mixed with bone allograft in humans is reported to result in periodontal regeneration in both Class II furcations and interproximal intrabony defects in human Class II furcation defects (Nevins et al., 2003).

The regenerative outcomes in maxillary sinus augmentation procedures were tested when recombinant human platelet-derived growth factor-BB was combined with particulate anorganic bovine bone mineral (Nevins et al., 2009). The surgical outcomes in all treated sites were uneventful at 6 to 8 months, with sufficient regenerated bone present. Large areas of dense, well-formed lamellar bone were seen throughout the intact core specimens, and a number of cores demonstrated efficient replacement of the normally slowly resorbing anorganic bovine bone mineral matrix particles with newly formed bone.

3.5 Mesenchymal stem cell

Long-term success of dental implants has been demonstrated when placed simultaneously with or after a sinus augmentation procedure (Gonshor et al., 2011). However, optimal bone formation can be from 6 to 9 months or longer with grafting materials other than autogenous bone (Pieri et al., 2008). Various osteoconductive materials have been applied to augment the sinus floor, but these materials are cell-free and may require more time for bone healing (Pieri et al., 2008).

Bone marrow contains a population of rare progenitor cells capable of differentiating into bone, cartilage, tendon, and other connective tissues, and these mesenchymal stem cells can be purified and culture-expanded from animals and humans and have been shown to regenerate functional tissue when delivered to the site of musculoskeletal defects in experimental animals (Bruder et al., 1998). Cells can be also be achieved intraorally from the maxillary tuberosity and the periosteum of the mandible (Turhani et al., 2005; Springer et al., 2006) The study was done to assess whether differences occur in bone formation after maxillary sinus floor elevation surgery with bovine bone mineral mixed with autogenous bone or autogenous stem cells (Rickert et al., 2010). Mesenchymal stem cellseeded on xenograft particles can induce the formation of a sufficient volume of new bone to enable the reliable placement of implants within a time frame comparable to that of applying either solely autogenous bone or a mixture of autogenous bone and xenograft; this technique could be an alternative to using autografts (Rickert et al., 2010).

Sinus augmentation procedures using either an allograft cellular bone matrix, containing native mesenchymal stem cells and osteoprogenitors, or conventional allograft showed similar results (Gonshor et al., 2011). Histomorphometric analysis of the allograft cellular bone matrix grafts revealed average vital bone content of 32.5% ± 6.8%, but results for the conventional allograft showed an average vital bone content of 18.3% ± 10.6% at an average healing period of 3.7 ± 0.6 months (Gonshor et al., 2011).

An ovine split-mouth study was applied to compare bovine bone mineral alone and in combination with mesenchymal stem cells regarding their potential in sinus augmentation (Sauerbier et al., 2010). The authors concluded that the high percentage of vital bone content, after a relatively short healing phase, may encourage a more rapid initiation of implant placement or restoration when a cellular grafting approach is considered (McAllister et al., 2009; Sauerbier et al., 2010).

4. Conclusion

Sinus augmentation procedures have been used clinically with very high success rates. Bone-substitute materials are reported to be as effective as autogenous bone when used alone or in combination with autogenous bone. It may be concluded that bone substitutes can be successfully used for sinus augmentation, reducing donor-site morbidity. Attempts have been made to accelerate bone formation with different scaffolds, growth factors, and mesencymal stem cells. Further studies are needed to find an optimal approach that can enhance bone formation in sinus augmentation procedures.

5. References

Arora, N. S., T. Ramanayake, et al. (2010). "Platelet-rich plasma in sinus augmentation procedures: a systematic literature review: Part II." Implant Dent 19(2): 145-157.

Avila, G., R. Neiva, et al. (2010). "Clinical and histologic outcomes after the use of a novel allograft for maxillary sinus augmentation: a case series." Implant Dent 19(4): 330-341.

Badr, M., P. Coulthard, et al. (2010). "The efficacy of platelet-rich plasma in grafted maxillae. A randomised clinical trial." Eur J Oral Implantol 3(3): 233-244.

Bae, J. H., Y. K. Kim, et al. (2010). "Sinus bone graft using new alloplastic bone graft material (Osteon)-II: clinical evaluation." Oral Surg Oral Med Oral Pathol Oral Radiol Endod 109(3): e14-20.

Boyapati, L. and H. L. Wang (2006). "The role of platelet-rich plasma in sinus augmentation: a critical review." Implant Dent 15(2): 160-170.

Boyne, P. J. and R. A. James (1980). "Grafting of the maxillary sinus floor with autogenous marrow and bone." J Oral Surg 38(8): 613-616.

Browaeys, H., P. Bouvry, et al. (2007). "A literature review on biomaterials in sinus augmentation procedures." Clin Implant Dent Relat Res 9(3): 166-177.

Bruder, S. P., A. A. Kurth, et al. (1998). "Bone regeneration by implantation of purified, culture-expanded human mesenchymal stem cells." J Orthop Res 16(2): 155-162.

Bystedt, H. and L. Rasmusson (2009). "Porous titanium granules used as osteoconductive material for sinus floor augmentation: a clinical pilot study." Clin Implant Dent Relat Res 11(2): 101-105.

Chaushu, G., O. Mardinger, et al. (2009). "The use of cancellous block allograft for sinus floor augmentation with simultaneous implant placement in the posterior atrophic maxilla." J Periodontol 80(3): 422-428.

Danesh-Meyer, M. J., M. R. Filstein, et al. (2001). "Histological evaluation of sinus augmentation using platelet rich plasma (PRP): a case series." J Int Acad Periodontol 3(2): 48-56.

De Leonardis, D. and G. E. Pecora (2000). "Prospective study on the augmentation of the maxillary sinus with calcium sulfate: histological results." J Periodontol 71(6): 940-947.

Del Fabbro, M., G. Rosano, et al. (2008). "Implant survival rates after maxillary sinus augmentation." Eur J Oral Sci 116(6): 497-506.

Dohan, D. M., J. Choukroun, et al. (2006). "Platelet-rich fibrin (PRF): a second-generation platelet concentrate. Part II: platelet-related biologic features." Oral Surg Oral Med Oral Pathol Oral Radiol Endod 101(3): e45-50.

Dohan Ehrenfest, D. M., G. M. de Peppo, et al. (2009). "Slow release of growth factors and thrombospondin-1 in Choukroun's platelet-rich fibrin (PRF): a gold standard to achieve for all surgical platelet concentrates technologies." Growth Factors 27(1): 63-69.

Froum, S. J., S. S. Wallace, et al. (2006). "Comparison of mineralized cancellous bone allograft (Puros) and anorganic bovine bone matrix (Bio-Oss) for sinus augmentation: histomorphometry at 26 to 32 weeks after grafting." Int J Periodontics Restorative Dent 26(6): 543-551.

Galindo-Moreno, P., G. Avila, et al. (2007). "Evaluation of sinus floor elevation using a composite bone graft mixture." Clin Oral Implants Res 18(3): 376-382.

Gonshor, A., B. S. McAllister, et al. (2011). "Histologic and histomorphometric evaluation of an allograft stem cell-based matrix sinus augmentation procedure." Int J Oral Maxillofac Implants 26(1): 123-131.

Gruber, R. M., A. Ludwig, et al. (2008). "Sinus floor augmentation with recombinant human growth and differentiation factor-5 (rhGDF-5): a pilot study in the Goettingen miniature pig comparing autogenous bone and rhGDF-5." Clin Oral Implants Res.

Guarnieri, R., R. Grassi, et al. (2006). "Maxillary sinus augmentation using granular calcium sulfate (surgiplaster sinus): radiographic and histologic study at 2 years." Int J Periodontics Restorative Dent 26(1): 79-85.

Haas, R., D. Haidvogl, et al. (2002). "Freeze-dried homogeneous and heterogeneous bone for sinus augmentation in sheep. Part I: histological findings." Clin Oral Implants Res 13(4): 396-404.

Hallman, M. and A. Thor (2008). "Bone substitutes and growth factors as an alternative/complement to autogenous bone for grafting in implant dentistry." Periodontol 2000 47: 172-192.

Ho, S. K., S. A. Peel, et al. (2010). "Augmentation of the maxillary sinus: comparison of bioimplants containing bone morphogenetic protein and autogenous bone in a rabbit model." J Can Dent Assoc 76: a108.

Hu, Z., S. A. Peel, et al. (2010). "The expression of bone matrix proteins induced by different bioimplants in a rabbit sinus lift model." J Biomed Mater Res A 95(4): 1048-1054.

Johansson, L. A., S. Isaksson, et al. (2010). "Maxillary sinus floor augmentation and simultaneous implant placement using locally harvested autogenous bone chips and bone debris: a prospective clinical study." J Oral Maxillofac Surg 68(4): 837-844.

Kalish, B. P., G. S. Schuster, et al. (2008). "Influence of matrix-suspended demineralized bone on osseous repair using a critical-sized defect in the rat (Rattus norvegicus) calvarium." J Oral Implantol 34(2): 83-89.

Kim, S. G., C. H. Chung, et al. (2002). "Use of particulate dentin-plaster of Paris combination with/without platelet-rich plasma in the treatment of bone defects around implants." Int J Oral Maxillofac Implants 17(1): 86-94.

Koch, F. P., J. Becker, et al. (2010). "A prospective, randomized pilot study on the safety and efficacy of recombinant human growth and differentiation factor-5 coated onto beta-tricalcium phosphate for sinus lift augmentation." Clin Oral Implants Res 21(11): 1301-1308.

Kolerman, R., H. Tal, et al. (2008). "Histomorphometric analysis of newly formed bone after maxillary sinus floor augmentation using ground cortical bone allograft and internal collagen membrane." J Periodontol 79(11): 2104-2111.

Lee, H. J., B. H. Choi, et al. (2007). "Maxillary sinus floor augmentation using autogenous bone grafts and platelet-enriched fibrin glue with simultaneous implant placement." Oral Surg Oral Med Oral Pathol Oral Radiol Endod 103(3): 329-333.

Maria Soardi, C., S. Spinato, et al. (2010). "Atrophic maxillary floor augmentation by mineralized human bone allograft in sinuses of different size: an histologic and histomorphometric analysis." Clin Oral Implants Res.

Marukawa, K., K. Ueki, et al. (2010). "Use of self-setting alpha-tricalcium phosphate for maxillary sinus augmentation in rabbit." Clin Oral Implants Res.

Mazor, Z., R. A. Horowitz, et al. (2009). "Sinus floor augmentation with simultaneous implant placement using Choukroun's platelet-rich fibrin as the sole grafting material: a radiologic and histologic study at 6 months." J Periodontol 80(12): 2056-2064.

McAllister, B. S., K. Haghighat, et al. (2009). "Histologic evaluation of a stem cell-based sinus-augmentation procedure." J Periodontol 80(4): 679-686.

Mirzayan, R., V. Panossian, et al. (2001). "The use of calcium sulfate in the treatment of benign bone lesions. A preliminary report." J Bone Joint Surg Am 83-A(3): 355-358.

Moore, W. R., S. E. Graves, et al. (2001). "Synthetic bone graft substitutes." ANZ J Surg 71(6): 354-361.

Nevins, M., M. Camelo, et al. (2003). "Periodontal regeneration in humans using recombinant human platelet-derived growth factor-BB (rhPDGF-BB) and allogenic bone." J Periodontol 74(9): 1282-1292.

Nevins, M., D. Garber, et al. (2009). "Human histologic evaluation of anorganic bovine bone mineral combined with recombinant human platelet-derived growth factor BB in maxillary sinus augmentation: case series study." Int J Periodontics Restorative Dent 29(6): 583-591.

Nkenke, E. and F. Stelzle (2009). "Clinical outcomes of sinus floor augmentation for implant placement using autogenous bone or bone substitutes: a systematic review." Clin Oral Implants Res 20 Suppl 4: 124-133.

Norton, M. R., E. W. Odell, et al. (2003). "Efficacy of bovine bone mineral for alveolar augmentation: a human histologic study." Clin Oral Implants Res 14(6): 775-783.

Park, J. B. (2009). "Use of bone morphogenetic proteins in sinus augmentation procedure." J Craniofac Surg 20(5): 1501-1503.

Park, J. B. (2010). "Implant installation with ridge augmentation using autogenous bone harvested from an adjacent site." J Oral Implantol 36(5): 409-413.

Pecora, G. E., D. De Leonardis, et al. (1998). "Short-term healing following the use of calcium sulfate as a grafting material for sinus augmentation: a clinical report." Int J Oral Maxillofac Implants 13(6): 866-873.

Pekkarinen, T., T. S. Lindholm, et al. (2005). "The effect of different mineral frames on ectopic bone formation in mouse hind leg muscles induced by native reindeer bone morphogenetic protein." Arch Orthop Trauma Surg 125(1): 10-15.

Pieri, F., E. Lucarelli, et al. (2008). "Mesenchymal stem cells and platelet-rich plasma enhance bone formation in sinus grafting: a histomorphometric study in minipigs." J Clin Periodontol 35(6): 539-546.

Rickert, D., S. Sauerbier, et al. (2010). "Maxillary sinus floor elevation with bovine bone mineral combined with either autogenous bone or autogenous stem cells: a prospective randomized clinical trial." Clin Oral Implants Res.

Sauerbier, S., K. Stubbe, et al. (2010). "Mesenchymal stem cells and bovine bone mineral in sinus lift procedures--an experimental study in sheep." Tissue Eng Part C Methods 16(5): 1033-1039.

Schaaf, H., P. Streckbein, et al. (2008). "Topical use of platelet-rich plasma to influence bone volume in maxillary augmentation: a prospective randomized trial." Vox Sang 94(1): 64-69.

Schilephake, H. (2002). "Bone growth factors in maxillofacial skeletal reconstruction." Int J Oral Maxillofac Surg 31(5): 469-484.

Sicca, C. M., M. V. Corotti, et al. (2008). "Comparative histomorphometric and tomographic analysis of maxillary sinus floor augmentation in rabbits using autografts and xenografts." J Biomed Mater Res B Appl Biomater 86(1): 188-196.

Springer, I. N., P. F. Nocini, et al. (2006). "Two techniques for the preparation of cell-scaffold constructs suitable for sinus augmentation: steps into clinical application." Tissue Eng 12(9): 2649-2656.

Stacchi, C., G. Orsini, et al. (2008). "Clinical, histologic, and histomorphometric analyses of regenerated bone in maxillary sinus augmentation using fresh frozen human bone allografts." J Periodontol 79(9): 1789-1796.

Tadjoedin, E. S., G. L. de Lange, et al. (2003). "Deproteinized cancellous bovine bone (Bio-Oss) as bone substitute for sinus floor elevation. A retrospective, histomorphometrical study of five cases." J Clin Periodontol 30(3): 261-270.

Tarnow, D. P., S. S. Wallace, et al. (2010). "Maxillary sinus augmentation using recombinant bone morphogenetic protein-2/acellular collagen sponge in combination with a mineralized bone replacement graft: a report of three cases." Int J Periodontics Restorative Dent 30(2): 139-149.

Terheyden, H., S. Jepsen, et al. (1999). "Sinus floor augmentation with simultaneous placement of dental implants using a combination of deproteinized bone xenografts and recombinant human osteogenic protein-1. A histometric study in miniature pigs." Clin Oral Implants Res 10(6): 510-521.

Thor, A., K. Wannfors, et al. (2005). "Reconstruction of the severely resorbed maxilla with autogenous bone, platelet-rich plasma, and implants: 1-year results of a controlled prospective 5-year study." Clin Implant Dent Relat Res 7(4): 209-220.

Toffler, M., N. Toscano, et al. (2010). "Osteotome-mediated sinus floor elevation using only platelet-rich fibrin: an early report on 110 patients." Implant Dent 19(5): 447-456.

Triplett, R. G., M. Nevins, et al. (2009). "Pivotal, randomized, parallel evaluation of recombinant human bone morphogenetic protein-2/absorbable collagen sponge and autogenous bone graft for maxillary sinus floor augmentation." J Oral Maxillofac Surg 67(9): 1947-1960.

Turhani, D., E. Watzinger, et al. (2005). "Three-dimensional composites manufactured with human mesenchymal cambial layer precursor cells as an alternative for sinus floor augmentation: an in vitro study." Clin Oral Implants Res 16(4): 417-424.

Urban, I., N. Caplanis, et al. (2009). "Simultaneous vertical guided bone regeneration and guided tissue regeneration in the posterior maxilla using recombinant human platelet-derived growth factor: a case report." J Oral Implantol 35(5): 251-256.

Valentini, P., D. Abensur, et al. (1998). "Histological evaluation of Bio-Oss in a 2-stage sinus floor elevation and implantation procedure. A human case report." Clin Oral Implants Res 9(1): 59-64.

Wallace, S. S. and S. J. Froum (2003). "Effect of maxillary sinus augmentation on the survival of endosseous dental implants. A systematic review." Ann Periodontol 8(1): 328-343.

Wang, E. A., V. Rosen, et al. (1990). "Recombinant human bone morphogenetic protein induces bone formation." Proc Natl Acad Sci U S A 87(6): 2220-2224.

Wen, B., M. Karl, et al. (2011). "An evaluation of BMP-2 delivery from scaffolds with miniaturized dental implants in a novel rat mandible model." J Biomed Mater Res B Appl Biomater.

Xiao, Y. T., L. X. Xiang, et al. (2007). "Bone morphogenetic protein

Recombinant human bone morphogenetic protein induces bone formation." Biochem Biophys Res Commun 362(3): 550-553.

Yamada, Y., S. Nakamura, et al. (2008). "Injectable tissue-engineered bone using autogenous bone marrow-derived stromal cells for maxillary sinus augmentation: clinical application report from a 2-6-year follow-up." Tissue Eng Part A 14(10): 1699-1707.

Zerbo, I. R., A. L. Bronckers, et al. (2005). "Localisation of osteogenic and osteoclastic cells in porous beta-tricalcium phosphate particles used for human maxillary sinus floor elevation." Biomaterials 26(12): 1445-1451.

Zijderveld, S. A., I. R. Zerbo, et al. (2005). "Maxillary sinus floor augmentation using a beta-tricalcium phosphate (Cerasorb) alone compared to autogenous bone grafts." Int J Oral Maxillofac Implants 20(3): 432-440.

Permissions

All chapters in this book were first published by InTech Open; hereby published with permission under the Creative Commons Attribution License or equivalent. Every chapter published in this book has been scrutinized by our experts. Their significance has been extensively debated. The topics covered herein carry significant findings which will fuel the growth of the discipline. They may even be implemented as practical applications or may be referred to as a beginning point for another development.

The contributors of this book come from diverse backgrounds, making this book a truly international effort. This book will bring forth new frontiers with its revolutionizing research information and detailed analysis of the nascent developments around the world.

We would like to thank all the contributing authors for lending their expertise to make the book truly unique. They have played a crucial role in the development of this book. Without their invaluable contributions this book wouldn't have been possible. They have made vital efforts to compile up to date information on the varied aspects of this subject to make this book a valuable addition to the collection of many professionals and students.

This book was conceptualized with the vision of imparting up-to-date information and advanced data in this field. To ensure the same, a matchless editorial board was set up. Every individual on the board went through rigorous rounds of assessment to prove their worth. After which they invested a large part of their time researching and compiling the most relevant data for our readers.

The editorial board has been involved in producing this book since its inception. They have spent rigorous hours researching and exploring the diverse topics which have resulted in the successful publishing of this book. They have passed on their knowledge of decades through this book. To expedite this challenging task, the publisher supported the team at every step. A small team of assistant editors was also appointed to further simplify the editing procedure and attain best results for the readers.

Apart from the editorial board, the designing team has also invested a significant amount of their time in understanding the subject and creating the most relevant covers. They scrutinized every image to scout for the most suitable representation of the subject and create an appropriate cover for the book.

The publishing team has been an ardent support to the editorial, designing and production team. Their endless efforts to recruit the best for this project, has resulted in the accomplishment of this book. They are a veteran in the field of academics and their pool of knowledge is as vast as their experience in printing. Their expertise and guidance has proved useful at every step. Their uncompromising quality standards have made this book an exceptional effort. Their encouragement from time to time has been an inspiration for everyone.

The publisher and the editorial board hope that this book will prove to be a valuable piece of knowledge for researchers, students, practitioners and scholars across the globe.

List of Contributors

Cássio do Nascimento and Rubens Ferreira de Albuquerque Jr.
Faculty of Dentistry of Ribeirão Preto, Department of Dental Materials and Prosthodontics Brazil

Tetsu Takahashi
Division of Oral and Maxillofacial Reconstructive Surgery, Kyushu Dental College Japan

Elnaz Moslehifard
Department of Prosthodontics, Tabriz University of Medical Sciences, Tabriz, Iran

Christopher Ogunsalu
Human Anatomy and Forensic Dentistry Department of Basic Medical Sciences Faculty of Medical Sciences, University of the West Indies, Mona Jamaica
Caribbean Institute of Oral and Maxillofacial Implantology and Surgery Jamaica

Takashi Sawada
Department of Ultrastructural Science, Tokyo Dental College, Japan

Sadayuki Inoue
Department of Anatomy and Cell Biology, McGill University, Canada

Dragana Gabrić Pandurić, Marko Granić, Mato Sušić and Davor Katanec
Department of Oral Surgery, School of Dental Medicine, University of Zagreb Croatia
Department of Oral Surgery, Clinical Hospital Center Zagreb Croatia

Christiane Kunert-Keil and Tomasz Gedrange
University of Greifswald, Department of Orthodontics, Germany

Tomasz Gredes
University of Wroclaw, Department of Orthodontics, Poland

Khalid S. Hassan
Department of Preventive Dental Sciences, Division of Periodontics, College of Dentistry, University of Dammam, Saudi Arabia
Faculty of Dental Medicine, Al-Azhar University, Assiut Branch, Egypt

Adel S. Alagl
Chairman of Department of Preventive Dental Sciences, College of Dentistry, University of Dammam, Saudi Arabia

Ayse Gulsahi
Baskent University Faculty of Dentistry, Ankara, Turkey

Jun-Beom Park
Department of Molecular Medicine and Biopharmaceutical Sciences, Graduate School of Convergence Science and Technology, Seoul National University, Seoul, Korea

Index

www.ingramcontent.com/pod-product-compliance
Lightning Source LLC
LaVergne TN
LVHW062233200926
848484LV00006B/1529